# Global HIV/AIDS Politics, Policy, and Activism

# Global HIV/AIDS Politics, Policy, and Activism

## Persistent Challenges and Emerging Issues

Volume 3
*Activism and Community Mobilization*

Raymond A. Smith, Editor

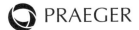 PRAEGER

AN IMPRINT OF ABC-CLIO, LLC
SANTA BARBARA, CALIFORNIA • DENVER, COLORADO • OXFORD, ENGLAND

**Library of Congress Cataloging-in-Publication Data**

Global HIV/AIDS politics, policy and activism : persistent challenges and emerging issues / Raymond A. Smith, editor.
        3 volumes ; cm
    Includes bibliographical references and index.
    ISBN 978-0-313-39945-9 (set : hardback : acid-free paper) —
ISBN 978-0-313-39946-6 (set : ebook)
    1. AIDS (Disease)   2. HIV infections.   3. Public health—International cooperation.
I. Smith, Raymond A., 1967–
    RA643.75.G56   2013
    362.19697'92—dc23        2013002498

ISBN:   978-0-313-39945-9
EISBN: 978-0-313-39946-6

17  16  15  14  13   1  2  3  4  5

This book is also available on the World Wide Web as an eBook.
Visit www.abc-clio.com for details.

Praeger
An Imprint of ABC-CLIO, LLC

ABC-CLIO, LLC
130 Cremona Drive, P.O. Box 1911
Santa Barbara, California 93116-1911

This book is printed on acid-free paper ∞
Manufactured in the United States of America

# Contents

## Volume 3
### Activism and Community Mobilization

# Introduction: Politics, Policy, and Activism in the Fourth Decade of AIDS

*Raymond A. Smith*

As this three-volume bookset was being launched in early 2011, the world was about to mark the 30th anniversary of the initial identification of the AIDS epidemic on January 5, 1981, prompting many both to look back and to look forward. In 1980, HIV had been circulating heavily in human populations for more than a decade, but not enough cases had yet clustered together to be recognizable as a single syndrome of acquired immunodeficiency. By 1990, AIDS had gone from an unknown condition to one that was near-universally recognized, but that remained untreatable and continued spreading uncontrollably—a crisis widely considered the most severe and acute health challenge facing the globe. Yet by 2000, advances in antiretroviral (ARV) treatment had begun transforming the idea that AIDS was an automatic "death sentence" to a paradigm viewing HIV infection as a severe but chronic illness—albeit only for those in the developed world who had access to ARVs. At the same time, truly effective HIV prevention seemed still a distant hope and progress on technologies such as vaccines and microbicides was stalled.

When the 19th International AIDS Conference convened in Washington, DC in July 2012, the mood was perhaps the most hopeful it had been in a decade, with compelling new evidence available that ARV treatment of HIV-positive individuals could dramatically reduce the likelihood of their transmitting the virus. These findings heralded the potential to eventually grind the epidemic to a halt through a combination of expanded treatment coverage and new biomedical approaches to prevention. At the same time, the severe global economic downturns of the previous five years were raising serious concerns that wealthy donor nations were faltering in their commitments to provide the funds and technical support that had been so crucial to the "rollout and scale-up" of ARV programs in the developing world, and that the governments of those developing nations had not yet achieved the ability to sustain the programs on their own. Still, an impressive infrastructure of global organizations, national institutions, and community partnerships had become solidly established around the world; in the United States, the first-ever National HIV/AIDS Strategy was reenergizing the domestic battle against the epidemic.

It was against this backdrop in the history of the epidemic that this bookset, *Global HIV/AIDS Politics, Policy, and Activism: Persistent Challenges and Emerging Issues,* was developed. My work as editor was heavily influenced by my early experiences in the mid-1990s in developing the first-ever *Encyclopedia of AIDS: A Social, Political, Cultural, and Scientific Record of the HIV Epidemic* (Fitzroy-Dearborn Publishers, 1998; Penguin paperback, 2001). My thinking on these evolving issues was further spurred by a book I co-authored (with Patricia Siplon) entitled *Drugs into Bodies: Global AIDS Treatment Activism* (Praeger, 2006). Another important influence was a 2009 conference I co-organized on HIV/AIDS social movements at the HIV Center for Clinical and Behavioral Studies, a research institute with which I have long been affiliated in the Division of Gender, Sexuality, and Health at the New York State Psychiatric Institute and Columbia University.

As indicated by the subtitle, the *Encyclopedia of AIDS* was a volume of exceptional breadth, attempting to be truly global and "encyclopedic" in its coverage of everything from music and literature about AIDS, to the treatment and prevention of HIV, to the key political struggles and policy debates. Even by the mid-1990s, it was a daunting task to begin to capture all of these dimensions in a single work; by 2012 the same undertaking would be nearly impossible. This bookset, therefore, has a much tighter focus, specifically on the political and policy dimensions of the epidemic. Yet, as the 45 chapters of these three volumes attest, the contemporary politics, policy debates, and activist campaigns of the global HIV/AIDS epidemic are themselves huge and sprawling topics. To best capture the most relevant range of "persistent challenges and emerging issues," a heavily inductive approach was taken to assembling the chapters in these volumes. The contents of the *Encyclopedia of AIDS* had begun with an a priori list of topics gleaned from a broad survey of the existing literature on HIV/AIDS. For this bookset, I took much the opposite approach. Beyond setting the broad parameters of "politics, policy, and activism," I did not seek authors to write on particular topics. Instead, I widely circulated a call for submissions, which sought to tap the expertise of the academic and advocacy communities working in this area, and asked them to propose what they considered to be the most relevant and pressing persistent challenges and emerging issues in global HIV/AIDS politics, policy, and activism.

The resulting three volumes reflect a rich, eclectic, and wide-ranging set of issues written by an international team of more than 70 authors. The majority of the contributors are based in English-speaking countries (United States, South Africa, Canada, United Kingdom, Ghana, Australia, New Zealand) but also hail from Brazil, Cambodia, Colombia, Jordan, the Netherlands, Norway, Peru, Portugal, and Qatar. Most are university professors, though a significant number are from major nongovernmental organizations (NGOs) and related advocacy and activist groups. The contributors represent a variety of disciplines, including political science, law, economics, sociology, psychology, anthropology, public health, and various biomedical fields, and bring with them a range of styles and methodological approaches appropriate to their specific topics and disciplines.

The thematic focus is also very geographically diverse, with 16 chapters categorized as "global/transnational" and the rest focused on countries/ regions including Brazil, Russia, South Africa, the Middle East, Ghana, Colombia, the Southern Africa region, India, Cambodia, China, Peru, the United States, the United Kingdom, Zambia, Sudan, and Lebanon. All of the chapters are previously unpublished (with the exception of the chapter on Russia, which was previously published only in Norwegian) and therefore purpose-written for this bookset. The manuscript of each chapter went through a thorough editorial process, typically including comments from one or more of the other contributors to the volume. However, this editorial process did not constitute traditional peer review per se, and therefore the chapters are not presented here as peer-reviewed works.

Likewise, no attempt was made for these volumes to be encyclopedic in their coverage, nor is any claim made that they are so. Rather, what these volumes do reflect are a concerted effort to capture the scale and scope of the actions (or inactions) of political systems and governments around the world, the realities of policy and policymaking amid widely differing national and regional epidemics, and the ongoing opportunities for—and limits of— activism and community mobilization. Some chapters cover more than one of these areas and could plausibly have fit into another volume, but were ultimately placed into the volume for which they were the best fit.

Volume 1 consists of 14 chapters focused primarily on "Politics and Government," Volume 2 contains 14 chapters on "Policy and Policymaking." Volume 3 has 17 chapters addressing themes of "Activism and

Community Mobilization." Within each volume, there are two parts, the first dedicated to global- and transnational-level dimensions, and the second to country- and regional-level analyses. Within each part, chapters are roughly sequenced so that they begin with the broadest themes and move progressively toward narrower and more specific topics or case studies. In the chapter descriptions below, the portions in quotation marks were provided by the authors as part of a chapter abstract.

## VOLUME 1: POLITICS AND GOVERNMENT

The 14 chapters of the first volume have a particular emphasis on how political actors and processes, and governmental responses, have continued to shape and be shaped by the challenges of HIV/AIDS. Part 1 on "The Global and Transnational Politics of HIV Prevention and Treatment" includes chapters focused on challenges related to sustaining funding of HIV treatment and care, on the use of law and diplomacy as tools to address HIV, and on the persistent impact of stigma in attempts to address the epidemic. Part 2 on "Country- and Regional-Level Politics of HIV Prevention and Treatment" includes chapters on the role of politics and government in the Middle East and North Africa (MENA) region, Brazil, Russia, Ghana, Colombia, and sub-Saharan Africa.

### Part 1: The Global and Transnational Politics of HIV Prevention and Treatment

Focusing on the top-priority question of continued funding for global HIV/AIDS treatment programs, Patricia Siplon argues in *The Troubled Path to HIV/AIDS Universal Treatment Access: Snatching Defeat from the Jaws of Victory?* that the "response to the global AIDS pandemic stands at an important decision point. Following a sustained global AIDS movement, much of it focused on treatment activism, resources have multiplied to address the pandemic while treatment costs have plummeted. However, these gains are currently threatened by intellectual property challenges to the availability of affordable medications; increasing criticism of AIDS funding; and a general pullback by donors. Recent scientific breakthroughs suggesting that treatment is also a highly effective form of prevention and a global activist movement in support of new global financing mechanisms may help address these threats, but the ultimate outcome remains to be determined."

Further exploring the questions of sustainable funding for global AIDS treatment programs, Ricardo Jorge Ribeiro Pereira "analyzes the prospect of sustainability as an envisaged goal for PEPFAR in its current phase" in *Sustainability in the Post-PEPFAR Period: Examples from Botswana, Ethiopia, and South Africa.* Pereira notes that "sustainability is normatively achieved through 'ownership' of initiated programs by the recipient countries, and is informed by the performance of major institutions such as the national government and by perceptions advanced by PEPFAR implementers. Through large-scale government engagement and liberal governance frameworks, Botswana and South Africa set out to achieve sustainability. Yet, both countries' prospects are challenged by severe social inequalities. The Ethiopian government is equally committed, yet sustainability is undermined by persisting low levels of development."

The issue of global governance of the HIV/AIDS epidemic is the focus of the next chapter, co-authored by Mandeep Dhaliwal, Tenu Avafia, Emilie Pradichit, Jeffrey O'Malley, and Vivek Divan. Their chapter, *The New Deal for the Global AIDS Response: Evidence and Human Rights–Based Legal Environments: The Global Commission on HIV and the Law,* discusses the "outcomes and effects of the Global Commission on HIV and the Law in revitalizing the focus on law as a central tool in an effective HIV response. The commission has responded to legal and policy challenges that have not only persisted but have also recently gained some impetus from the increased criminalization of persons living with HIV, both in the framing of new laws and in their prosecution, the continued and widespread abuse of police powers, to an ever-growing treatment gap in relation to new-generation antiretroviral treatment, access to which is impeded by the current intellectual property regime. The commission has also addressed emerging issues, such as novel approaches to dealing with drug use as against the hitherto punitive measures that have incurred great social and public health costs. Through its findings and recommendations the commission has provided guidance to lawmakers and implementers on the importance of a rights-based approach in effectively responding to HIV. The commission has emphasized the necessity for an honest appraisal of prejudice, fear, and false morality, which have confounded the AIDS response for decades. Informed by its inclusive and dynamic Regional Dialogues process, the commission has generated unprecedented evidence on the manner in which law impacts the lives of people, their health, and the critical role that legal empowerment can play in protecting the individual and benefiting society as a whole." The authors, who have been professionally affiliated with the commission, assert that "The commission's messages should form the basis of the next generation of HIV responses, where governments approach HIV through multiple lenses of health, equity, and justice."

Further expanding the theme of global connection, the next chapter is *The Politics of Global Health Diplomacy: Conceptual, Theoretical, and Empirical Lessons from the United States, Southeast Asia, and Latin America.* Eduardo J. Gómez explains that "global health diplomacy (GHD) has emerged as an important area of scholarly research. In essence, GHD seeks to combine domestic health policy processes with foreign policy objectives. This chapter explains the rise and evolution of this new literature, as well as two of its main research areas: that is, international negotiations for health policy, such as access to ARV medication for AIDS, as well as the creation of bilateral policy for foreign policy objectives, such as increasing a nation's international reputation and legitimacy—a.k.a. 'soft power.' Several case studies from the United States, Southeast Asia, and Latin America are used to illustrate the potential utility of this approach. This chapter closes with a discussion about the potential that this new research agenda has to advance our understanding of the politics and policy behind the AIDS epidemic as well as future areas of research."

The persistent challenge of bias and discrimination in the context of the global health response is the focus of Peris Sean Jones in *The "Dirty Work" of Public Health: Politics, Policy, Prejudice, and Human Rights in a Time of HIV/AIDS.* Jones argues that "from the very first appearance of cases concerning what would become known as AIDS-related illness in the early 1980s, a persistent challenge has been how policy responses are weighted toward either the public interest or the human rights of individuals and groups. Broader political factors and modes of public health determine the shape and direction of the response far beyond actual biology and physiology." The objective of the chapter is "to consider how AIDS presented a critical juncture in responses to epidemics. AIDS was a signifier of older, more coercive traditions in public health but, critically, potentially a catalyst for creating new modalities of public health and decision making: in rethinking public health policy more generally. Some key considerations in the chapter include: Why does HIV/AIDS generate such an intensity of feeling? What is public health? Are public health approaches simply knocked off course due to the rights-based backlash against 'putting people in circles and talking about control,' or is the backlash warranted? And, as the technology to treat AIDS continues to develop, a rapidly emerging issue is how antiretroviral medication is altering the borderline between rights and public and political interests."

Part 1 is rounded out with a discussion of *The Subtle Politics of AIDS: Values, Bias and Persistent Errors in HIV Prevention* by Justin O. Parkhurst, in which he argues that "the field of HIV prevention is intensely political, often split along ideological and moral lines. But ideologies and belief systems can further bias the understanding of epidemiological and public health evidence, leading to what is termed here a 'subtle politics of AIDS.'" This chapter takes a cognitive-political approach, "applying the 'heuristics and biases approach' from the cognitive sciences alongside critical policy analysis methods to explore a range of epidemiological mis-understandings that have persisted in the global AIDS and development community. These errors can derive as much from (contestable) normative values as from gaps in epidemiological evidence."

## Part 2: Country- and Regional-Level Politics of HIV Prevention and Treatment

Focusing on a region of the world that has traditionally had low rates of HIV but also has been in rapid flux in recent years, Laith R. Abu-Raddad, Sema K. Sgaier, and Ghina M. Mumtaz contributed a chapter on *The HIV Response in the Middle East and North Africa (MENA) Region: An Epidemic and Its Dilemmas.* The authors explain that "the Middle East and North Africa is witnessing emerging HIV epidemics among injecting drug users, men who have sex with men, and female sex workers and their clients. These rising epidemics compel policy changes to control HIV transmission. Decision makers, though, face dilemmas in the development of an effective HIV response. These include political and sociocultural sensitivities surrounding high-risk populations, limited availability of concrete data to warrant a sense of urgency to act, and limited human and financial resources. However, the region also offers opportunities for an effective HIV response. HIV epidemics are generally in an early phase, civil society has proved effective in avoiding sensitivity in dealing with stigmatized populations, and a common denominator focused in a public health perspective is increasingly feasible. There is a window of opportunity to deal with the HIV epidemic that should not be missed."

Shifting specifically to the world's most heavily impacted region in *The Diagonal Approach: Programming to Combat HIV While Strengthening Primary Health Care Systems in Africa,* Samuel Kalibala notes that "advocacy efforts have resulted in unprecedented HIV funding through various global health initiatives. Many HIV interventions require a functioning primary health care (PHC) system. However, wholesale use of HIV funding to strengthen entire PHC systems in Africa may not be prudent given the lack of evidence for cost-effectiveness of this 'horizontal approach' and the danger of diluting the advocacy focus on HIV. This chapter proposes the 'diagonal' approach, which uses HIV funds to strengthen key areas of PHC while maintaining some verticality and allows studies on feasibility and cost-effectiveness to inform further refining of the approach."

William McColl II brings the focus to the United States, arguing that "the United States has responded to the HIV/AIDS crisis by providing increasing funds for domestic HIV prevention, treatment, and research. Funding at both the federal and state levels has strongly relied on both discretionary funding such as the Ryan White Program and entitlement funding such as Medicaid for low-income people. Beginning in 2001 discretionary domestic funding began to slow growth rates relative to the epidemic." In his chapter, *Funding HIV Prevention, Treatment, and Care in the United States: The Limits of Politics in Responding to a Deadly Epidemic,* McColl makes the case that "today, domestic funding for HIV programs is endangered in part due to the recession beginning in 2007, ongoing deficit reduction efforts, and political change. Additionally, programs face major changes with the implementation of the Patient Protection and Affordable Care Act and the development of antiretroviral-based prevention technologies." His chapter focuses on "the major challenges to the current domestic funding structure while seeking to provide a roadmap to secure a stronger continuum of funding for national HIV prevention, treatment, and care services."

Continuing a focus on the United States in *A National HIV Prevention Strategy for the United States: Troubling Echoes of Earlier VD Control Programs,* William Ward Darrow explains that "in July 2010, President Obama released his National HIV/AIDS Strategy for the United States. In contrast to the first Public Health Service strategy of 1985, which promised no new HIV infections in the United States after 2000, the 2010 strategy provides a vision 'where new HIV infections are rare' and everyone 'will have unfettered access to high-quality, life-extending care, free from stigma and discrimination.'" Both strategies, he asserts, "are mired in a biomedical model that fails to address the fundamental causes of AIDS, respect human rights, ensure input from community members, empower the disenfranchised, and obtain information necessary to implement effective programs."

Examining politics in another major country and HIV epicenter, the chapter *Understanding Brazil's Strategic Response to HIV/AIDS: History, Politics, and International Relations* by Eduardo J. Gómez notes that "in recent years, Brazil has been considered by many to have the best model response to combating the AIDS epidemic." In this chapter, he explains how and why Brazil successfully earned this title, arguing that "Brazil's strategic response to the international health community, as well as the penetration of proactive social health movements and government aspirations to increase its international reputation, created incentives to strategically use the international community toward its benefit. That is, while Brazil worked closely with international financial donors, such as the World Bank, to help initiate and consolidate its national AIDS prevention policies and administration, the government has repeatedly resisted international financial assistance and advice challenging its domestic commitment to the universal distribution of AIDS treatment and controversial prevention policies. Therefore the key to Brazil's success has been its ability to simultaneously acquire the national AIDS program's financial needs from the international community while safeguarding the program's preexisting domestic AIDS policy commitments to those in need."

Shifting to another of the world's leading powers, Aadne Aasland, Arne Backer Grønningsæter, and Peter Meylakhs pose the question: *More Are Testing Positive—but Is Everything Negative?* In this chapter on Russia and the HIV epidemic (originally published in Norwegian but appearing here in English for the first time), the authors state that "despite enhanced attention to HIV and AIDS among the authorities in Russia, accompanied by growing public funds to fight the epidemic, the number of HIV-infected people continues to increase." Their chapter "focuses on factors in Russian society that contribute to explaining Russia's lack of progress in curbing the epidemic. Based on interviews with a variety of actors at federal, regional, and local levels, the authors examine coordination and cross-sectoral collaboration, the distribution of tasks and responsibilities between the different levels, and the tension between general health promotion and targeted measures directed at the most vulnerable groups. The important role of civil society is also discussed. Stigma and discrimination in connection with HIV, which are widespread in Russian society, create obstacles for both targeting and coordination."

Within sub-Saharan Africa, the region with the most manageable HIV/AIDS epidemic has been West Africa, though that region still faces considerable challenges. In *HIV Prevention in the West African Context: Barriers and Facilitators in Ghana,* Lafleur Small and Nyonuku Akosua Baddoo state that "there is a growing body of international research, focused on developing countries, which highlights political, economic, and social factors that influence the spread of HIV/AIDS and consequently serve as either barriers or facilitators to successful HIV prevention programs. Sub-Saharan Africa has become the global epicenter of the HIV/AIDS pandemic. However, Ghana is considered a low-level-epidemic HIV/AIDS country with national prevalence rates that oscillated between 2 and 3 percent from 2004 to 2010. As a low–middle-income country, with poor population health and a fledging health care system, Ghanaian citizens' experience increased barriers to successful HIV/AIDS prevention. In Ghana, facilitators to successful HIV reduction strategies are influenced by government impetus to achieve several Millennium Development Goals (MDGs). Relatively low rates of HIV/AIDS prevalence in Ghana are a result of a well-coordinated national response and governmental activism. Other facilitators include HIV prevention programs targeting school-aged children and young adults, and emerging forms of church-based and folk art activism. However, social and cultural barriers limit the strengthening of existing female gender–based activism in Ghana."

The final chapter of Volume 1 takes a somewhat different methodological approach than the preceding chapters, and also examines the often-overlooked issue of linkages between HIV/AIDS and various forms of "security." In *A People-Centered Approach to the Links among HIV/AIDS, Conflicts, and Security in Colombia,* Fernando Serrano-Amaya "discusses the links between HIV/AIDS and armed political conflicts." He argues that "such links have been made using a limited idea of security that has redefined HIV/AIDS as a threat to the functioning of states. Other approaches to security and other ways to explore the connections between HIV/AIDS and conflicts have received less attention. Using a peace studies perspective, the nature of lived experiences of HIV/AIDS in areas of conflict is explored with reference to two cases from Colombia. The conclusions discuss the possibilities and limits of doing HIV activism in war zones."

## VOLUME 2: POLICY AND POLICYMAKING

The 14 chapters of the second volume have a particular emphasis on persistent challenges and emerging issues in critical areas of public policy and in the process of public policymaking. Part 1 on "Global and Transnational Policy Debates over HIV Prevention and Treatment" includes chapters on intellectual property, medical male circumcision, global data collection, U.S. international policies, and HIV-related stigma. Part 2 on "Country- and Regional-Level Policy Debates over HIV Prevention and Treatment" is comprised of chapters focused on China, India, Cambodia, and the United States, as well as various parts of the sub-Saharan Africa region.

## Part 1: Global and Transnational Policy Debates over HIV Prevention and Treatment

Volume 2 begins with a focus on *The Shifting Sands of Intellectual Property Law and Policy: Implications for the Future of HIV Treatment and Public Health* by Boyan Konstantinov, Tenu Avafia, Mandeep Dhaliwal, and Jeffrey O'Malley. The authors state that "the unprecedented scale-up of antiretroviral treatment for people living with HIV in the past decade would not have been possible without the drastic price reduction in treatment regimens from the year 2000 to the present day. The decrease in treatment price can be largely attributed to competition from generic pharmaceutical manufacturers, predominantly from India, the efforts of treatment activists, and the economies of scale as the numbers of treatment increased. Today, the vast majority of people on this life-saving treatment for HIV rely on generic medicines. Despite the initial success, the sustainability of current and future treatment programs is under jeopardy from global developments in intellectual property policy and law." The chapter explores the "paradigm shift in intellectual property and access to medicines that occurred with the introduction of the WTO Agreement on Trade-Related Aspects of Intellectual Property Rights, the most recent changes and trends in this field, and the need to develop an agenda for the global South that balances intellectual property and the human right to the highest attainable standards of health."

The next chapter explores another complex public health challenge in *Medical Circumcision and the Politics of No Alternative: Why the Public Health Imperative Scored a Victory against HIV/AIDS*. Co-authors Ilaria Regondi, Kaymarlin Govender, Kerisha Naidoo, and Gavin George state that "medical male circumcision (MMC) is one of the latest biomedical interventions to be advocated by the international community as a key HIV/AIDS prevention strategy. Despite its association with exogenous cultural and religious customs, the practice has been relatively well received in non-Western contexts." This chapter examines the reasons for this and "posits that a range of historical, scientific, and cultural factors have facilitated such an endorsement. While MMC could be seen as the product of a convergence of discourses, we caution against the widespread implementation of this HIV prevention intervention without due consideration for addressing the localized complexities of the epidemic, including the challenges of community participation that are regarded as being central to the broad spectrum of HIV-related interventions."

Chapter 3 is titled *Count Us In: The Need for More Comprehensive Global Data on HIV/AIDS Prevention, Testing, and Knowledge among LGBT Populations.* Gemma Oberth and Phillipa Tucker argue that "lesbian, gay, bisexual, and transgender (LGBT) people face particular barriers in accessing quality prevention and treatment for HIV and AIDS, which current data collection and reporting are simply not reflecting or addressing. Although global indicators exist for men who have sex with men (MSM) and male sex workers, there is no data collection framework for women who have sex with women (WSW) or for transgender individuals (TG). With increasing cause for alarm—both epidemiologically and from a human rights perspective—it is clear that accountability and transparency around the response to HIV and AIDS among LGBT people need inclusion."

Sean Cahill, Robert Valadéz, and Nathan Schaefer shift to a U.S. focus, but on a topic with global and transnational implications in their chapter *Promoting HIV Prevention and Research with Men Who Have Sex with Men (MSM) through U.S. Foreign Policy.* They note that "men who have sex with men (MSM) remain disproportionately affected by the HIV epidemic worldwide. However, stark differences exist from country to country, both in the epidemiologic trends of HIV among MSM, but also in the structure of different countries' responses. Some intergovernmental funding mechanisms are beginning to shape how MSM-specific HIV prevention and treatment resources are managed, at times controversially. Homophobia and antigay stigma continue to have dramatic influences on how HIV is transmitted, monitored, and combated. New and emerging biomedical interventions (e.g., sero-sorting, preexposure prophylaxis, circumcision) are altering the HIV landscape among MSM across the world."

Michelle Beadle-Holder explores several themes with global and transnational significance in *HIV/AIDS-Related Stigma as the Root of HIV Criminalization and Bias against Sex Workers.* This chapter "draws upon the concept of stigma and political mobilization to explore how people experience and resist contemporary forms of marginalization and discrimination associated with HIV/AIDS. It examines the ways in which specific laws, policies, and ideas grounded in preexisting stigma contribute to HIV/AIDS-related stigma and discrimination. The chapter also examines the strategies that groups such as the Positive Justice Project and Global

Network of Sex Work Projects employ to challenge HIV/AIDS-related-stigma and discrimination."

## Part 2: Country- and Regional-Level Policy Debates over HIV Prevention and Treatment

Focusing on perhaps the most vulnerable sector with the global HIV/AIDS epidemic, Morten Skovdal and Catherine Campbell discuss *Public Engagement and Policymaking for Caregiving Children of the HIV Epidemic in Sub-Saharan Africa*. This chapter "maps out the policy spaces that influence policymaking for children of the HIV epidemic at both local and global levels and reflects on a public engagement project, which sought greater policy recognition of children's caregiving. Two key dilemmas emerged, pertaining to the unintended consequences of creating a new HIV-related social welfare category (i.e., 'caregiving children'), and fears that a recognition of caregiving children can be used to justify child labor. The dilemmas are discussed and highlight the need for a critical framework for policy analysis and action—one that considers the mismatch of local realities and global legislation processes."

The next chapter continues a focus on policy dilemmas in sub-Saharan Africa in *The Intersection of Disability and HIV in Eastern and Southern Africa*. Jill Hanass-Hancock presents "a summary of data in regard to the growing evidence on the interrelationships of disability and HIV, responses from civil society as well as an analysis of National Strategic Plans on HIV (NSP)." This chapter "illustrates how regional and international advocacy work raised awareness for the interrelationship of disability and HIV, influenced major international HIV events, and led to the development of a disability-inclusive framework, which was launched at the International Conference on AIDS and STIs in Africa (ICASA) conference in December 2011. The framework contributes to the review process and the inclusion of disability in HIV planning in the future and ultimately prepares the region for the long-term impact of disability and HIV."

*A Chinese-Style AIDS Exceptionalist Paradigm: Reflection on China's Recent HIV/AIDS Policy Reform* by Wenjue Lu Knutsen brings the focus of Volume 2 to the world's most populous country. The author argues that "China's HIV/AIDS policy has progressed significantly since 2002. Government regulations were issued and various programs launched. China's current policy resembles an AIDS exceptionalist paradigm that is characterized by treating HIV/AIDS as fundamentally different from other communicable diseases. This study questions whether an exceptionalist paradigm is suitable for China, especially when an opposite trend of normalization is emerging internationally." This chapter provides an overview of China's HIV/AIDS policy, the application of AIDS exceptionalism to China, and an analysis of benefits and disadvantages of applying AIDS exceptionalism to China. It concludes that a hybrid approach may be most suitable for China.

Continuing with the world's second-most populous nation, Mangala Subramaniam discusses *The Medicalization of HIV/AIDS Policy: The Case of India*. She explains that "although the proportion of women who acquire HIV/AIDS from heterosexual contact has grown across countries, there has only been a slow shift in the focus of HIV/AIDS prevention strategies that consider more gender-specific interventions. Models for understanding and addressing HIV/AIDS have their limits; specifically, their reliance upon individualistic models that presuppose agency of subjects fails to consider the subjects' social structural context." She argues that "the emphasis on the overly medicalized nature of HIV prevention in organizational efforts marginalizes gender in efforts to arrest infection rates. Medical knowledge does not simply flow; it is dependent on communicative processes structured by inequities of power and resources based on social differences often overlooked in preventive efforts."

Shifting to another region of Asia, Ian Lubek and his team of collaborators focused their chapter on *HIV/AIDS and Alcohol Risks in Cambodia: Confronting Challenges and Policymaking through Research-Guided Actions*. This chapter describes how researchers, practitioners, and interns from social sciences, medicine, public health, and global development have collaborated in Cambodia with local health providers, employers, NGOs, grassroots stakeholders, and volunteers to confront HIV/AIDS and the co-risk of alcohol overuse. They state that "results from research-driven interventions engage the local community and also seek to effect national and global policy and practices. The grassroots NGO SiRCHESI (Siem Reap Citizens for Health, Educational, and Social Issues) uses local health workers and peer educators to provide interventions and evaluate their impact. These health-promotion interventions involve contacts with local partners, global business headquarters, government policymakers, and relevant decision makers. Strategies are discussed for changing policy or practices by directly 'making data matter' or 'indirectly' by providing the data to others (e.g., press, unions, international organizations) whose mandates involve greater activism than permitted to Cambodian NGOs."

With a focus on the country with the world's highest burden of HIV infections, Rebecca Hodes contributes the chapter entitled *"You Know What a Bad Person You Are?" HIV, Abortion, and Reproductive Health Care for Women in South Africa.* This research examines the "provision of comprehensive reproductive healthcare to women with HIV in South Africa, with a focus on the highly contested issue of abortion. It explores how the emergence and escalation of the HIV epidemic and the later implementation of the national antiretroviral (ARV) treatment program influenced the public provision of reproductive healthcare for women with HIV. It also examines the effects of government's failure to implement health protocols and policies to provide adequate reproductive health-care for women with HIV. This has resulted in the punitive treatment of patients by healthcare workers and in further coercive practices such as forced abortion and sterilization. Despite the copious data generated about the medical and sociological effects of the HIV pandemic, little research has been conducted on abortion and HIV. This chapter builds on the work of public health scholars, medical historians and bioethicists to document and analyze persistent challenges in the provision of reproductive health services to HIV-positive women in South Africa."

Also focused on South Africa, the chapter *Constraints on the Potential Effectiveness of HIV/AIDS Early Treatment Policy in South Africa* by Josué Mbonigaba explains that "the South African government has, since 2007, made a serious commitment to deal with HIV/AIDS by changing both its treatment and prevention policies. One of the latest policies consists of enrolling patients on treatment at a CD4 count below 350 (early treatment), rather than at CD4 counts below 200 (late treatment)." This chapter explores "the likely effects of such a policy on funding, the state of the health care system, risk behaviors, and HIV transmission, finding that each may well work against the effectiveness of early treatment. Whether the findings prove valid will depend on long-term changes in funding and significant decreases in HIV transmissions, which basically determine the future of HIV/AIDS prevention and treatment."

In *HIV Prevention Fatigue and HIV Complacency: Ongoing Challenges in Advanced Industrialized Nations,* Tasleem J. Padamsee and Hugh Klein state that "referring in general to the difficulties of maintaining continuous vigilance to HIV/AIDS issues at individual, cultural, and policy levels, prevention fatigue and prevention complacency represent important challenges in Western nations at the vanguard of coping with HIV/AIDS." The authors address "the origins and prevalence of HIV prevention fatigue and HIV complacency in industrialized nations, the effects of these phenomena among gay men and others at significant risk of HIV infection, and important areas for future research," and conclude by "considering the roles activists and national-level policymakers can play in addressing these challenges."

Rounding out Volume 2 is *HIV Prevention Policies at the Intersection of Gender, Race, and Class in the United States* by Karen L. Baird. In this broad recap of women and HIV/AIDS in the United States, the author notes that "in the early days of the epidemic, women remained invisible or were viewed as 'vessels' or 'vectors.' In time, HIV/AIDS research began to focus on how women become infected. Transmission to women was initially by injection drug use (IDU), but in the mid-1990s, the dominant mode of transmission became heterosexual sex. Few prevention programs were developed for women, and the few that were developed focused on women changing their 'risky' sexual behavior and ignored contextual and structural issues that shaped their risk. Though researchers have now clearly documented the connections of poverty, violence and abuse, and gender inequality—to name only a few—to HIV risk, prevention policies, programs, and funding rarely incorporate such concerns. This omission is one of the primary reasons why the HIV/AIDS rates for women have remained unchanged over the last decade."

## VOLUME 3: ACTIVISM AND COMMUNITY MOBILIZATION

The 17 chapters of the third volume have a particular emphasis on the various social movements that have been such critical factors in focusing attention on the global HIV/AIDS crisis. Part 1 on "Global and Transnational HIV/AIDS Activism and Community Mobilization" includes several broad chapters sketching persistent challenges and emerging issues confronting activists and communities. Part 2 on "Country- and Regional-Level HIV/AIDS Activism and Community Mobilization" is comprised of chapters focused on China, India, Cambodia, and the United States, as well as various parts of the sub-Saharan Africa region.

### Part 1: Global and Transnational HIV/AIDS Activism and Community Mobilization

Volume 3 begins with a chapter intended to provide an anchor for subsequent chapters on the issue of HIV/AIDS activism. *Social Movement Responses to HIV/AIDS in the United States and Globally: Intersecting Chronological, Strategic, and Health Movement Frames* by Raymond A.

Smith, Richard G. Parker, Jonathan Garcia, and Robert H. Remien "builds upon the existing literature on the role of social movements, particularly with regard to health-related social movements, to propose three intersecting frames by which to understand the role of social movement responses to HIV/AIDS in the United States and globally. The first frame relates to the basic chronological/historical unfolding of responses to the epidemic. The second focuses on the strategic choices of movement activity made by activists, in particular whether to pursue 'structural' or 'cultural' forms of activism. The third frame then overlays the chronological development and strategic choices with a typology of health social movements in order to illuminate the shifting and overlapping rationale(s) for HIV/AIDS social movement activity."

This broad portrait of activism is continued, with a cross-national emphasis on treatment activism, in *AIDS Treatment Advocacy in the United States, Brazil, and South Africa: Diverse Actors, Strategies, and Sectors.* Author Susan M. Chambré argues that "public representations of AIDS treatment advocacy privilege the critical role of AIDS activists— individuals and organizations that forward their claims by demonstrating and engaging in acts of civil disobedience rather than more conventional political strategies." This chapter examines "the nature of AIDS treatment advocacy in three political contexts, the United States, Brazil, and South Africa, pointing out that obtaining extensive and in some cases universal access to antiretrovirals was the result of collaboration among activists, advocates who used conventional political strategies, and institutional advocates working within the state. The campaigns that resulted in expanded access involved multiple institutional targets, including the state and corporations. Future challenges remain, however, in maintaining the fragile coalition that finances access in developing nations."

On a complementary note, San Patten, Joanne Mantell, and Zena Stein focus on prevention activism in *Discord and Harmony in Biomedical HIV Prevention Technologies: Advancements through Advocacy.* They state that "the expectation that we would soon see a technological breakthrough against AIDS with an effective and universal vaccine rose with the discovery of the causal agent, but gradually faded as the peculiar properties of HIV emerged. The social and personal changes in many lives required to prevent sexual transmission—celibacy or lifetime mutual monogamy—seemed almost unattainable, with the male condom being the only available alternative in the first decades of the pandemic. With women virtually unable to regard the use of that tool as under their control, active minds turned to other technological possibilities. Currently, several new biomedical approaches to HIV prevention are at various stages in the research and development pipeline, and many have proof-of-concept as viable means of preventing sexual transmission of HIV, but their emergence has taken decades, and the work is not complete."

*Building "HIV/AIDS-Competent Communities" in Resource-Poor Settings: Creating Contexts That Enable Effective Community Mobilization* by Catherine Campbell and Morten Skovdal shifts from activism to broader community engagement. They argue that "while community empowerment is a pillar of HIV/AIDS policy, less attention is given to creating contexts that support communities in putting new skills and capacities into action." Conceptualizing "community HIV/AIDS competence" to address this challenge, the authors "discuss two very different case studies (in South Africa and Kenya), which sought to facilitate local HIV/AIDS competence through (1) empowering marginalized groups to respond more effectively to HIV/AIDS, (2) building local support for such efforts, and (3) facilitating supportive partnerships with donors, policy-makers, NGOs, and public-sector agencies outside of the community." The authors pay particular attention to the local–global relationships that provide the most enabling context for the strengthening of local community responses to HIV/AIDS.

Examining the critical interface between science and activism, Emily Bass, Julien Burns, Mitchell Warren, and Deirdre Grant are the co-authors of *Citizen Scientists and Activist Researchers: Building and Sustaining HIV Prevention Research Advocacy in the "Era of Evidence."* They argue that "the field of biomedical prevention research (e.g., development of and advocacy for new prevention strategies such as a microbicide, preexposure prophylaxis, an AIDS vaccine, voluntary medical male circumcision) has undergone a profound change since 2005, as a cascade of positive results has emerged from various efficacy trials. Advocates working in this field who had previously emphasized the need to understand the potential benefit of yet-to-be-identified strategies are now working in a highly complex actual landscape in which each positive trial result raises specific questions about next steps, advocacy goals, and essential communication. The broad contours of strategies and priorities of biomedical prevention research before and after the 'era of evidence' are described, with an emphasis on some of the emerging tactics and imperatives for key stakeholder groups seeking to optimize the benefits of new prevention options."

Rounding out Part 1, Nicoli Nattrass turns to a perennially thorny topic in *Contesting Conspiracies: Science, Activism, and the Ongoing Battle against AIDS Denialism.* This chapter "examines different ways in which

HIV scientists and AIDS activists have mobilized scientific evidence and engaged in credibility battles with AIDS denialists." The chapter "highlights the AIDS policy debacle in South Africa under President Mbeki and how the fight against long-standing AIDS denialist Peter Duesberg has involved both scientific rebuttals and credibility battles, including attempts by scientists and AIDS activists to deny his work the imprimatur of science. The conclusion discusses how credibility battles against AIDS denialism have extended in new ways in the Internet era, for example publicizing the deaths of iconic AIDS denialists, arguing that the struggle for evidence-based medicine is alive and well in the Internet era."

## Part 2: Country- and Regional-Level HIV/AIDS Activism and Community Mobilization

Part 2 begins with a topic and a region only rarely addressed in the HIV/AIDS activist literature: *The Challenges of Forming Associations of People Living with HIV in Low-Prevalence and High-Stigma Contexts: The Case of Sudan and Lebanon.* Jocelyn DeJong, Iman Mortagy, and Rana Haddad Ibrahim state that "civil society groups formed by people living with HIV/AIDS have been critical in shaping the response to HIV. However, most of the research on such movements is based on the experience of high-income countries or countries with high HIV prevalence. Countries in the Middle East and North Africa have seen the emergence of associations for people living with HIV, but there has been little analysis of their role or impact." This chapter compares findings from two qualitative studies in Sudan and Lebanon on the experience of forming these associations and draws lessons from other countries with a similar HIV context.

Addressing the role of large-scale philanthropy, Robert Lorway presents *How to Exit an Epidemic: Philanthrocapitalism, Community Mobilization, and the Domestication of Sexual Dissidence in South India.* The chapter argues, "as the Gates-sponsored India AIDS initiative known as Avahan transitions toward the public system, controversies erupt over how the state will sustain the successes demonstrated by Avahan. Those who have the most at stake are the sex workers whose lives have been dramatically altered by community mobilization programs, which govern their access to prevention services. This chapter analyzes intervention techniques deployed in Karnataka State, highlighting where market-oriented logics combine with epidemiological surveillance approaches." He argues that "the business rationalities at work in community mobilization schemes, along with enumerative techniques of accountability, operate to domesticate sexual dissidence, stifling the transformative potential of sex worker social movements."

Focusing on a different sector of civil society and an often-overlooked population, Wessel van den Berg, Dean Peacock, and Tim Shand provide *Mobilizing Men and Boys in HIV Prevention and Treatment: The Sonke Gender Justice Experience in South Africa.* They state that "the fact that men represent a 'blind spot' in the global AIDS response is self-evidently bad for men's health. Put bluntly, men get sick and die unnecessarily. It is also bad for other men, for women, their families and communities, and for public health systems. When men do not know their HIV status they are less likely to change their sexual practices and are less likely to use condoms, and are thus much more likely to infect their partners. They are also less likely to access treatment and more likely to need ongoing care and support—initially at home where the burden of care is usually borne by women, and then later by public health officials who attend to men with alarmingly compromised immune systems who are hard to treat and who often require expensive treatment to restore to health."

Continuing on the theme of HIV/AIDS primarily in South Africa, *Crisis and Chronicity: How Treatment Is Changing Activism in South Africa and Beyond* by Christopher J. Colvin examines the impact of antiretroviral treatment (ART) on AIDS activism. It begins with a case study of South Africa's Treatment Action Campaign and its response to the provision of ART in the public sector. It then reviews some of the ways treatment and prevention activism have changed in the context of a chronic HIV epidemic. The final section explores recent changes in global public health, many of which were the result of AIDS activism. The author makes the case that "like treatment access, this context shapes the political conditions of possibility for AIDS activists looking to convert short-term struggles and gains into a longer-term health social movement to respond to HIV."

In *AIDS Mobilization in Zambia: Agency versus Structural Challenges,* Amy Patterson presents the argument that "organizations of people living with HIV (PLWHAs) are part of Africa's nascent civil society, providing services government often cannot or will not provide and advocating for issues that affect people infected with or affected by HIV and AIDS." The chapter focuses on the advocacy role of PLWHA groups in Zambia. Advocacy can occur through formal political institutions such as legislative bodies, or through informal entities such as local community groups." It focuses on grassroots advocacy, as it investigates how urban-based PLWHA groups in Zambia seek to influence local decision making to gain policies and programs that will benefit them. The author asserts that while "scholars have examined national-level advocacy by PLWHA groups in Africa, there has been limited research on how PLWHA groups mobilize at the community level, and there is tension between individual agency and structural challenges to mobilization." The chapter argues that for a small number of groups, "political efficacy, leadership, and linkages to external supporters facilitated advocacy, though most groups faced economic, political, cultural, and organizational challenges that limited this activism."

In *From Dissidence to Partnership and Back to Confrontation Again? The Current Predicament of Brazilian HIV/AIDS Activism,* Carlos Guilherme do Valle discusses "how Brazilian HIV/AIDS activism emerged and reconfigured itself in the last 25 years and shows the complex ways by which nongovernmental organizations and networks have defined their relations among themselves and with governmental agencies and health policies on the AIDS epidemic." The chapter "highlights issues, such as the creation of spaces of participation and political articulation among HIV/AIDS activist groups and networks, the historical definition of models of identity construction in relation to illness, the political disputes around the distribution of new antiretroviral drugs, the criminalization of HIV transmission, and challenges to the sustainability and political autonomy of Brazilian HIV/AIDS activism. The main focus is on the conflictive and interdependent relations between activism and AIDS policy in Brazil."

Continuing an emphasis on Latin America, Antonio Torres-Ruiz offers a chapter titled *The NGO-ization of HIV/AIDS Activism in Mexico: Not So Scandalous After All?* He argues that "several analyses of the process of NGO-ization of social movements, including those engaged in the struggle against HIV/AIDS, tend to emphasize its negative effects on the relations between civil society and the state, and warn us about the shrinking distance between the two, the resulting lack of autonomy for the former, and the detrimental impact on a vibrant public sphere." In contrast, this chapter "offers a more nuanced assessment and some optimistic insights to counter such warnings, which are based on a close analysis of the NGO-ization of HIV/AIDS activism in Mexico."

Shifting emphasis from the developing to the developed world, Richard Boulton offers the chapter *Children, HIV, Stigma, and Activism in the UK: Treading the Line between Innocence and Vulnerability, Vice and Virtue.* The chapter "explores formations of stigma found in relation to children with HIV in the UK and the ensuing effect this has on activism, arguing that the stigma of children with HIV is interlaced with ideas of innocence associated with childhood. This has implications for the way that activism is formed around the condition and has a bearing on the ways that children, parents, and families are organized into activist groups. In general, families don't wish to acknowledge their HIV or associate with it. This results in limited possibilities for a united voice and the organization of activism or activist groups and puts combating stigma at the top of the agenda for charities campaigning for children with HIV."

Placing an emphasis on a controversial topic in the law, *"We Are Not Criminals": Activists Addressing the Criminalization of HIV Nondisclosure in Canada* by Daniel Grace and Tim McCaskell "presents a short introduction to the issue of criminalizing HIV transmission, exposure, and/or nondisclosure in local and macro-regional contexts." The chapter reviews key transnational texts and activist work in this field. With this background provided, the chapter presents "the specific forms of activism work being conducted by the Ontario Working Group on Criminal Law and HIV Exposure (CLHE) as a focused case study of activism in Ontario, Canada." Through an explication of the local activism of this group, the chapter "makes visible important successes, context-specific issues, and lessons learned by this complex example of HIV activism. This focus allows connections to be made to broader global activist movements that are working across borders to address the social construction and criminal prosecution of a viral underclass."

Next, William Ward Darrow examines another dimension of community engagement in *Community Mobilization, Community Planning, and Community-Based Research for HIV Prevention in the United States*. He argues that "organized community efforts lie at the heart of public health. Members of gay and bisexual communities organized to confront the AIDS crisis through collective action when federal health authorities failed to respond in the early 1980s. CDC initiated a national program of community planning in 1993 to take advantage of grassroots organizing efforts, but this laudable attempt to collaborate collapsed in the early 2000s. HIV-prevention efforts in the United States continue to be severely hampered by a biomedical model of reductionism, a top-down bureaucratic approach to problem solving, and an emphasis on scientific efficacy instead of comprehensive program effectiveness."

In the concluding chapter of the bookset, Jeff Maskovsky focuses on an exceptional case study in *Diversifying AIDS Activism: Lessons Learned from ACT UP/Philadelphia*. This chapter discusses "the diversification of AIDS activism during the period from 1997 to 2012, in particular the case of ACT UP/Philadelphia, a group that thrived during this period, in part thanks to increased participation by low-income African Americans."

The chapter "emphasizes two interconnected aspects of ACT UP/Philadelphia's diversification. The first is the internal dilemmas that diversity posed for the group and the concrete changes that it made to its radical democratic practice in order to overcome them. The second is the extent to which diversity enhanced the political effectiveness of the group's grassroots campaigns." The author's broader argument is that, "although ACT UP/Philadelphia was unable to overcome entrenched race- and class-based inequalities, it managed them in ways that helped to sustain the AIDS activist movement. This, in turn, created an important space of political participation for low-income African Americans, for whom movement participation restored essential civil rights, a sense of social value, and, for many, life itself."

## ACKNOWLEDGMENTS

The editor would like to acknowledge the efforts of all of the contributors to these volumes, as well as all of their colleagues and staff within their institutions, both for their own chapters as well as for their invaluable comments on the work of other chapter authors. He would also like to thank his colleagues in the Division of Gender, Sexuality, and Health and at the HIV Center for Clinical and Behavioral Studies at the New York State Psychiatric Institute and Columbia University, as well as colleagues in the political science programs at Columbia and New York University. Special thanks go out to Alicia Merritt, Debbie Carvalko, and the editorial and production teams at Praeger; to the project's editorial assistants, Samantha Gilbert, Michael Luke, Peter Capp, and Danielle Benson; and to the bookset's associate editor, Brandon Aultman.

# PART 1
# GLOBAL AND TRANSNATIONAL HIV/AIDS ACTIVISM AND COMMUNITY MOBILIZATION

# 1

# Social Movement Responses to HIV/AIDS in the United States and Globally: Intersecting Chronological, Strategic, and Health Movement Frames

*Raymond A. Smith, Richard G. Parker, Jonathan Garcia, and Robert H. Remien*

The ebbs and flows of social movements, political and cultural revolutions, have been analyzed through a variety of lenses in an attempt to understand the incentives for collective action against grievances, the structural moments that foster mobilization, and cultural framings that shape advocacy and activism. Social movements are sometimes considered the venue through which "people who lack regular access to institutions . . . act in the name of new or unaccepted claims, and . . . behave in ways that fundamentally challenge others or authorities" (Tarrow, 1998; see also McAdam, Tarrow, & Tilly, 2001). The study of contentious politics has focused on finding reasons why and mechanisms through which individuals mobilize for a common cause.

Health-related grievances and inequalities have harnessed a variety of diverse responses from societies, but only recently have social scientists begun to study the particularities of social movements focused on health and the ways in which these impact on health policies and practices. The forms in which cultural meanings and embodied realities of illness influence these movements add complexity to understandings of contentious politics in relation to health issues—particularly in recent decades, under conditions of increasing globalization, as the importance of civil society organizations and the rise of transnational activism has been felt in relation to health policy and the organization of health programs. Movements such as the environmental breast cancer movement, the reproductive health and rights movement, and the HIV/AIDS activist movement have all begun to be studied using ethnographic methods, oral histories, and other social movement research approaches in order to understand how personal experiences lead individuals to acquire collective identities and to take action in response to a variety of factors affecting their health and well-being.

In this chapter, we briefly review a number of the key theories through which social movements have been studied in the social sciences, and then we look at how these theories can be applied to health social movements. We then look more closely at the specific case of one of the earliest and most influential health-related movements—the HIV/AIDS social movement—and at the different ways in which it has been organized historically around paradigms of access to health, constituency-based mobilization, and politicized embodiment. The vast majority of mainstream medical and public health research in relation to HIV/AIDS has focused on individual behavior and behavioral change, and only more recently on the structural and environmental factors that condition it. We argue that social movement research approaches might offer key insights that make it possible to move beyond the frequently cited impasse between individual behaviors and structural barriers to behavioral change.

This is potentially a particularly important contribution given the increasing emphasis on structural interventions, those that "work by altering the context within which health is produced or reproduced. Structural interventions locate the source of public-health problems in factors in the social, economic and political environments that shape and constrain individual, community, and societal health outcomes" (Blankenship, Bray, & et al., 2000, p. 11). We identified two dimensions along which structural interventions can vary. They may locate the source of health problems in factors relating to availability, acceptability, or accessibility; and they may be targeted at the individual, organizational, or environmental levels (Blankenship, Bray, et al., 2000).

We seek to explore the ways in which social movement theories and methods applied to examine social responses to HIV/AIDS in empirical, historical circumstances may highlight some of the factors that bring about changes in response to the epidemic in the real world. We argue that such detailed empirical studies of historical events and lived experience of people responding to the epidemic under "real-world conditions" may ultimately offer far greater insight into processes of change in response to HIV/AIDS than the kinds of controlled-trials that have tended to dominate both biomedical and behavioral research on the epidemic.

The study of social movements has been an important area of research across a range of social science disciplines—particularly in sociology, but also in anthropology, political science, social psychology, and related disciplines—and it is impossible to do justice, in the space available here, to the full range of theories and approaches that have emerged in this highly active field of research. Given our focus on the relative lack of research attention on social movements in relation to health, and on HIV/AIDS in particular, we focus here above all on some of the key approaches that we think may have greatest potential importance in relation to these issues. We pay special attention to a distinction between *rationalist* and *structuralist approaches,* the study of what have been described as *new social movements,* and research on *cultural frames* and *collective identities.*

## RATIONALISTS AND STRUCTURALISTS

Rationalist theories of action, as initially articulated by Mancur Olson, question why individuals would participate in social movements, considering what Olson (1965) terms the "collective action problem" primarily based on microeconomic logic. The question of *why* individuals participate in collective action when they can "free ride" on the efforts of others—rationally creating disincentives for participation unless there is differential individual gain or "selective incentives"—spurred the study of social movements, primarily by sociologists and political scientists. In this case, both civil society and the state constitute a complex of stakeholders with self-interests, including politicians, social elites, labor unions, and those concerned with identity-related grievances. The increased study of social movements along these lines led to the development of theories focused on resource mobilization and political opportunities. This approach has continued to be applied in many areas of the social sciences, often with important modifications such as the introduction of imperfect information and political entrepreneurship (Moe, 1980) and a focus on the instrumental value of expressive and social incentives (Chong, 1991). Yet many social movement researchers have found the rigorously parsimonious assumptions of Olson's rationalist theory as insufficient, particularly for issues and movements that are not solely or directly related to economic issues.

Increasingly the study of social movements has been expanded by focusing on the availability and successful mobilization of resources, such as connections to elites, financial support, and social networks. McCarthy and Zald (1973) introduced what they described as "resource mobilization theory," which posits that the motivation to form and join social movements is partially a result of the availability of such organizational resources. They argued "that there is always enough discontent in any society to supply the grass-roots support for a movement if the movement is effectively organized and has at its disposal the power and resources of some established elite group" (McCarthy & Zald, 1973, p. 1215). The role of "outsiders" or "conscience adherents"—who will not directly benefit from the goals of the movement—in organizing movements is crucial to their theory of mobilization. According to McCarthy and Zald (1973), entrepreneurs build social movement organizations when they see an opportunity in a resource-rich sector of the population group that shares a set of values.

Resource mobilization theory has been critiqued because it pays little attention to the importance of indigenous leadership, cultures, and the overall atmosphere of contention. McAdam (1982) and Tilly (1978) argued that the study of mobilization should take into account preexisting informal social networks among individuals, and that the political constraints on social movements should not be considered constant (Tarrow, 1998). In response to the last critique, work has increasingly focused on how the political process frames the opportunities for collective action to emerge and succeed. Charles Tilly's work has been especially influential in suggesting that in addition to the internal resources of movements that affected their capacity to act, external factors are crucial in explaining when collective action occurred (Tilly, 1978). Other writers have placed more emphasis on the institutional structures of government that shape how the political opportunity structure affects the ability of social movements to mobilize and affect strategies (Kitschelt, 1986). Kitschelt (1986), for example, has emphasized how open a political system is to inputs and the capacity of a system to implement policies as crucial in explaining the strength (and effects) of social movements, while Tarrow (1996) has emphasized (1) the opening up of political access, (2) unstable alignments among political actors, (3) the appearance of influential allies, and (4) the emergence of divisions among elites as key in explaining participation in collective action. Therefore, looking at structural political changes, such as democratization, helps us understand when and how social movements will most likely gain momentum. Such research has highlighted the fact that for social movements to be effective, they must be operating in an environment in which government actors have the capacity to produce change but at the same time remain vulnerable to pressure from societal actors, including activists and protestors, offering important insights into the social and political conditions that appear to be necessary for successful social movements.

## NEW SOCIAL MOVEMENTS

The last third of the twentieth century was a time of great social and political upheaval, with many countries either emerging from colonial or neocolonial rule or returning to formal democratic governments after years of authoritarian rule (Lind, 1992; Joseph, 1997; Jones, 1998; Bunce, 1997). In these political transitions, social movements—and institutions such as labor unions—played a critical role in setting the agenda for contention. During the rise and continuance of dictatorships in many countries during the 1960s and 1970s, various social movements organized around class issues and achieving control of the state as a means to transform society, yet with only a few notable exceptions, these movements did not gain control of the state, and many suffered extreme repression (O'Kane, 2000; Findji, 1992; Ortiz, 1987; Warren, 1989; Linz, 2000).

With the wave of democratization, through the 1980s, new theories of political mobilization and social transformation began to emerge to explain these processes in different developmental contexts. Political energy in many so-called developing countries (especially in Latin America, but also in many countries in Africa, Eastern Europe, and Asia) became concentrated again on electoral politics and state policies, and some social researchers began to question whether social movements might be losing their political militancy and becoming co-opted by the state, especially through populist governments, as well as being subject to the political economic forces of globalization and neoliberalism (Findji, 1992; Ortiz, 1987; Turner, 1995; Robbins, 2004; Bunce, 1997, 2000; Jones, 1998; Joseph, 1997; Van Rooy, 2000; Kriesi et al., 1998).

Many different kinds of social movements emerged during the mid/late 1970s and early 1980s, which rather than framing their concerns in terms of the state and revolution, were more limited in focus and local in scope. Theories of these "new social movements" emerged primarily to explain political processes occurring in Western Europe, but they were rapidly diffused throughout the globe. In the change from "old" to "new" social movements, there was an important shift of attention away from a primary concentration with political economic regimes as vast sources of domination and repression—allowing for the politicization of issues such as peace and the preservation of the environment (Warren, 1998; Elmerdorf, 1997; Hochstetler, 1997). Just as social movements have changed over the years, so have the ways in which social scientists have studied them. When the "new social movements" first appeared in the late 1970s and early 1980s, many analysts championed their emancipatory and radical potential (Burdick, 1992a; Alvarez, 1998; Jelin, 1990, 1998; Gillet, 2003).

More recently, the field of social movement research, including work carried out by many of the first articulators of "new social movement" theory, seems to be adopting a more balanced approach that moves beyond either/or assessments and employs broader definitions of what counts as "political" (Offe, 1999; Inglehart, 1999; Kriesi, 1989; Wignaraja, 1993; Burdick, 1992a; Jelin, 1998). Much recent work on emerging fields of contention is focusing primarily on social justice issues, while another important focus has been on other forms of mobilization that are more associated with so-called "identity politics," including feminist, racial and/or ethnic, and lesbian/gay movements (Bernstein 2005; Laraña, Johnston, et al., 1994). These movements empirically "have combined political goals with more cultural oriented efforts" (Polletta & Jasper, 2001, p. 287). With their emphasis on the politicization of everyday life and new ways of doing politics, these movements strongly shaped the democratization process and the development of civil society in many countries.

## THE ROLE OF CULTURE AND COLLECTIVE IDENTITY

Both the resource mobilization and the political opportunity theories are "rational," behavioral theories in which the costs and benefits to mobilizing affect whether collective action occurs. However, these theories gloss over several crucial questions of collective action theory, such as how individuals come to recognize their common interests. McAdam (1982) has argued for the necessity of incorporating cultural factors into analyses based on political opportunities and organizational strength. People must recognize their similar interests and realize the possibility for successful insurgency before collective action can occur: "cognitive liberation" and particularly the shift from "individual attribution" to "system attribution" is a key part of his model (McAdam, 1982, pp. 49–51). Some analysts have argued that it is the shift from general blame attribution to specific blame attribution that is important to explaining participation in political protest (see Javeline, 2003)—but in some cases the change target is in the cultural realm rather than policy change (Polletta & Jasper, 2001). Tilly's work on "repertoires of contention" highlights the importance of cognitive framing in explaining *how* individuals coordinate and organize specific strategies for collective action (Tilly, 1985, p. 747). Thus, identification through cultural framing is one way scholars have attempted to explain how people develop a collective identity and why they enter social movements.

On the other hand, theories of "collective identity" have analyzed the ways in which cultural representations are contested (Polletta & Jasper, 2001, p. 283). Rather than focusing solely on the state or on political reform as the targets of collective action, cultural interpretations of the self and affective bonds, as well as providing strategies for policy reform and "expanded political representation," have "impacts outside the formal political sphere" (Polletta & Jasper, 2001, p. 284). Polletta and Jasper (2001) argue that rather than the interpretation of collective identity as strategy that divides individuals, it can be better understood as expressions of culture through symbols, narratives, rituals, and clothing, for example. Thus, communities can be created based on politicized personal attributes, struggles, and claims. But so-called identity politics has also been criticized for its tendency to create fault lines, rather than basing mobilization on social justice and solidarity.

Much recent work on the nature of identity has sought to deepen this discussion by focusing on the constructed and constantly changing character of social identities. This, in turn, has made it possible to begin to theorize changing constructions of identity in relation to both the experience of oppression as well as resistance to it (Castells, 1997). Such a view has been most clearly articulated by Alain Touraine and Manuel Castells, who have sought to examine changes in the formation of social, cultural, and political identities under conditions of rapid globalization (Castells, 1997; Touraine, 2000). Castells (1997) has distinguished between what he describes as *legitimizing identities,* which are "introduced by the dominant institutions of society to extend and rationalize their domination vis-à-vis social actors"; *resistance identities,* which are "generated by those actors that are in positions/conditions devalued and/or stigmatized by the logic of domination"; and *project identities,* which are formed "when social actors, on the basis of whatever cultural materials are available to them, build a new identity that redefines their position in society and, by so doing, seek the transformation of overall social structure" (Castells, 1997, p. 8).

This framework is particularly helpful in seeking to understand many of the largely identity-based social movements that have received growing research attention in recent years. Ethnic and racial movements have rallied around these attributes in order to address discrimination and social inequities, as well as to create opportunities for racial equality in the future through affirmative action campaigns. However, some have criticized these movements for contributing to the social "essentialization" of particular ethnicities and races having biologically or innate characteristics (Solomos, 1998). In the case of health issues, such as sickle cell anemia, which is largely specific to people of African descent, or Tay-Sachs, which mostly affects Ashkenazi Jews, the struggles for research and funding attention from medicine and politicians can perhaps be justifiably essentialist. However, when we consider broader health inequalities based on racial disparities, there is a range of sociocultural issues related to stigma and discrimination, as well as economic issues that determine access to quality health care.

One interesting movement toward a solidarity-oriented approach to identity politics was through the denomination of "queer" causes to counteract some of the hegemonic elements of the gay rights movement, which was first dominated by middle-class white men (Bernstein, 2005). By "reappropriating the word 'queer' and redefining it to mean anything that contradicts dominant cultural norms . . . queer activists attempted to form a multiracial, multigendered movement of people with diverse sexualities" (Bernstein, 2005, p. 56; see also Seidman, 1993; Epstein, 1998). The constant attempt to classify sexual diversity within one social movement, as seen in how the movement for sexual diversity grew to include lesbians, bisexuals, transgender, transvestites, transsexuals, queers, and intersex persons, resulted in a growing acronym, LBTTTQI. Even though there has been a tendency toward amalgamating causes related to sexuality, it is questionable whether links based on grievances or shared cultural experiences can be strong enough to understand this "solidarity" as a sexual rights movement (Corrêa, Petchesky, & Parker, 2008). Considering that the agenda of social movements related to sexuality has been more focused (probably because of the heterosexist norms that become the major targets of those advocating for sexual rights) on the protection of women from violence than on the celebration of nonheterosexual sexualities (Garcia & Parker, 2006), in the same way, advocating for same-sex marriage can follow heteronormative patterns that do not reflect other sexual and affective relationship arrangements (Warner, 2000; Walters, 2001).

Identities often do not capture the multidimensional character of individuals and groups. Simply put, individuals have multiple and sometimes contradicting identities. These divisions have caused contention between and within social movements, as well as creating the necessity of choosing which battles it makes the most sense to fight. Should a Latino man decide to fight against racial discrimination and health inequities, or should he fight for gay rights that his Latino community sometimes violates? The contextual factors, such as poverty and community ties, shape the ways in which these choices are made, impacting on the person's agency. In the case of the feminist movements, there are sometimes divides between lesbian feminists and straight feminists due to social stigma and diverging agendas/priorities, for example. Because of the need to make strategic claims or to create culturally bonded communities, social movements have hegemonic positions or structures, wherein voices at the extremes are possibly silenced. The dominant position of a movement does not necessarily evolve through democratic deliberation, as hegemonic structures within a social movement can be determined by factors such as links to elites or funding agendas, among other factors.

Identity-based mobilization and resulting competition for political-economic agenda setting have led to the increasing bureaucratization of collective action, and social movements have sometimes been mistaken for networks of nongovernmental organizations. Although social movements are dominantly driven by "social movement organizations," which include NGOs, mobilization is also driven by collective moods, shared experiences, and ideologies that are not necessarily institutionalized. The growth in nongovernmental organizations has paradoxically led to questions of whether the state is co-opting civil society, as it is a main funding source for these institutions in some countries. The expansion of civil society, via the proliferation of NGOs, has been useful for operationalizing ways to address social problems, but financial constraints and state involvement have changed the meaning of "civil society." These tensions, in turn, have potentially important implications that may have a special salience in turning to the study of social movements and social mobilization in relation to issues of health.

## HEALTH-RELATED SOCIAL MOVEMENTS

Social scientists have recently brought some of the historical debates about why and how people engage in contentious politics to analyze mobilization around health issues (Brown et al., 2004; Zoller, 2005; Keefe, Lane, et al., 2006; Williamson, 2007; Archibald, 2008). Indeed, two major currents of social movement activity, concerning reproductive rights and disability, have encompassed significant health-related dimensions. The movement for rights regarding abortion and reproductive decision making directly addresses the medical condition of pregnancy and involves such issues as the doctor-patient relationship and access to abortion and family planning services. However, it is notable that the dominant discourse in this movement has been framed around issues of personal autonomy and women's equality rather than more narrowly as a health issue. Similarly, the broadly based disability rights movement is concerned with access to quality health care, but only as one issue alongside a range of others such as discrimination in employment and housing, accessibility in transportation and public accommodations, and access to supportive services (Stroman, 2003).

In this sense, the reproductive rights and disability movements that address health issues are related to but still distinct from "health social movements" (HSMs), which are

> collective challenges to medical policy and politics, belief systems, research and practice that include an array of formal and informal organisations, supporters, networks of cooperation, and media. HSMs' challenges are to political power, professional authority and personal and collective identity. HSMs, as a class of social movements, are centrally organised around health, and address issues including the following general categories: (a) access to, or provision of, health care services; (b) health inequality and inequity based on race, ethnicity, gender, class and/or sexuality; and/or (c) disease, illness experience, disability and contested illness. (Brown et al., 2004, p. 52)

Health social movements have been driven by politicized collective identities of suffering, by incentives to better the health of particular groups—defined by race and gender, for example—and by more general forms of mobilization on behalf of access to health care, which brings in the central element of poverty (Brown et al., 2004). This is an evolving area of study that has recently begun to engage in dialogue with theories related to resource mobilization, political opportunity structures, cultural framings, and emotions as explanations for individual and community engagement. These theories address how individuals have been motivated to mobilize when they encounter the forces of biomedicine, government agencies, and international donors, sometimes as both friends and foes.

Brown et al. (2004) further distinguish among three overlapping yet distinct categories of HSMs. *Health access movements* are perhaps the most straightforward in seeking more equitable and better quality care, such as the broad-based campaigns for a single-payer insurance system. *Constituency-based movements* are more narrowly focused on issues related to the health care needs of a particular social group, such as the greater inclusion of women in clinical trials or attempts to improve health care facilities on

Native American reservations. *Embodied health movements,* by contrast, "address disease, disability or illness experience by challenging science on etiology, diagnosis, treatment and prevention" (Brown et al., 2004, p. 50).

In the collection of articles published in 2004 by Brown and colleagues in the *Sociology of Health & Illness,* several articles appear that are helpful in our discussion of how a variety of illnesses have led to the creation of collective identities, have grappled with science and biomedicine, as well as worked in collaboration or as adversaries with corporations, states, and donor agencies (Brown et al., 2004; Beard, 2004, Klawiter, 2004; Kolker, 2004; Hess, 2004). There is a broad range of health issues for which lobbies, communities, and individuals have formed HSMs to bring grievances against the state or cultural norms, such as in the case of breast cancer, tobacco use, abortion, Alzheimer's disease, needle exchange, obesity, and mental health—among other health issues that have become politicized. One of the earliest, most significant, and most influential of these HSMs has been the HIV/AIDS movement, which was launched shortly after the emergence of AIDS in 1981 through the creation of such activist groups as Gay Men's Health Crisis (GMHC) and the People with AIDS Coalition (PWAC), and which reached a peak in the late 1980s and early 1990s through the pioneering work of the AIDS Coalition to Unleash Power, better known as ACT UP.

Before creating mobilizing on behalf of health-related rights, grievances, or for the change of cultural understandings and stigma, the creation of a collective identity is one way in which health issues have become significant in research and sociocultural and political agendas. Self-help and mutual-aid organizations have played a role in creating spaces for sharing common experiences with health problems (Archibald, 2008; Katz, 1993). These groups can provide psychological support and expose services that are not provided by the health care system and perhaps raise awareness about the need for social change, but most do not enter social movements in an aggressive way. Certainly sharing stories of the lived experience of illness is significant in creating connections through cultural symbols, emotions, and identifying common grievances.

Social mobilization can also evolve from support and from borrowing repertoires of contention from other health social movements:

Many social movements (e.g., the women's movement, disability rights, the environment movement) and their affiliated organizations have achieved enough institutional standing that they can extend legitimation to others and provide resources necessary for their expansion, directly, in the form of intermovement alliances or spillover. (Archibald, 2008, p. 86; see also Meyer and Whittier, 1994)

The organizational formation and fostering of collective identities also involves the resourceful support of health professionals (and organizations such as the American Medical Association) and, more importantly, elites from the state. But this process of transforming the personal experience, a private affair, into a public issue, as in the case of the Alzheimer's movement (Beard, 2004) encounters and attempts to combat stigma and discrimination. In this movement, the involvement of organizations such as the Alzheimer's Association, family, and friends were key spokespersons for those with the illness. Although personal experience has been an important element in the Alzheimer's movement, it has taken a more "macro national approach easily converted into an interest group aimed at making policy changes from within existing social structures" (Beard, 2004, p. 799).

Unlike in the case of the Alzheimer's movement, challenges to hegemonic biomedical constructions of science, funding, and research agendas have been central fields of contention in the AIDS movement (Epstein, 1996; Patton, 1991; Treichler, 1999) and the breast cancer movement (Keefe, Lane, et al., 2006; Klawiter, 2004; Kolker, 2004; McCormick, Brown, et al., 2003), and to some extent in the mental health movement (Brown, 1984; Rogers & Pilgrim, 1991; Crossley, 2006). Instead of being movements where the power dynamic was primarily organized top-to-bottom, activists from the grassroots have expended considerable energy and emotional concern in a bottom-up approach. Due to the power held by "experts" in health social movements, activists have had to engage with scientific material, learning how to question the validity of scientific claims made by experts and making coherent arguments that articulate their demands both to grassroots activists and policymakers.

This type of collective action is resonant of claims against cultural norms of domination based on the power of knowledge. As much as they consider medicine and politicians as targets, the relationship among activists, doctors, cultural icons, and politicians shifts depending on the movements' agendas. While biomedicine is seen as a hegemonic force, it is also considered necessary for treatment and for validating social movement claims. Political agendas determine funding for research, which can then be used by activists and academics to make evidence-based arguments—making political alliances with funding agencies crucial. In a sense, movements such as the environmental breast cancer movement were what Kolker (2004) and McCormick, Brown, et al., (2003) term "boundary movements," in which the distinctions between the worlds of science/knowledge and that of activists are blurred, through processes of contestations as well as due to the contemporary availability of information through sources such as the Internet. This blurring also reveals that the scientific is also political, because even though scientists and researchers claim to pursue objectivity and truth, funding fads, congressional interests, and lobbies determine what is studied and result in data on which empirically based arguments are based.

In describing the narrative of a woman with breast cancer, Klawiter (2004, p. 845) offers the concept of the "disease regime as a way of conceptualizing the structure shaping of illness experience," as in the "regime of breast cancer." Drawing from four years of ethnographic research, 40 interviews, and oral histories from patients, activists, educators, scientists, support group leaders, and volunteers, she comments on the ways in which the breast cancer social movement emerged and how its interactions with institutions shape the experience of the person living with the illness. Due to breast cancer activism in the 1990s, there was an increase in breast cancer organizations, funding, and a shift in discourse, cognitive framing, and collaboration with the environmental movement (Klawiter, 2004, p. 846). Breast cancer became the social cause of hegemonic institutions and corporations, creating symbols such as pink ribbons and decreasing the stigma attributed to the disease. In fact, she describes a moment of solidarity among breast cancer, lesbian, feminist, and environmental activists—drawing from the repertoires of contention of political protests, educational forums, and exhibits, and calling for increased funding for research. However, there were wings of this movement, particularly composed of activists linked to the feminist movement, that questioned and rejected the "idea of putting a pretty bow on an ugly reality" (Klawiter, 2004, p. 848). The "disease regime" of breast cancer activism is a result of an interactive power dynamic among discourses, policies, funding, cultural grammar, and networks, creating an impact on the collective identities of women with breast cancer (and supporters) as well as on the representations of lived, emotional experiences.

In the following section, we explore more closely the ways in which AIDS activism and research have paralleled—and also fundamentally shaped—understandings of social movements worldwide. Rationalist explanations of political opportunity structures can help us understand how the political will of elites and their responses to various social divisions have facilitated or impeded the development of prevention policies and programs; shaped sexual cultures, religion, and gender relations; impacted stigma and discrimination against persons living with HIV/

AIDS; influenced the resources available from international and national donors and the mechanisms through which they support research and intervention; mobilized the increase in nongovernmental organizations carrying out services and prevention in civil society; and shaped the roll-out of treatment campaigns. Framing the AIDS social movement as a contestation of science and pharmaceutical industries reveals that class is still at the heart of issues related to access to health and understanding of health systems. At the same time, the identity-based and cultural issues related to gender, sexuality, and race that are brought forth by "new social movement theory" add a level of complexity to arguments that social movements are a result of class domination. By outlining the history of how activists, academics, health systems, donor agencies, and governments have approached the fight against HIV, we delineate several paradigmatic shifts that have been significant in the responses from civil society and social movements. These paradigmatic shifts from individual-based approaches to collective action, much like the layers of theories of social movements reviewed, show that a combination of their insights are necessary to understand the reality of HIV/AIDS social movements.

Below we present a framework for thinking about HIV/AIDS-related social movements that employs three intersecting frames. The first relates to the basic chronological/historical unfolding of responses to the epidemic. The second focuses on the strategic choices of movement activity made by activists, in particular whether to pursue "structural" or "cultural" forms of activism. The third frame then overlays the chronological development and strategic choices with the Brown et al. (2004) typology of health social movements (introduced above) in order to illuminate the shifting and overlapping rationale(s) for social movement activity.

## THE CHRONOLOGICAL FRAME

The first frame, focused chronologically, emphasizes the history of the epidemic as it has evolved over time and plays out against a background of several overlapping stages of roughly five years each. These included: (1) a stage of basic scientific discovery and early social responses following emergence of the epidemic in 1987; (2) a period of growing public panic about possible "casual transmission" alongside organized protest politics; (3) a relative "normalization" of the epidemic in the early 1990s as it became better understood by both the public and by public health organizations; (4) a great upswell in optimism following major treatment advances first introduced in 1996; (5) international solidarity in increasing treatment access in the developing world through the early 2000s; and (6) the period since about 2006, which has seen less activism and more of a focus on the technical demands of the rollout and scale-up of treatment programs.

From 1981 through the mid-1980s, the epidemic was characterized by emergence and discovery, beginning with the initial classification of AIDS as a clinical syndrome, the identification of HIV as the etiologic agent, the licensing of an HIV antibody test, and a focus on palliative and prophylactic care in the absence of any effective forms of treatment for HIV itself (see Epstein, 1996). Early community responses included the formation of the Gay Men's Health Crisis (GMHC) as a service provider, and the People with AIDS Coalition (PWAC) as a vehicle for group self-empowerment. In 1985, the First International AIDS Conference was held in Atlanta, recognizing the virus as a worldwide threat. In the developing world, Brazil was one of the first countries to have a strong response from civil society, where mobilization was based on ideals of "solidarity" and "citizenship" rather than on singular identities (Daniel & Parker, 1993; Berkman et al., 2005; Parker, 2009). This sense of global solidarity was symbolized through the creation of World AIDS Day in 1987. Community-based responses also emerged in Uganda with the foundation of TASO in 1987, showing that where there are few medical resources, volunteerism resulting from solidarity among persons living with HIV/AIDS, including friends and family, can impact access to health (Kalibala & Kaleeba, 1989; Kaleeba et al., 1997).

The next several years, in the early 1990s, were marked both by broad panic in the public and, in reaction, an intense period of protest politics by activists. This is the time that begins with the death of Rock Hudson and resulting fears of a generalized epidemic, which led to calls for coercive approaches to public health and also to widespread social stigmatization. But this period was equally marked by the rise of the activist group ACT UP, wide-scale protests against government agencies and pharmaceutical companies, and also the first public displays of the AIDS Memorial Quilt. Beginning in 1992, there was a diffusion of activism supported by an increase in numbers of NGOs, and networks such as the Global Network of People Living with AIDS (GNP+), the International Community of Women Living with HIV/AIDS, and the Society for Women and AIDS in Africa were developed to represent the specific needs of people with HIV in the context of their particular communities and nations. The early architecture of a global AIDS activism movement was thus being built upon groups such as the International Council of AIDS Service Organizations

(ICASO) along with parallel regional networks. At the same time, transnational identity-based movements, such as those focused on issues related to gays/lesbians, sex workers, and women's groups (Altman, 1999), were integral components of the HIV/AIDS social movement. At the symbolic level, the proliferation of "red ribbons" throughout the world signaled a broader acceptance and awareness.

In 1996, the formation of the Joint United Nations Program on AIDS (UNAIDS) signified the increased involvement of the United Nations in the fight against an AIDS pandemic beyond more limited, though important, contributions made by the World Health Organization. These programmatic responses from the international community were due in part to the realization that health systems, which were deeply compromised by structural adjustment programs of the World Bank and the International Monetary Fund, were not equipped to mitigate the spread of HIV. The medical breakthrough years of 1996 to 1999 saw the advent of combination antiretroviral medications that drastically reduced HIV-related mortality and morbidity and transformed AIDS, for some, into a chronic but survivable illness, albeit with exceptionally demanding medical regimens and significant side effects. In South Africa, the Treatment Action Campaign began a concerted effort to press the postapartheid regime to take urgent action against the world's most concentrated and wide-scale epidemic.

Against this backdrop, the period since about 2000 was marked by an emphasis on disparities in access to treatments. The 13th International AIDS Conference in South Africa brought forth issues expounded by Thabo Mbeki of AIDS "denialism" and skepticism about the global scientific and activist responses to AIDS. In the developing world, health disparities have been underlined by the entrenchment of HIV in poorer, more vulnerable populations. At the same time in the developing world, a great deal of activism has focused on ensuring the affordability and availability of ARVs to all who need them despite the impediments of pharmaceutical patents and measures taken by governments to protect corporate profits. In the 20th century, international activism has interacted greatly with the development of funding streams such as the Global Fund to Fight AIDS, Tuberculosis and Malaria, in 2002, and the Bush administration's PEPFAR. There was both optimism and skepticism that the international effort could reach its goal to extend treatment to "3 by 5" (3 million people by 2005). While in the 21st century AIDS activism has prioritized addressing social, economic, and political issues, there has been a primary focus on treatment, showing the predominance of biomedicine in the history of the responses to AIDS. Finally, since about 2006, the global activist movement has become fragmented, as some sectors of civil society have engaged in the implementation of treatment access and scale-up, while others have focused on a range of more localized struggles related to specific populations and groups (Parker, 2011).

## THE STRATEGIC FRAME

The second frame regards the strategies employed by activists, which we divide broadly into "structural" and "cultural" activism. Structural activism targets social, political, and economic factors that regulate the availability, acceptability, and accessibility of resources (Blankenship, Bray, et al., 2000). Key attention has focused on questions of poverty, as well as on the impact of race and racism, gender power inequalities, and homophobia, creating what has been described as a kind of synergistic effect involving multiple forms of oppression and shaping HIV-related risk through diverse forms of voluntary as well as involuntary risk practices (Parker, Pasarelli, Terto Jr., Pimenta, Berkman, & Muñoz-Laboy, 2003; Baer, Singer, et al., 1997; Singer et al., 1990; Farmer, 1990, 1992, 1999; Schoepf, 1991, 1995; Singer, 1994, 1998; Kreniske, 1997; Bond & Vincent, 1997; Parker, Easton, et al., 2000; Parker, 2001).

Examples of structural activism include harm reduction social movements, which have used science to prove that there is a public health benefit to needle exchange because it reduces risk for HIV and hepatitis C infection, while not increasing the propensity for drug use (Tempalski et al., 2007; Bluthenthal, 1998). Needle exchange programs that are protected from police invasion are examples of interventions that make contextual resources available to reduce vulnerability. In a handful of countries, laws that decriminalize sex work altered political and social standards related to the acceptability of this "occupation"—while taking into account the ways in which prevention work can be more effective if sex workers are more accessible to public health systems (Vanwesenbeeck, 2001; Kempandoo & Doezema, 1998).

In the case of HIV/AIDS, structural activism has targeted centers of power including government agencies such as the FDA and the CDC, as well as transnational pharmaceutical companies, the biomedical establishment, scientific frameworks for clinical trials and other forms of research, and major media outlets. Community-based organizations have played in the global response to HIV/AIDS, which has included providing social services, developing prevention activities, fighting for the rights of persons with HIV/AIDS, shaping media and public conceptions of the illness, and lobbying for the creation of more effective governmental policy in relation to the epidemic (Altman, 1994, 1999; Bolton & Singer, 1992; Castro & Farmer, 2005; Parker and Aggleton, 2003; Farmer, Connors, et al., 1996).

The latter strategy of cultural activism relates the ways in which HIV/AIDS social movements have attempted to transform systems of meaning related to the epidemic. Framing HIV as an "ideological virus" (Daniel & Parker, 1993) contests an interpretation of a purely biological illness, highlighting the ways in which this was a social epidemic, where addressing social mores was inherently part of the struggle for rights. These can include the "self-help" and communal advancement agendas often found as integral components of social movement activities. Cultural activism has ranged from community-driven campaigns to eroticize safer sex to the use of powerful symbols such as the reclaimed Nazi pink triangle as the symbol of ACT UP in the well-known "Silence = Death" image that became the logo of ACT UP (Crimp, 1988).

HIV/AIDS social movements have used both structural and cultural activism consistently throughout the epidemic, and at times have employed both simultaneously. Most often, however, the choice of strategies was determined by whether activists believed that action by government (or other power centers) was necessary to achieve their goals and had a plausible potential for success, or whether government activity was either not conducive or inappropriate for the goal to be achieved. This choice relates, in part, to what Kirp and Bayer (1992) identified as two principal approaches to HIV/AIDS by public health policymakers in several countries: a traditional "contain-and-control" approach using the coercive power of the state and a newer "cooperation-and-inclusion" approach that encouraged social participation.

Thus, activists chose *not* to try to prompt government action when this would be likely to induce a "contain-and-control" response such as mass quarantine, compulsory testing, mandatory partner notification, aggressive contact tracing, or enforcement of sodomy laws. Here, the dichotomization between prevention and treatment gains some salience, since prevention has been far more controversial and thus much more prone to regressive contain-and-control strategies, involving as it does questions of illicit drug use, anal intercourse, and human sexuality in general. Around such issues, cultural activism was far more commonplace, perhaps most notably in the case of the "invention" of safer sex and its voluntary proliferation through communities of gay men. Cultural activism also prevailed in areas in which the government had no productive role, such as the use of candlelight processions and name-recitation vigils to memorialize the dead. By contrast, the desirability, at least in principle, of providing treatment of "sick people" is uncontroversial and near universally shared. As a result, government action with regard to the drug and approval development process, the provision of access to health care, and antidiscrimination protections were all sought, and obtained, by AIDS activists.

## THE HEALTH SOCIAL MOVEMENT FRAME

For the third frame, we return to Brown et al. (2004) who, in their discussion of health social movements, distinguish among three overlapping yet distinct categories: *constituency-based movements, embodied health movements,* and *health access movements* (Brown et al., 2004, p. 8). While Brown and colleagues (2004) acknowledge overlaps among these three categories, they largely present them as relatively discrete categories. Given the extraordinary global breadth and impact of the HIV epidemic and the multiple and variable activist responses to it, we believe that over time, HIV/AIDS-related social movements have reflected all three categories of the Brown et al. typology.

It is at this point that the three frames presented above intersect. First, the chronological frame intersects with the Brown et al. typology in that the earliest social movements were principally constituency-based; later movements increasingly incorporated dimensions of the embodied experience; and ultimately HIV/AIDS-related social movements have had a powerful impact on the broader issue of access to health care for all. Within each of the three categories, HIV/AIDS social movements had to make situational decisions relating to the second frame: whether and when to pursue structural activism, cultural activism, or some combination of both.

### Constituency-Based Movement

The HIV/AIDS-related social movement can clearly be identified as having begun as a *constituency-based* movement. Indeed, AIDS itself was originally, after its first emergence in 1981, known as GRID or "gay-related immune deficiency." The association of HIV/AIDS with homosexuality in general and with anal sex between men in particular (Treichler, 1999) has persisted down to the current day, with some good reason. In the developed world, gay men—or more broadly "men who have sex with men" (MSM)—remain the single most highly impacted group, although this is not true in all parts of the developing world, particularly sub-Saharan Africa. The first and most sustained organizational and activist responses in many countries also developed from within the lesbian, gay, bisexual, and transgender (LGBT) community; in fact, the oldest and perhaps the preeminent U.S. AIDS service organization was named "Gay Men's Health Crisis." ACT UP, the flagship AIDS protest organization, was launched at a public meeting at New York's LGBT Community Center and took as its symbol the pink triangle originally used by the Nazis to identify homosexuals in concentration camps. Both GMHC and ACT UP were co-founded by the incendiary gay playwright and novelist Larry Kramer, who was but one of the many gay artists who shaped the initial cultural response to the epidemic.

This strong early linkage between a disease and a discrete, socially disfavored population largely shaped the ongoing conceptualization of AIDS itself. Indeed, the central role of gay men in the early AIDS epidemic in the United States and many other Western countries, both as subjects and objects, has also continued to shape the AIDS politics and policy. Negative reactions to homosexuality, ranging from violent homophobia to public squeamishness about gay sex, easily transmuted into AIDS-phobia, which carried with it the stigma and bias linked to homosexuality compounded by that relating to sexually communicable disease in general. At the same time, powerful skepticism and even hostility toward official authority dampened gay men's willingness to engage with government agencies. Particularly in the realm of HIV prevention, most activism centered on actions that the community could take itself, most importantly inculcating norms of safer sexual behavior and, later, harm reduction models in drug use. With regard to the state, prevention demands revolved around negative liberty, or the "right to be left alone," such as the decriminalization of sodomy and the ability to maintain public sex environments. Privacy concerns also became far more central than with regard to most diseases, reflecting longstanding fears of a largely hidden community long subjected to police entrapment, societal disapproval, and discrimination. Indeed, many of the trappings of the gay "closet" were reflected in discourse and policy about AIDS, in which testing HIV positive and disclosing this to others was viewed as parallel to the experience of "coming out." All of these influences led to policies shaped by "AIDS exceptionalism" in which public health approaches to HIV/AIDS would be far more confidential and voluntary than had traditionally been the case for earlier communicable diseases such as tuberculosis or polio.

Of course, from the earliest days of the epidemic, it became clear that gay men were not the only "constituency" being affected but the early notion of "risk groups" remained powerful. By 1982, in the United States, AIDS was seen as limited to a derisively termed "4H Club" of "homosexuals, hemophiliacs, heroin users, and hookers," with "Haitians" and "hospital workers" also sometimes included in an expanded listing. This narrow perspective would have significant policy consequences, perhaps most notably a strong tendency to overlook the care and prevention needs of those who fell outside the narrowly constructed risk groups. The single most significant manifestation of this was the systematic neglect of women in terms of enrollment in timely diagnosis and treatment, enrollment in clinical trials, access to experimental drugs, and counseling on prevention. A particularly egregious example of this was the exclusion of invasive cervical cancer, an AIDS opportunistic infection obviously limited only to women, from the list of AIDS-defining illnesses. It was only concerted activism on the part of the AIDS Law Project that persuaded the CDC to revise the case definition and thus drastically improve diagnosis and treatment among women.

The CDC case definition revision, by also adding extrapulmonary TB, also worked to the benefit of HIV-positive injecting drug users, who were the ones most likely to contract this particular opportunistic infection. However, in general, injecting drug users mostly did not succeed in coalescing into a distinctive activist constituency in the United States. This lack of effective collective action can be attributed to multiple factors, including the marginal legal status of injecting drug users due to prohibitionist and coercive drug policies, the social and economic problems that often face people struggling with addiction, and perhaps also because injecting drug use did not form a sufficiently stable identity basis for sustained, organized collective organization. Other groups were somewhat more successful, a notable example being people with hemophilia. Already often linked by family ties in the context of a genetic disease and already organized around issues such as research advocacy and community blood drives, hemophiliac organizations were able to mobilize their preexisting constituency-based activism toward HIV issues after the large majority of people with hemophilia were infected via pooled blood plasma supplies.

More broadly, people of color, who today represent the largest number of people in the United States with HIV, were also slow to organize at the communal level. This is due, in part, to LGBT social networks, which in the 1980s and 1990s were largely white and middle class and thus marginalized people of color. This led to a construction of AIDS as a "white" disease, both in the minds of communities of color who sought to avoid the stigma of homosexuality, drug use, and "promiscuity," as well as within LGBT communities. One telling example was an early campaign by GMHC about the AIDS-related skin cancer Kaposi's sarcoma, which described it only as it appeared on skin of light complexion.

Perhaps ironically, it was a heterosexual African American man, basketball star Magic Johnson, whose HIV-positive diagnosis and subsequent public press conference in 1991 did more than any other event to loosen the linkage between HIV/AIDS and specific risk groups. At about this time, the paradigm that "everyone is at risk for HIV" began to proliferate in public health campaigns, popular culture, and via symbols such as the red AIDS ribbons, which became ubiquitous in the early 1990s. This universalizing message did help to destigmatize the disease, may have helped prevent a more generalized epidemic, and worked to build political support for broader access to HIV treatments, such as through the ADAP program. At the same time, critics have argued that the "de-gaying" of the epidemic has also led to the misallocation of prevention funds and programs away from the individuals and groups at greatest need, contributing to recent rises in HIV incidence among young gay men, particularly men of color.

Globally, the most salient constituencies have been gay activist groups and women's groups, as well as organizations focusing on sexual and reproductive health more generally. Social movements not only led to the dissemination of collective action in the global North related to the particular vulnerabilities of women, for example, but transnational social movements in Latin America, Asia, and Africa have also formed constituencies for target populations. Constituency-based contention is often driven by interests and grievances of a particular segment of the population. When observed through a global lens, poverty and inequality often define distinct social groups that can only gain control through collective action. South Africa and Brazil provide two examples of countries where social movement organizations have global and regional constituencies. In South Africa, where the epidemic is generalized, it affects not only "target" risk groups but also the broader population, mostly self-identified heterosexuals. Powerful social movement organizations, such as the Treatment Action Campaign, have revolutionized not only the ways in which HIV and AIDS are conceptualized medically and culturally, but they have also focused on universalizing and destigmatizing treatment throughout Africa. The battles fought on behalf of increasing the antiretroviral rollout have been influenced heavily by grassroots organizations that pressure the government through constituency-based mobilization.

In Brazil, social movement organizations from the gay movement, the feminist movement, and the sanitary reform movement, among others, pressured the Brazilian government and the Brazilian National AIDS Program to act boldly in the international arena in order to make HIV prevention and treatment more affordable in resource-poor settings. Brazil has been forging South-South collaborations to export technology and medications that are more affordable, especially throughout Latin America and Lusophone Africa, making treatment access movements part of a "global constituency-based movement." This intersects with Brown et al.'s (2004) definition of "health access" movements. However, there is a crucial constituency-related dimension to treatment access because there are differences among concentrated and generalized epidemics in their patterns of contention taken on behalf of comprehensive approaches to combating HIV. In concentrated epidemics it is more feasible to target particular groups that are most vulnerable; however, a broader "health access" conceptualization of collective action is more pertinent to countries with generalized epidemics.

Throughout the world, the biomedicalization of AIDS research funding and interventions has been countered by constituencies focused on identity politics (facilitating constituencies) rather than on the human right to comprehensive approach to combating HIV and AIDS epidemics. Constituency-based movements have not focused sufficiently on the right to HIV prevention because of political reasons and because of debates within the scientific community related to primary prevention (risk avoidance) as opposed to risk management. The lived experiences of people with HIV and AIDS affect community and constituency formation, but the bodily experience of living with HIV and AIDS has also led to the "embodied" social movements described in the next section.

## Embodied Health Movement

Another critical dimension of HIV/AIDS-related activism can be found in its reflection of the embodied experience of people living with HIV/AIDS, as well as to a lesser extent of those close to them and those at risk for HIV. Although immune disorders of various types have a long history, AIDS itself emerged as a ravaging and completely new disease syndrome in the early 1980s. As a result, in some very real ways people living with AIDS had a level of expertise derived from their "embodied" experience, which made them more "experts" on the disease than most medical practitioners.

In the earliest days, people with AIDS tended to be diagnosed late and to die quickly and there was no way to identify HIV until the antibody test in 1985. As a result, the embodied experience was not central at first—the response was initially at the level of the gay community, whose members nearly all perceived themselves as being at heightened risk. Better preventive care (e.g., aerosolized pentamidine for PCP), earlier detection of HIV, and ART monotherapy started to increase the numbers of people with HIV among the activist ranks. The "embodied" aspect of the AIDS movement was initiated as early as 1983 with the founding of the People with AIDS Coalition (PWAC) and subsequently the National Association of People with AIDS (NAPWA). Although nearly all of its founders and early members were gay men, the organizing principle for this group was not sexual orientation but rather the status of having AIDS, which at the time was still being identified through the actual physiological experience of symptoms such as swollen glands and night sweats rather than by antibody or CD4 tests.

The signature event of the PWA self-empowerment movement was the articulation, at the Fifth Lesbian and Gay Health Conference in Denver in 1983, of the "Denver Principles" (People with AIDS Coalition, 1983). This list of four demands and recommendations issued by the new ad hoc PWAC group could only have been made by people who were living through the experience of the illness itself. Its preamble stated: "We condemn attempts to label us as 'victim,' which implies defeat, and we are only occasionally 'patients,' which implies passivity, and dependence upon the care of others. We are 'people with AIDS.'" The first principle calls upon health care professionals to overcome their biases and to treat people with AIDS as "whole people and address psychosocial issues as well as biophysical ones." The second warns against the scapegoating or blaming of PWAs. The third, perhaps most important principle urges PWAs to "form caucuses to choose their own representatives, to deal with the media, to choose their own agenda, and to plan their own strategies . . . to be involved at every level of AIDS decision making . . . [and to] be included in all AIDS forums with equal credibility." The final point identifies various rights of people with AIDS, including to full and satisfying sexual and emotional lives, access to quality medical treatment and social services without discrimination, full explanations of treatments, privacy and confidentiality, and finally "to die and to LIVE in dignity."

The articulation of the Denver Principles was enormously influential in shaping subsequent discourse about HIV/AIDS, and was clearly a progenitor of the burst of activism that began in 1987 with the formation of the AIDS Coalition to Unleash Power (ACT UP). In a now-historic speech, playwright Larry Kramer caught the attention of his audience by flatly stating most of them might be dead in five years, and then asked a simple, pointed question: "Do we want to start a new organization devoted solely to political action?" Large numbers of the activist core of ACT UP and related later groups, such as the Treatment Action Group and Housing Works, have been people who were themselves living with HIV and as such were fighting not only for a "cause" but with hopes of concrete health benefits to themselves. Many of the same people who advocated drug development and access were themselves either using the drugs or hoped to use them. A flyer at the first major ACT UP action—a protest on Wall Street that in some ways presaged the 2011 Occupy movement— called for "immediate abolishment of cruel double-blind studies wherein some get the new drugs and some don't"; "immediate release of these drugs to everyone with AIDS"; and "immediate availability of these drugs at affordable prices." One of the simplest but most compelling demands of ACT UP, as an embodied movement, was the slogan: "Drugs into Bodies!"

In some very real ways, the "embodied" experience might also be said to extend to those who were not necessarily HIV-positive themselves, much less diagnosed with AIDS. Many activists might not themselves have been infected, but the threat of infection remained a visceral reality. Even among those who regularly practiced safer sex, the limitation and precautions of "protected" sex, most notably condom use and refraining from exchange of bodily fluids, HIV was in a very real sense an experience of the body. The experience of AIDS as an assault on the body also extended to increasing numbers of partners, family, and other caregivers who nursed dying people, and later grieved them. A significant portion of AIDS-related literature, often highly autobiographical and suffused with political anger, focused on the experience of caregivers and survivors. The AIDS Memorial Quilt clearly reflected the loss of specific individuals and their unique lives rather than a more abstract group identity. The quilt may have primarily been a social and cultural phenomenon, but it also contained a powerful political critique and call for change—it is no coincidence that the most iconic images of the quilt are from its first unfurling in Washington, DC, when it covered most of the National Mall leading up to the Capitol Building.

At the same time, the sheer novelty and tremendous scale of AIDS placed medical professionals and their preexisting assumptions at a disadvantage relative to those with a lived, embodied experience of the disease. Thus, to a degree previously unseen among most disease-impacted populations, people with HIV/AIDS and their close allies were able to become experts in their own right on many aspects of the disease. In perhaps the definitive study of how "knowledge" about AIDS has been constructed, Steven Epstein (1996) noted, "Over the course of the epidemic, members of the AIDS movement have taught themselves details of virology, immunology, and epidemiology. . . . They have established their credibility as people who might legitimately speak in the language of medical science, in particular with regard to the design, conduct, and interpretation of clinical trials used to test the safety and efficacy of AIDS drugs." But the claims to expert authority and a "place at the table" of people with AIDS were often backed up by—or accompanied by—protests, demonstrations, and zaps aimed at structures of power.

HIV/AIDS activism also led to greater "ownership" of the sexual body. In some cases throughout the world, sex workers have come together to formulate cultural counter-identities, a movement that was both emancipatory and transgressive of social norms that criminalize and dehumanize sex workers (Kempandoo & Doezema, 1998). Founded in 1985, the NGO EMPOWER in Thailand is an example of how cultural activism allies with media, some elements of government, and private establishments such as bars to promote AIDS activism and the rights of those who do not conform to hegemonic "clean" sexual representations and practices, primarily sex workers (Brier 2009). EMPOWER has been recognized by winning the UNAIDS Red Ribbon Award in 2008, not only for its local action—especially related to artistic exhibits and interventions at bars, schools, and colleges—but also for building international networks supporting HIV prevention in sex worker communities. Using cultural venues, the organization has harnessed strong forces to mitigate police violence against sex workers and open political discussions about the human rights of sex workers.

In another example, the Bambanani Group, a group of women living with AIDS in South Africa, in collaboration with Médecins Sans Frontières started the body-mapping project in 2002 to develop a new way for women living with HIV/AIDS to come to terms with their diagnosis, communicate with their families, and prepare for the future. These paintings are not about "absence," but about "lives, loves and losses of women who participated in a unique therapeutic process" (Thom, 2003, p. 1). Although the body maps were originally "viewed as an alternative method for people to tell their stories and deal with issues relating to their HIV status," they have "evolved into a research tool, which helped participants to sketch, paint and find words" for their inner selves (Morgan, 2003, p. 8). The paintings are rife with symbolism representing feelings such as love, fear, sadness, hope, and pain, and political messages calling for treatment access.

## Health Access Movement

As seen above, the HIV/AIDS social movement has been centrally organized around constituencies and around the embodied experience of people living with AIDS and those close to them. But over time, it has had a much broader impact on access to quality health care for all. Some of this was possible because of some unusual properties of the HIV epidemic. Whereas most diseases strike particularly at the very young and the very old, HIV has tended to most affect those in the middle of their lives, when they have a great deal to lose but also the ability to organize. The middle-class, white, and often well-educated gay men who have been the "ground zero" of HIV/AIDS in the developed world were able to bring resources to bear that other marginalized groups might not be able to, including financial contributions, professional skills, "cultural capital" in the creative professions, and, to some extent, influential social networks.

This position of relative strength enabled AIDS activists to challenge long-established elements of the biomedical and public health organizations, which had a profound effect on the nature and availability of health care for all. With everyone starting from the same minimal baseline of knowledge, AIDS activists were able to create parallel structures, including their own information networks, conferences, publications, and recommendations. These networks undermined the methodical but slow process of drug development and improved accelerated access to experimental drugs; at times they went even further and sponsored their own "underground" drug trials. AIDS activists also challenged the practice of delaying the release of new drug development data until it could appear in a prestigious, peer-review journal, creating pressure for faster release while establishing alternative publications and other channels for information-sharing. They also demanded the establishment of, and then demanded seats on, a range of advisory committees, institutional review boards, consumer panels, and other decision-making bodies run by government agencies, hospitals, pharmaceutical companies, and other power centers.

Perhaps the most singular accomplishment was to alter the formerly hierarchical balance of power in the doctor-patient relationship by encouraging people with AIDS to be active "health consumers." Often better informed about drug trials, side effects, and cutting-edge research than some of their physicians, AIDS activists were able to move from a paternalistic to a partnership model of health care. This proactive approach has since been adopted by other groups such as people with breast cancer, Alzheimer's disease, chronic fatigue syndrome, and other conditions. This underscores, once again, the critical role of the example of AIDS activism for a broad range of health social movements in general and health access movements in particular.

More recently, AIDS activists have taken the concept of the "amateur expert" into new realms that are on the surface unrelated to AIDS—global intellectual property law and policy. After the introduction into the developed world of effective ARV combinations, much of the need to pressure government to produce new and better drugs ceased; indeed, since the major breakthrough of protease inhibitors in 1996, pharmaceutical companies have produced and government agencies have quickly approved an ever-growing armamentarium of different classes of ARV drugs. However, global intellectual property rights, specifically in the form of patents on newer ARVs, soon emerged as a major obstacle to widespread affordability of and access to life-saving medications in sub-Saharan Africa and other areas. This arcane area involves principally the World Trade Organization (WTO) along with the major international instrument governing patents, a multilateral agreement called the Trade-Related Aspects of Intellectual Property Rights (or TRIPS) treaty. Drawing upon the same intellectual reserves that enabled them to battle the biomedical and public health establishments in the developed world, AIDS activists focused much of their attention in the early to mid-2000s on establishing that the AIDS crisis clearly should invoke the waiver allowed in Article 31 of TRIPS for a "national emergency or other circumstances of extreme urgency or in cases of public non-commercial use." By reviving the theatrical street protests of the 1980s alongside keen analysis of such issues as the actual costs of pharmaceutical manufacturing, AIDS activists have contributed substantially to recent major expansions in access to ARVs throughout the developed world.

Treatment access movements show the importance of social movements as structural interventions in the process of policy formation, policy implementation, and cultural adaptation (Gamson, 1989; Von Schoen Angerer et al., 2001). Issues faced by treatment access activists and sometimes discussed in the literature include the stigmatization and discrimination associated with treatment (Castro and Farmer, 2005; Parker & Aggleton, 2003), gender inequality and violence that prohibit access (Farmer, Connors et al., 1996; Msimand, 2003), cultural and traditionalist norms that sometimes frame HIV/AIDS medications as "Western" and "foreign" (Schneider, 2002), and the effects of globalization and disputes of intellectual property and patent rights (Petchesky, 2003; Smith & Siplon, 2006).

Treatment access movements highlight the importance of poverty and social class as major determinants of access to medication—yet they also call attention to how these factors are complicated by the politics of identity and the intricate intercourse between the local and the global. Using a variety of mechanisms for action, treatment activists have not only used the constitutional right to health in places such as Brazil and South Africa to frame the imperative for universal and free access, but they have complemented legal advocacy with grassroots empowerment interventions to reduce stigma and create a demand for medications on the ground (Robbins, 2004). In Brazil, for example, policymakers who were also activists in the early 1990s confronted the World Bank's claim that the universal provision of antiretrovirals was "antieconomical" by showing that providing treatment was actually a cost-saving strategy in the medium-term (Parker, 1997). Nongovernmental organizations, such as the Brazilian Interdisciplinary AIDS Association (ABIA), have engaged in an international dialogue to pressure drug companies to either lower drug prices or to lose their share of the market to generic, in-country production (Reis, Terto Jr., & Pimenta, 2009). With pressure from the Brazilian AIDS social movement, President Lula da Silva's administration effectively broke Merck's patent for the AIDS medication Efavirenz, in 2007, setting a precedent for placing collective health over intellectual property rights.

In South Africa, through civil disobedience campaigns and by distributing antiretrovirals through nongovernmental organizations, the movement has shown government that treatments are safe and their provision feasible, making service provision an integral component in the movement's repertoire of strategies. One of the most prominent NGOs working in South Africa is the Treatment Action Campaign (TAC), which has worked both in contention and collaboration with the South African government to implement the rollout of antiretrovirals. The TAC has confronted stigma and discrimination in local communities, implementing "treatment literacy" programs to increase adherence to medicines, while it has battled with international pharmaceutical companies to allow for the generic production of medicines to reduce costs. Treatment access movements are more recently proliferating in countries around the world (Von Schoen Angerer et al., 2001; Petcheskey, 2003) through the transnational linkages characteristic of social movements in an era of globalization (Tarrow, 1998), and these movements are attempting to move away from the fragmentation associated with the politics of identity by reframing their mission in terms of social justice and the universal human right to health (Farmer, 1999; Parker, 1996a).

## CONCLUSION: LOOKING FORWARD

As this broad overview has indicated, there are multiple vantage points from which to analyze HIV/AIDS social movements, activism, and community mobilization. This dimension of the global response to HIV/AIDS has, arguably, been on the wane since the mid-2000s, when governments and international organizations began to respond to pressure from activists— as well as from the epidemiological realities facing them—and to provide expanded access to treatment. As noted above, the second wave of HIV/AIDS activism in the late 1990s and early 2000s was largely successful. As described by Parker (2011): "[t]here is still much to be done in terms of advocating for broader access among poor and marginalized populations across the global South. There is also a strong sense, however, that the ideological battle has been won—that the majority of the organizations and institutions responsible for administering the global response to the epidemic fully recognize the necessity of access and that the key struggles now lie in implementation."

Such success, however, poses challenges of its own, as energy and attention have flowed away from more overtly political struggles with a focus on global solidarity toward more location-specific needs and technical challenges. HIV/AIDS activists increasingly find themselves not only "at the negotiating table" but also organizationally embedded within the key institutions that now determine how HIV prevention and treatment are being administered. As Parker (2011) also noted, "this growing involvement of activists and civil society representatives in a range of new program activities and service provision functions has almost inevitably led to at least some decrease in more confrontational political activism, as activist energy (and technical expertise) has been incorporated into what some analysts came to describe as the growing global AIDS industry. . . . While the direct action and political confrontation that characterized earlier periods of mobilization in response to the epidemic have not completely disappeared, they have certainly been reduced, in both frequency and intensity, and in some ways domesticated."

This waning of activist energies also poses dangers in a time of financial crisis and reduced resource availability. Although HIV/AIDS was successfully positioned as a budgetary priority in the United States and in many other countries around the world, this focus has been slipping in many places. Ironically, the successful incorporation of HIV/AIDS into the agenda of many social movements may be leading some policymakers and member of the public alike to view HIV/AIDS as less of an urgent problem in itself. Rather, it may be increasingly seen as just another problem faced by millions of people, alongside hunger, displacement, gender oppression, sexual oppression, racial discrimination, and so forth. Similarly, as health systems become more aware of the multiple vulnerabilities of populations that are linked to HIV, funds are being reallocated to fight other diseases as well.

Still, there is reason to believe that HIV/AIDS activism may yet see another wave of activity. All social movements undertake their work through a series of ebbs and flows, and the HIV/AIDS movement has been no exception. At two major inflection points, at least, in the three decades of the global epidemic, activists and community members have galvanized to action both to defend against threats and to seize new opportunities. First in the late 1980s in the search for effective treatments, and in the late 1990s and early 2000s in the pursuit of greater global equity, HIV/AIDS activists have galvanized highly effective movements to meet the challenges of the day. Today's ebb must some day give way to tomorrow's flow, as the world's most severe crisis poses continuing challenges and faces emerging issues.

## BIBLIOGRAPHY

Abreu, H. (1992). *Movimentos sociais: Crise e perspectivas* [Social movements: Crisis and perspectives]. Porto Alegre: FASE/CIDADE.

Allen, D. (1991/1992). Reflections on "O Movimento Negro": The black movement. *Journal of Caribbean Studies, 8*(3), 167–193.

Alonso, A., & Koreck, M. (1989). Silences: "Hispanics," AIDS and sexual practices. *Differences, 1,* 101–124.

Altman, D. (1994). *Power and community organizational and cultural responses to AIDS.* London: Taylor and Francis.

Altman, D. (1999). Globalization, political economy, and HIV/AIDS. *Theory and Society, 28,* 559–584.

Alvarez, S. (1998). Latin American feminisms "go global": Trends of the 1990s and challenges for the new millennium. In S. Alvarez, E. Dagnino, & A. Escobar (eds.), *Cultures of politics/politics of culture: Re-visioning Latin American social movements* (pp. 293–324). Boulder: Westview Press.

Archibald, M. E. (2008). Institutional environments, sociopolitical process, and health movement organizations: The growth of self-help/mutual-aid. *Sociological Forum, 23*(1), 85–115.

Baer, H., Singer, M., et al. (1997). AIDS: A disease of the global system. In H. Baer, M. Singer, & I. Susser (eds.), *Medical anthropology and the world system: A critical perspective* (pp. 159–188). Westport, CT: Bergin & Garvey.

Beard, R. L. (2004). Advocating voice: Organisational, historical and social milieux of the Alzheimer's disease movement. *Sociology of Health and Illness, 26*(6), 797–819.

Berkman, A., Garcia, J., Muñoz-Laboy, M., Paiva, V., & Parker, R. (2005). A critical analysis of the Brazilian response to HIV/AIDS: Lessons learned for controlling and mitigating the epidemic in developing countries. *American Journal of Public Health, 95* (7), 1162–1172.

Bernstein, M. (2005). Identity politics. *Annual Review of Sociology 31,* 47–74.

Blankenship, K. M., Bray, S. J., et al. (2000). Structural interventions in public health. *AIDS 14* (Suppl 1), S11–S21.

Bluthenthal, R. N. (1998). Syringe exchange as a social movement: A case study of harm reduction in Oakland, California. *Substance Use and Misuse, 33*(5), 1147–71.

Bolton, R., & Singer, M. (eds.) (1992). *Rethinking AIDS prevention: Cultural approaches.* Philadelphia: Gordon and Breach.

Bond, G., & Vincent, J. (1997). AIDS in Uganda: The first decade. In G. Bond, J. Kreniske, I. Susser, and J. Vincent (eds.), *AIDS in Africa and the Caribbean* (pp. 85–98). Boulder: Westview Press.

Brier, J. (2009). *Infectious ideas: U.S. political responses to the AIDS crisis.* Chapel Hill: University of North Carolina Press.

Brown, P. (1984). The right to refuse treatment and the movement for mental health reform. *Journal of Health Policy, Politics, and Law, 9,* 291–313.

Brown, P., Zavestoki, S., et al. (2004). Embodied health movements: New approaches to social movements in health. *Sociology of Health and Illness, 26*(1), 1–50.

Bunce, V. (1997). Comparative democratization: Big and bounded generalizations. *Comparative Political Studies, 33*(6/7), 703–734.

Bunce, V. (2000). Presidents and the transition in Eastern Europe. In K. Von Mettenheim (ed.), *Presidential institutions and democratic politics* (pp. 161–176). Baltimore: Johns Hopkins University Press.

Burdick, J. (1992a). Rethinking the study of social movements: The case of Christian base communities in urban Brazil. In A. Escobar & S. Alvarez (eds.), *The making of social movements in Latin America* (pp. 171–184). Boulder: Westview.

Burdick, J. (1992b). Brazil's black consciousness movement. *Report of the Americas, 25*(4), 23–27.

Cardoso, R., & Corrêa, L. (1987). Movimentos sociais na América Latina [Social movements in Latin America]. *Revista Brasileira das Ciências Sociais, 3*(1), 27–37.

Cardoso, R., & Corrêa, L. (1992). Popular movements in the context of the consolidation of democracy in Brazil. In A. Escobar and S. Alvarez (eds.), *The making of social movements in Latin America* (pp. 291–302). Boulder: Westview Press.

Carrier, J. (1989). Sexual behavior and the spread of AIDS in Mexico. *Medical Anthropology, 10,* 129–142.

Carrier, J. (1995). *De los otros: Intimacy and homosexuality among Mexican men.* New York: Columbia University Press.

Carrier, J., & Magaña, R. (1991). Use of ethnosexual data on men of Mexican origin for HIV/AIDS prevention programs. *The Journal of Sex Research, 28*(2), 189–202.

Castells, M. (1997). *The power of identity.* Malden, MA: Blackwell.

Castro, A., & Farmer, P. (2005). Understanding and addressing AIDS-related stigma from anthropological theory to clinical practice in Haiti. *American Journal of Public Health, 95*(1), 53–59.

Chong, D. (1991). *Collective action and the civil rights movement.* Chicago: University of Chicago Press.

Cook, M. L. (1997). Regional integration and transnational politics: Popular sector strategies in the NAFTA era. In D. A. Chalmers (ed.), *The new politics of inequality in Latin America: Rethinking participation and representation* (pp. 516–540). Oxford: Oxford University Press.

Corrêa, S., Petchesky, R., & Parker, R. (2008). *Sexuality, health and human rights.* London and New York: Routledge.

Crimp, D. (ed.) (1988). *AIDS: Cultural analysis/cultural activism.* MIT Press.

Crossley, N. (2006). *Contesting psychiatry: Social movements in mental health.* Abingdon: Routledge.

Daniel, H., & Parker, R. (1993). *Sexuality, politics and AIDS in Brazil: In another world.* London: The Falmer Press.

Elbaz, G. (1997). Adolescent activism for postmodern HIV/AIDS: A new social movement. *The Urban Review, 29*(3), 145–174.

Elmerdorf, G. F. (1997). Mexico's environmental and ecological organizations and movements. *SALALM Papers, 36,* 123–129.

Epstein, S. (1996). *Impure science: AIDS, activism, and the politics of knowledge.* Berkeley: University of California Press.

Epstein, S. (1998). Gay and lesbian movements in the United States: Dilemmas of identity, diversity and political strategy. In B. D. Adam, J. W. Duyvendak, & A. Krouwel (eds.), *The global emergence of gay and lesbian politics: National imprints of a worldwide movement* (pp. 30–90). Philadelphia: Temple University Press.

Escobar, A., & Alvarez, S. (eds.) (1992). *The making of social movements in Latin America.* Boulder: Westview Press.

Farmer, P. (1990). The exotic and the mundane: Human immunodeficiency virus in Haiti. *Human Nature, 1*(4), 415–446.

Farmer, P. (1992). *AIDS and accusation: Haiti and the geography of blame.* Berkeley and Los Angeles: University of California Press.

Farmer, P. (1999). *Infections and inequalities: The modern plagues.* Berkeley, Los Angeles, and London: University of California Press.

Farmer, P., Connors, M. et al. (eds.) (1996). *Women, poverty and AIDS: Sex, drugs, and structural violence.* Monroe, ME: Common Courage Press.

Findji, M. T. (1992). From resistance to social movement: The indigenous authorities movement in Colombia. In S. Alvarez and A. Escobar (eds.), *The making of social movements in Latin America* (pp. 134–149). Boulder: Westview.

Fisher, W. F. (1997). Doing good? The politics and antipolitics of NGO practices. *Annual Review of Anthropology, 26,* 439–464.

Gamson, J. (1989). Silence, death and the invisible enemy: AIDS activism and social movement "newness." *Social Problems, 36*(4), 351–365.

Ganchoff, C. (2004). Regenerating movements: Embryonic stem cells and the politics of potentiality. *Sociology of Health and Illness, 26*(6), 757–774.

Garcia, J., & Parker, R. (2006). From global discourse to local action: The makings of a sexual rights movement? *Horizontes Antropológicos, 12*(26), 13–41.

García, M. P. (1992). The Venezuelan ecology movements symbolic effectiveness, social practices, and political strategies. In A. Escobar and S. Alvarez (eds.), *The making of social movements in Latin* America (pp. 150–170). Boulder: Westview.

Gillet, J. (2003). The challenges of institutionalization for AIDS media activism. *Media, Culture and Society, 25,* 607–624.

Gonzales, L., & Hasenbalg, C. (1982). O movimento negro na ultima década [The black movement in the last decade]. In L. Gonzales and C. Hasenbalg (eds.), *Lugar de negro* (pp. 9–68). Rio de Janeiro: Marco Zero.

González Block, M., & Liguori, A. (1992). *El SIDA en los estratos socioeconómicos de México.* Cuernavaca: Instituto Nacional de Salud Pública.

Gorman, E. (1991). Anthropological reflections on the HIV epidemic among gay men. *The Journal of Sex Research, 28*(2), 263–273.

Green, J. (1994). The emergence of the Brazilian gay liberation movement 1977–. *Latin American Perspectives, 2*(1), 38–55.

Grueso, L., Rosero, C., et al. (1998). The process of black community organizing in the southern Pacific Coast region of Colombia. In S. Alvarez, E. Dagnino, & A. Escobar (eds.), *Cultures of politics/politics of culture: Re-visioning Latin American social movements* (pp. 196–219). Boulder: Westview Press.

Henriksson, B., & Mansson S. (1995). Sexual negotiations: An ethnographic study of men who have sex with men. In H. ten Brummelhuis & G. Herdt (eds.), *Culture and sexual risk: Anthropological perspectives on AIDS* (pp. 157–182). Amsterdam: Gordon and Breach.

Herdt, G. (1997). Intergenerational relations and AIDS in the formation of gay culture in the United States. In M. Levine, P. Nardi, & J. Gagnon (eds.), *Changing times: Gay men and lesbians encounter HIV/AIDS* (pp. 245–281). Chicago and London: The University of Chicago Press.

Herdt, G., & Boxer, A. (1991). Ethnographic issues in the study of AIDS. *The Journal of Sex Research, 28*(2), 171–187.

Herdt, G., & A. Boxer (1992). Sexual identity and risk for AIDS among gay youth in Chicago. In T. Dyson (ed.), *Sexual behaviour and networking: Anthropological and socio-cultural studies on the transmission of HIV* (pp. 153–202). Liège, Belgium: Derouax-Ordina.

Herdt, G., Leap, W., et al. (1991). Anthropology, sexuality and AIDS. *The Journal of Sex Research, 28*(2), 167–169.

Herdt, G., & Lindenbaum, S. (eds.) (1992). *The time of AIDS: Social analysis, theory, and method.* Newbury Park, CA: Sage.

Hess, D. J. (2004). Medical modernization, scientific research fields and the epistemic politics of health social movements. *Sociology of Health and Illness, 26*(6), 695–709.

Hochstetler, K. (1997). The evolution of the Brazilian environmental movement and its political roles. In D. A. Chalmers, C. M. Vilas, S. B. Martin, K. Piester, & M. Segarra (eds.), *The new politics of inequality in Latin America: Rethinking participation and representation* (pp. 192–216). Oxford: Oxford University Press.

Inglehart, R. (1999). Values, ideology and cognitive mobilization in new social movements. In M. Waters (ed.), *Modernity: Critical concepts* (pp. 373–410). London: Routledge.

Javeline, D. (2003). The role of blame in collective action: Evidence from Russia. *American Political Science Review, 97,* 107–121.

Jelin, E. (ed.) (1990) *Women and social change in Latin America.* London: Zed Books.

Jelin, E. (1998). Toward a Culture of Participation and Citizenship: Challenges for a More Equitable World. In S. Alvarez, E. Dagnino, & A. Escobar (eds.), *Cultures of politics/politics of culture: Re-visioning Latin American social movements* (pp. 405–414). Boulder: Westview Press.

Jones, D. M. (1998). Democratization, civil society, and illiberal middle class culture in Pacific Asia. *Comparative Politics, 30,* 147–170.

Joseph, R. (1997). Democratization in Africa after 1989: Comparative and theoretical perspectives. *Comparative Politics, 29,* 363–382.

Kaleeba, N., Kalibala, S., et al. (1997). Participatory evaluation of counseling: Medical and social services of the AIDS support organization (TASO) in Uganda. *AIDS Care 9*(1), 13–26.

Kalibala, S., & Kaleeba, N. (1989). AIDS and community-based care in Uganda: The AIDS support organization TASO. *AIDS Care, 1*(2), 173–175.

Katz, A. H. (1993). *Self-help in America: A social movement perspective.* New York: Twayne.

Keck, M. E., & Sikkink, K. (1998). *Activists beyond borders: Advocacy networks in international politics.* Ithaca, NY: Cornell University Press.

Keefe, R. H., Lane, S. D., et al. (2006). From the bottom up: Tracing the impact of four health-based social movements on health and social policies. *Journal of Health and Social Policy, 21*(3), 55–69.

Kempandoo, K., & Doezema, J. (eds.) (1998). *Global sex workers: Rights, resistance, and redefinition.* New York: Routledge.

Kirp, D., & Bayer, R. (eds.) (1992). *AIDS in the industrialized democracies: Passions, politics and policies.* New Brunswick, NJ: Rutgers University Press.

Kitschelt, H. (1986). Political opportunity structures and political protest. *British Journal of Political Science, 16*(1), 57–85.

Klawiter, M. (2004). Breast cancer in two regimes: The impact of social movements on illness experience. *Sociology of Health and Illness, 26*(6), 845–874.

Kolker, E. S. (2004). Framing as a cultural resource in health social movements: Funding activism and the breast cancer movement in the US, 1990–1993. *Sociology of Health and Illness, 26*(6), 820–844.

Kreniske, J. (1997). AIDS in the Dominican Republic: Anthropological reflections on the social nature of disease. In G. Bond, J. Kreniske, I. Susser, & J. Vincent (eds.), *AIDS in Africa and the Caribbean* (pp. 33–50). Boulder: Westview Press.

Kriesi, H. (1989). *New social movements and the new class in the Netherlands.* Chicago: University of Chicago Press.

Kriesi, H., Koopmans, R., et al. (1998). *New social movements in Western Europe: A comparative analysis.* Minneapolis, MN: University of Minnesota Press.

Krishna, A. (2002). Enhancing political participation in democracies: What is the role of social capital? *Comparative Political Studies, 35*(4), 437–460.

Laclau, E. & Chantel, M. (1985). *Hegemony and socialist strategy: Towards a radical democratic politics.* London: Verso.

Laraña, E., Johnston, H., et al. (eds.) (1994). *New social movements: From ideology to identity.* Philadelphia: Temple University Press.

Lind, A. C. (1992). Power, gender, and development: Popular women's organizations and the politics of needs in Ecuador. In A. Escobar & S. Alvarez (eds.), *The making of social movements in Latin America* (pp. 134–149). Boulder, CO: Westview Press.

Lindenbaum, S. (1997). AIDS: Body, mind, and history. In G. Bond, J. Kreniske, I. Susser, & J. Vincent (eds.), *AIDS in Africa and the* Caribbean (pp. 191–194). Boulder: Westview Press.

Lindenbaum, S. (1998). Images of catastrophe: The making of an epidemic. In M. Singer (ed.), *The political economy of AIDS* (pp. 33–58). Amityville, NY: Baywood.

Linz, J. (2000). *Totalitarian and authoritarian regimes.* London: Routledge.

Lumsden, I. (1991). *Homosexualidad, sociedade y estado en México.* Mexico City and Toronto: Canadian Gay Archives.

Lune, H., & H. Oberstein (2001). Embedded systems: The case of HIV/AIDS nonprofit organizations in New York City. *Voluntas: International Journal of Voluntary and Nonprofit Organizations, 12*(1), 17–33.

Maluwa, M., Aggleton, P., et al. (2002). HIV/AIDS-related stigma, discrimination and human rights. *Health and Human Rights, 6*(1), 1–16.

Mann, J., Tarantola, D., et al. (eds.) (1992). *AIDS in the world.* Cambridge, MA: Harvard University Press.

Mann, J., & Tarantola, D. (eds.) (1996). *AIDS in the world II: Global dimensions, social roots, and responses.* New York: Oxford University Press.

McAdam, D. (1982). *Political process and the development of black insurgency, 1930–70.* Chicago: University of Chicago Press.

McAdam, D., McCarthy, D., et al. (eds.) (1996). *Comparative perspectives on social movements: Political opportunities, mobilizing structures, and cultural framings.* New York: Cambridge University Press.

McAdam, D., Tarrow, S., and Tilly, C. (2001). Dynamics of contention. Cambridge: Cambridge University Press.

McCarthy, D., & Zald, M. (1973). *The trend of social movements in America.* New Jersey: General Learning Press.

McCormick, S., Brown, P., et al. (2003). The personal is scientific, the scientific is political: The public paradigm of the environmental breast cancer movement. *Sociological Forum, 18*(4), 545–576.

McKeganey, N., Friedman, S., et al. (1998). The social context of injectors. In G. Stimson, D. C. Des Jarlais, & A. Ball, *Drug injecting and HIV infection* (pp. 22–41). London: UCL Press.

Meyer, D. S., & Whittier, N. (1994). Social movement spillover. *Social Problems, 41,* 277–298.

Moe, T. (1980). *The organization of interests: Incentives and the internal dynamics of political interest groups.* Chicago: University of Chicago Press.

Morgan, J. (2003). *Long life . . . positive HIV stories.* Cape Town: Spinifex Press.

Msimand, S. (2003). HIV/AIDS, globalization and the international women's movement. *Gender and Development, 11*(1), 109–113.

Nash, J. (1989). Cultural resistance and class consciousness in Bolivian tin-mining communities. In S. Ekstein (ed.), *Latin American social* movements (pp. 82–202). Berkeley: University of California Press.

Nathanson, C. (2007). *Disease prevention as social change: The state, society, and public health in the U.S.* New York: Russell Sage Foundation.

Obbo, C. (1993). HIV transmission through social and geographic networks in Uganda. *Social Science and Medicine, 36,* 949–955.

Offe, C. (1999). New social movements: Challenging the boundaries of institutional politics. In M. Waters (ed.), *Modernity: Critical concepts* (pp. 336–372) London: Routledge.

O'Kane, R. H. T. (2000). *Revolutions: Critical concepts in political science.* London: Routledge.

Olson, M. (1965). *The logic of collective action.* Cambridge: Harvard University Press.

Ortiz, R. D. (1987). Indigenous rights of regional autonomy in revolutionary Nicaragua. *Latin American Perspectives, 14*(1), 43–66.

Paiva, V. (2000a). Gendered scripts and the sexual scene: Promoting sexual subjects among Brazilian teenagers. In R. Parker, R. Barbosa, & P. Aggleton (eds.), *Framing the sexual subject: The politics of gender, sexuality and power* (pp. 216–239). Berkeley: Los Angeles, and London: University of California Press.

Paiva, V. (2000b). *Fazendo arte com camisinha.* São Paulo: Summus Editorial.

Parker, R. (1988). Sexual culture and AIDS education in urban Brazil. In R. Kulstad (ed.), *AIDS 1988: AAAS symposia papers* (pp. 269–289). Washington: American Association for the Advancement of Science.

Parker, R. (1996a). Empowerment, community mobilization, and social change in the face of HIV/AIDS. *AIDS 10* (Suppl 3), S27–S31.

Parker, R. (1996b). Behavior in Latin American men: Implications for HIV/AIDS interventions. *International Journal of STD and AIDS 7* (Suppl 2), 62–65.

Parker, R. (1997). *Políticas, instituições e AIDS: Enfrentando a epidemia no Brasil* [Politics, institutions and AIDS]. Rio de Janeiro: Jorge Zahar/ABIA.

Parker, R. (2001). Sexuality, culture and power in HIV/AIDS research. *Annual Review of Anthropology, 30,* 163–179.

Parker, R. (2009). Civil society, political mobilization, and the impact of HIV scale-up on health systems in Brazil. *JAIDS: Journal of Acquired Immune Deficiency Syndromes, 52* (Suppl. 1): S49–S51.

Parker, R. (2011) Grassroots activism, civil society mobilization, and the politics of the global HIV/AIDS epidemic, *Brown Journal of World Affairs, 12*(2), 21–37.

Parker, R., & Aggleton P. (2003). HIV/AIDS-related stigma and discrimination: A conceptual framework and implications for actions. *Social Science and Medicine, 57*(1), 13–24.

Parker, R., Barbosa, R., et al. (2000). Framing the sexual subject. In R. Parker, R. Barbosa, & P. Aggleton, *Framing the Sexual Subject: The Politics of Gender, Sexuality and* Power (pp. 1–25). Berkeley, Los Angeles, and London: University of California Press.

Parker, R., & Carballo, M. (1990). Qualitative research on homosexual and bisexual behavior relevant to HIV/AIDS. *The Journal of Sex Research, 27,* 497–525.

Parker, R., Easton, D., et al. (2000). Structural barriers and facilitators in HIV prevention: A review of international research. *AIDS, 14* (Suppl 1), S22–S32.

Parker, R., Herdt, G., et al. (1991). Sexual culture, HIV transmission, and AIDS research. *The Journal of Sex Research, 28,* 77–98.

Patton, C. (1991) *Inventing AIDS.* New York: Routledge.

Parker, R., Passarelli, C. A., Terto, V., Pimenta, C., Berkman, A., & Munoz-Laboy, M. (2003). Introduction: The Brazilian respoonse to HIV/AIDS: Analyzing its components and assessing its transferability. Divulacao em Saude para Debate, 27, 140–142.

People with AIDS Coalition (1983). *The Denver Principles.* Accessed at http://www.actupny.org/documents/Denver.html, on January 25, 2012.

Petchesky, R. (2003). *Global prescriptions: Gendering health and human rights.* London: Zed Books.

Polletta, F., & Jasper, J. (2001). Collective identity and social movements. *Annual Review of Sociology, 27,* 283–305.

Reis, R., Terto Jr., V., and Pimenta, C. (eds.) (2009). *Intellectual property rights and access to ARV medicines: Civil society resistance in the global South.* Rio de Janeiro: ABIA.

Robbins, S. (2004). Long live Zackie, long live: AIDS activism, science and citizenship after apartheid. *Journal of Southern African Studies, 30*(3), 651–672.

Rogers, A., & Pilgrim, D. (1991). "Pulling down churches": Accounting for the British mental health users' movement. *Sociology of Health and Illness, 13*(2), 129–148.

Rosenberg, T. (2001). Look at Brazil. *New York Times.* Accessed at http://www.nytimes.com/2001/01/28/magazine/look-at-brazil.html?pagewanted=all&src =pm, on January 12, 2012.

Schneider, H. (2002). On the fault-line: The politics of AIDS policy in contemporary South Africa. *African Studies, 61* (1), 145–167.

Schoepf, B. (1991). Ethical, methodological and political issues of AIDS research in central Africa. *Social Science and Medicine, 33,* 749–763.

Schoepf, B. (1992). Sex and condoms: African healers and the reinvention of tradition in Zaire. *Medical Anthropology, 14,* 225–242.

Schoepf, B. (1995). Culture, sex research and AIDS prevention in Africa. In H. Ten Brummelhuis & J. Vincent (eds.), *Culture and sexual risk: Anthropological perspectives on AIDS* (pp. 29–51). Amsterdam: Gordon and Breach.

Seidman, S. (1993). Identity and politics in a "postmodern'"gay culture: Some historical and conceptual notes. In M. Warner (ed.), *Fear of a queer planet: Queer politics and social theory* (pp. 105–142). Minneapolis: University of Minnesota Press.

Singer, M. (1994). AIDS and the health crisis of the U.S. urban poor: The perspective of critical medical anthropology. *Social Science and Medicine, 39,* 931–948.

Singer, M. (ed.) (1998). *The political economy of AIDS.* Amityville, NY: Baywood.

Singer, M., Flores, C., et al. (1990). SIDA: The economic, social and cultural context of AIDS among Latinos. *Medical Anthropology Quarterly, 14,* 285–306.

Siplon, P. (2002). *AIDS and the policy struggle in the United States,* Washington, D.C.: Georgetown University Press.

Smith, R. A., & Siplon, P. (2006). *Drugs into bodies: Global AIDS treatment activism.* Westport, CT: Praeger.

Solomos, J. (1998). Beyond racism and multiculturalism. *Patterns of Prejudice, 32*(4), 45–62.

Starn, O. (1992). "I dreamed of foxes and hawks": Reflections on peasant protest, new social movements and the Rondas Campesinas of northern Peru. In A.

Escobar & S. Alvarez (eds.), *The making of social movements in Latin America* (pp. 89–111). Boulder: West View Press.

Stimson, G. V., & Choopanya, K. (1998). Global perspectives on drug injecting. In G. Stimson, D. C. D. Jarlais, and A. Ball (eds.), *Drug injecting and HIV infection* (pp. 1–21). London: UCL Press.

Stroman, D. (2003). *The disability rights movement: From deinstitutionalization to self-determination.* Lanham, MD: University Press of America.

Tarrow, S. (1996). State and opportunities. In D. McAdam, J. D. McCarthy, & M. Zald (eds.), *Comparative perspectives on social movements: Political opportunities, mobilizing structures, and cultural framings* (pp. 41–61). New York: Cambridge University Press.

Tarrow, S. (1998). *Power in movement: Social movements, collective action and politics.* Cambridge, England and New York: Cambridge University Press.

Tempalski, B., Flom, P. L., et al. (2007). Social and political factors predicting the presence of syringe exchange programs in 96 US metropolitan areas. *American Journal of Public Health, 97*(3), 437–447.

Terto Jr., V. (1996). Homossexuais soropositivos e soropositivos homossexuais: Questões da homossexualidade masculina em tempos da AIDS. In R. Parker & R. Barbosa (eds.), *Sexualidades brasileiras* (pp. 90–104). Rio de Janeiro: Relume-Dumará Editores.

Thom, A. (2003). Mapping souls. Available at www.csa.za.org/article/articleview/262/1/1/, accessed on December 12, 2003.

Tilly, C. (1978). *From mobilization to revolution.* New York: Random House.

Tilly, C. (1985). *Models and realities of popular collective action.* New York: Center for Studies of Social Change.

Touraine, A. (1981). *The voice and the eye: An analysis of social movements.* Cambridge: Cambridge University Press.

Touraine, A. (1985). An introduction to the study of social movements. *Social Research, 52*(4), 749–787.

Touraine, A. (1998). *The return of the actor.* Minneapolis, MI: University of Michigan Press.

Touraine, A. (2000). A method for studying social actions. *Journal of World-Systems Research, VI*(3), 900–918.

Treichler, P. (1999). *How to have theory in an epidemic: Cultural chronicles of AIDS.* Durham and London: Duke University Press.

Turner, T. (1995). An indigenous people's struggle for socially equitable and ecologically sustainable production: The Kayapo Revolt against extractivism. *Journal of Latin American Anthropology, 1*(1), 98–121.

Van Rooy, A. (2000). *Civil society and the aid industry.* London: Earthscan.

Vanwesenbeeck, I. (2001). Another decade of social scientific work on sex work: A review of research 1990–2000. *Annual Review of Sex Research, 12*, 242–289.

Von Schoen Angerer, T. A., Wilson, D. A., et al. (2001). Access and activism: The ethics of providing antiretroviral therapy in developing countries. *AIDS, 15* (Suppl 5), S81–S90.

Walters, S. D. (2001). *All the rage: The story of gay visibility in America.* Chicago: University of Chicago Press.

Warner, M. (2000). *The trouble with normal: Sex politics and the ethics of queer life.* Cambridge, MA: Harvard University Press.

Warren, K. (1989). *The symbolic of subordination: Indian identity in a Guatemala town.* Austin, TX: University of Texas Press.

Warren, K. (1998). Indigenous movements as a challenge to the unified social movement paradigm for Guatemala. In S. Alvarez, E. Dagnino, & A. Escobar (eds.), *Cultures of politics/politics of culture: Re-visioning Latin American social movements* (pp. 165–195). Boulder: Westview Press.

Watney, S. (2000). *Imagine hope: AIDS and gay identity.* London: Routledge.

Wignaraja, P. (1993). *New social movements in the South: Empowering the people.* London and Atlantic Highlands, NJ: Zed Books.

Williamson, C. (2008). The patient movement as an emancipation movement. *Health Expectation, 11,* 102–112.

Zoller, H. M. (2005). Health activism: Communication theory and action for social change. *Communication Theory, 15*(4), 341–364.

# 2

# AIDS Treatment Advocacy in the United States, Brazil, and South Africa: Diverse Actors, Strategies, and Sectors

*Susan M. Chambré*

Accounts of AIDS policymaking emphasize the central role of "AIDS activists." These are usually defined as the political outsiders who mount street demonstrations and who challenge, question, and in some cases publicly taunt and even threaten state officials. Influential discussions of AIDS policymaking in the United States begin their accounts in 1987, the year that ACT UP was founded (Epstein, 1996; Gould, 2009). A *New York Times* article marking the 20th anniversary of the epidemic was entitled "Advocates for Patients Barged In, and the Federal Government Changed" (Pear, 2001). Similarly, accounts of AIDS policy in South Africa note the central role of the Treatment Action Campaign (TAC). Just as the icon of AIDS activism in the United States has been Larry Kramer, Zackie Achmat, the South African activist, is portrayed as the major force in the rollout of antiretroviral therapy (ARV) in sub-Saharan Africa. When the United States withdrew its sanctions against South Africa, which had challenged international copyright agreements by importing generic AIDS medications, the shift in U.S. policy was attributed to a series of ACT UP protests and to Achmat's refusal to take lifesaving medications until they were universally available (Power, 2003). In contrast to the United States and South Africa, there is no such icon in Brazil, a country that is widely viewed as a model for AIDS policy in developing countries since prevention efforts have sharply reduced HIV transmission and there is universal access to treatment. The relatively limited amount of overt political protest in Brazil and the representations of its prominence in the United

States and South Africa suggest that there are different styles of political activism and advocacy in varied political contexts.

This chapter describes the evolution of access to lifesaving medications in these three political contexts. It indicates that a variety of political actors—activists engaged in protest, elite allies, and institutional advocates inside the state—collaborated in various ways to gain media attention, influence public opinion, and persuade state and corporate officials to expand access to AIDS treatment. The evolution of this and other policies is far more complex than is captured in the idea that activists "barged in." Policy development in a multi-institutional and transnational field of this sort depends on synchronizing the interests of an array of state, corporate, and civil society actors (cf. Armstrong and Bernstein, 2008) and a mixture of political strategies including lobbying, political protest, and effective utilization of the media and other modes of communication.

## THREE CONTEXTS

There are important similarities and differences among the United States, Brazil, and South Africa. All three are federalist systems in which the role of civil society was expanding during the time that they were confronting the AIDS epidemic. They were also undergoing significant political changes and experiencing the impact of economic globalization, which has contributed to the worldwide increase in nongovernmental organizations (Brown, Khagram, et al., 2000) and is related to greater claims and challenges to nonstate actors like firms (Milner and Moravcsik, 2009; Spar and La Mure, 2003). However, they differ in several important ways, most notably the timing of the epidemic, the policy response, the nature and styles of political advocacy, and the methods of organizing and financing health care, particularly access to medications. The United States has a stable rate of new infections; Brazil has a much smaller epidemic than was initially anticipated; and South Africa has the largest number of people currently living with HIV, totaling 5.6 million people in 2010, 37 percent of whom were estimated to receive ARV treatment, the largest such program in the world (HIV and AIDS in South Africa, n.d.).

Beginning in the late 1960s, the United States began to shift the direction of its human service financing, design and public delivery away from federal dominance toward devolution and privatization. This trend became especially pronounced with the election of President Reagan in 1980 and had a profound effect on the response to the AIDS epidemic in which the federal role was relatively limited until the mid-1980s and much of the policymaking was at the local level with enormous variations between cities and states. A related trend was a sharp increase in the number of civil society organizations and a growing professionalization of political advocacy (Skocpol, 2003).

The United States has a mixed economy of human services. This means that individuals pay out of pocket for a substantial share of health care costs and a great deal of coverage is provided by employers. Growing numbers of people are uninsured, a situation likely to change if and when the United States adopts more universal health care coverage. For older people, the disabled, and those with low incomes, access to social benefits, health care, and medications is based on eligibility for a patchwork of human service programs. The delivery of services is similarly complex with the nonprofit sector delivering a major portion of services along with a federalist model where payment for some programs and services is local or state while others are federally financed. The financing of AIDS medications varies according to class and location. Many patients pay out of pocket, others have prescription drug coverage, and people with lower incomes have their medications paid for by Medicaid or by the federally subsidized but state administered AIDS Drug Assistance Program (ADAP).

Brazil was also undergoing political change in the early 1980s with an end to dictatorship, a process of democratization, and an expansion of civil society organizations. Since 1988, health care has been a right. The federal government underwrites the cost of HIV prevention and health services while relying on a host of public and nonprofit organizations to deliver services. Brazil has a substantial pharmaceutical industry, which allows it to produce most of the antiretroviral treatment (ARVs) needed by its citizens.

South Africa responded to the AIDS epidemic far later than the two other societies. A complex set of factors contributed to this late start including a host of cultural factors, the fact that the country was emerging from its racist apartheid system, experiencing democratization, and an expansion of civil society (Friedman, 2006). The country established health care as a right in its 1996 constitution but has a far weaker public health system and relies more heavily on external financing from global funding mechanisms including foundations and international organizations like the Global Fund and the President's Emergency Plan for AIDS Relief (PEPFAR).

For Brazil and South Africa, the presence of external funding sources was critical to their ability to provide access to AIDS treatment. At the same time, another crucial development, not totally unrelated to advocacy, was the declining price of treatment (Kapstein and Busby, 2010), which allowed for the expansion of access to ARVs.

## THEORETICAL PERSPECTIVES

I draw on several frameworks developed by social movement and public policy theorists: resource mobilization, political process, strategic agency, and policy network theories. The goal of this chapter is to draw on various dimensions of these theories in order to develop a middle-range theory that explains common threads in AIDS policy development.

Resource mobilization studies focus on the importance and impact of drawing on and cultivating various types of political resources including elite financial support and legitimacy as well as media attention (McCarthy and Zald, 1977; Jenkins, 1983; Jenkins and Perrow, 1977). Recent work has correlated the impact of various types of strategies (e.g., protest vs. lobbying) on garnering media attention, and recent studies have examined claims against nonstate actors like corporations whose reputation and stock prices may be affected by social movement activity (Amenta, Caren, et al., 2009; Andrews and Caren, 2010; King and Soule, 2007).

Political process research focuses on the interaction between broad cultural, social, economic, and political factors and social movement activity. From this perspective, political opportunities and contexts both constrain and enable activities and, at the same time, involve a recursive process in which opportunities influence collective action and movement actions influence opportunities. Building on this framework are newer studies that emphasize individual agency, noting the importance of emotions and culture (Goodwin, Jasper and Polletta, 2001; Jasper, 2012). Recent work has conceptualized social movement actors as players in an elaborate iterative process who operate in various action fields or arenas (Goodwin and Jasper, 2012). Clearly, this approach has a great deal of promise in explaining health policy because political leaders are often motivated by personal interests and experiences (Blumenthal and Morone, 2009) and operate as policy entrepreneurs (Mintrom, 1997).

These two theories focus almost exclusively on social movements. They are extremely useful in identifying key variables and specifying their importance and interrelationships. However, they conceptualize allies as either elites or patrons; this overlooks the possibility that actors and organizations that are not part of a movement are, in fact, important collaborators in what tends to be a highly changeable and varied process (Clemens and Guthrie, 2011). This is particularly true for institutional advocates, bureaucrats, and politicians within the state, who share and sometimes articulate the same goals as a social movement (Banaszak, 2005; Santoro and McGuire, 1997). A theory developed by political scientists, the policy network framework, offers great promise by adding another dimension to our understanding of AIDS policymaking since it specifies the collaborative nature of a diverse set of actors with common interests as well as sometimes fragile issue-based coalitions, which might wax and wane over the course of time (Jordan, 1981).

## Finding a Cure: AIDS Advocacy in the United States

The earliest AIDS cases in the United States and in the world were reported in June 1981, and the first community-based organization, New York's Gay Men's Health Crisis, was established the following winter. By the mid-1980s, the growing number of new groups and organizations in New York City and throughout the nation led to the idea that there was an identifiable AIDS community with a distinctive culture that framed collective action (Chambré, 2006).

Finding a cure was a major agenda item. Early advocates, some of whom were gay rights movement veterans, focused on expanding the role of the state in funding scientific research. Members of the AIDS community thought that a cure was within reach if enough money and enough scientific talent were made available. The AIDS community influenced policies related to finding a cure during the 1980s in three important ways. First, they used preexisting political contacts and networked and lobbied for more public funding for research. Second, they engaged in collective action and established organizations that had the effect of destabilizing the drug testing system by expanding access to unapproved medications. Third, they engaged in direct action and employed highly contentious strategies to challenge the system of drug approval.

The growth of AIDS civil society organizations was rapid. Much of the effort was directed toward educating and providing social and emotional support to the growing numbers of people affected by this new and lethal disease. But there was a small critical mass of people, mostly veterans of the gay rights movement, which was involved in political advocacy and lobbying. Localized efforts like New York City's AIDS Network brought AIDS advocates and public officials together weekly. Some of the representatives of new community-based organizations collaborated with national groups like the American Association of Physicians for Human Rights and the Gay Rights National Lobby to lobby for federal funding for AIDS research.

These political strategies had an impact. New York State established an AIDS Institute in the Department of Health, which conducted scientific research and coordinated program and policy development. By July 1983, when there were 1,600 AIDS cases in the United States, federal AIDS funding exceeded the total spent for two other disease emergencies, Legionnaire's disease and toxic shock syndrome. With greater public awareness as a result of the widely publicized illness of film star Rock Hudson and celebrity interest in the issue, including support from film star Elizabeth Taylor, federal funding for AIDS research rose to $106.5 million in 1985 and private foundations were gearing up to support scientific research (Chambré, 2006). By then, 3,000 People with AIDS (PWAs) were enrolled in clinical trials, nearly one-third of the country's 10,000 cases (Cimons, 1985); 30 new drugs were under development; and six drugs were being tested in 1986 (Wyrick, 1986). Federal funding for AIDS research rose to $2 billion in 1988 (Chase, 1988).

The culture of the AIDS community emphasized patient empowerment and the importance of becoming active health care consumers who sought out approved, alternative, and unapproved medical treatments (Chambré, 1995). PWAs believed that access to unapproved treatments was a right; they were willing to take risks and take medicines not approved by the Food and Drug Administration (FDA) because, in the words of one PWA, "You're going to die from the disease one way or another so anything you can do to prolong your life is worth a try. It's my body. My choice. I can't wait for the FDA" (Braun et al., 1993).

These beliefs contributed to the development of an AIDS underground starting in 1984. Individuals and groups imported medications from outside the United States where drug approval requirements were less stringent. FDA officials and customs agents overlooked this smuggling and only seized drugs deemed to be toxic. Allowing people to import drugs for their own use became official policy in 1988 (Boffey, 1988a; Chase, 1985; Sirica, 1985). The AIDS underground also included guerilla laboratories and buyers clubs, which were also overlooked by the FDA and allowed people to purchase imported and unapproved drugs. In 1988, a dozen buyers clubs and more than 40 AIDS "clinics" in the United States and in Canada were selling bootlegged drugs (Kolbe, 1988; Reed, 1987; Span, 1992). This was an important form of resistance and advocacy designed to pressure the FDA to approve new drugs.

An important change had also taken place in the culture of disease in the United States. Clinical trials were no longer viewed as risky but as treatment and as a right (Annas, 1992). Participants in the AIDS community developed a network of community-based organizations that operated clinical trials. This was part of a broader change in the system of drug trials in which nonuniversity settings—once the major site for clinical trials—are now less dominant and more drug testing is conducted by for-profit organizations in a globalized industry (Fisher, 2009; Petryna, 2009). The Community Research Initiative (CRI) in New York was the first community-based testing organization. It opened in May 1987 and was a major site for testing aerosolized pentamidine, an early AIDS drug.

The efforts of the AIDS community to help people to gain access to unapproved and experimental treatments had the effect of destabilizing the traditional drug approval system with experimental groups receiving treatment and control groups getting placebos. Unlike past generations of patients who accepted the expertise of physicians and willingly participated in clinical trials in an effort to help themselves and to advance science, PWAs fiercely and aggressively fought for their own lives by traveling abroad and purchasing new medications from buyers clubs. They were also willing to compromise the scientific integrity of drug trials by having their capsules tested to see if they were new compounds or placebos. A 1989 *Washington Post* article noted, "So many AIDS patients are taking so many different kinds of untested drugs from underground suppliers that federal health officials now concede that many traditional methods of testing new drugs scientifically have broken down" (Specter, 1989).

By the late 1980s, growing numbers of people believed that a cure might already exist. This expectation was based on the fact that AZT, the first new AIDS medication, had been sitting on a shelf for years. This belief also contributed to a widely held understanding, expressed by Larry Kramer (1989), who pointed out, "The delays that are keeping these drugs from us are not scientific. They are bureaucratic. . . . We are being held prisoners by the Food and Drug Administration and the National Institutes of Health, by callous, greedy pharmaceutical companies, and by government regulations that leave us to die."

A second strand of AIDS advocacy was directed toward the FDA's slow approval process. Criticism of the FDA predated AIDS but the AIDS community gave the issue a new urgency. Public demonstrations of the AIDS community's concern about public policy date back to the spring of 1983 with a series of candlelight vigils in several cities (Chambré, 2006). Beginning in March 1987, ACT UP complemented the work of AIDS nonprofits like the buyers clubs and community-based clinical trial organizations using more strident and visible tactics to gain public interest. The first demand listed at ACT UP's first demonstration on Wall Street that month was

"Immediate release by the Federal Food & Drug Administration of drugs that might help save our lives."

On October 11, 1988, between 600 and 1,500 demonstrators from 15 ACT UP groups throughout the country demonstrated at the "Federal Death Administration" because "Many Federal agencies, not to mention local and state ones, have been derelict in the fight on AIDS. . . . Yet only one agency, the FDA, is actively blocking the delivery of promising drugs to PWAs and people with HIV infection" (ACT UP, 1987).

Two important changes followed these demonstrations: a reduction in the cost of AZT and, one week after the FDA demonstration, a commitment by the FDA to speed up drug approval after two stages of testing (to prove safety and efficacy) and granting conditional approval before the third stage (which required large clinical trials) if drug companies did postmarketing studies.

Both were apparent victories for the AIDS Coalition to Unleash Power (ACT UP). However, a closer look at the broader context and the role of elite allies challenges this idea. Some thoughtful observers note that price reductions for AZT were due to improved production costs (in 1987) and the perceived growth in the market (in 1989). It is quite clear that a host of actors—congressmen planning to investigate the manufacturer, editorials in major newspapers and in medical journals like JAMA, and efforts of various organizations in the AIDS community, like a lawsuit filed by the National Gay Rights Advocates and a threatened boycott of Burroughs Wellcome products—were also important sources of this change (Chase, 1987a, 1987b; Hilts, 1989a, 1989b; Lugliani, 1989). In addition, drug companies themselves recognized that the market for AIDS drugs was expanding with greater availability of public funding to underwrite the cost of treatment both for those receiving Medicaid as well as those with somewhat higher incomes who would later become eligible for public funding for medications under the federal ADAP program.

The FDA itself was ready for reform (Chambré, 2006). Criticism of slow drug approval came from many quarters including drug companies, which benefited from having drugs released faster; from scientists, FDA staff, cancer researchers, and the National Academy of Sciences; and from government officials like Vice President Bush who headed a task force that gave the issue legitimacy and the President's Commission on HIV whose 1988 report pointed out the need for more rapid pharmaceutical approval (Boffey 1988; Carpenter and Moore, 2007; Gevisser, 1988; Leary, 1989). News articles also gave ACT UP's claims visibility and legitimacy. In 1987, the *Wall Street Journal's* Marilyn Chase (1987c) pointed out,

"When Marie Shelby died of AIDS last year, she was also a victim of the way drugs are developed in this country."

The innovative role of institutional advocates working inside the state is also illustrated in the development of the parallel track. In June 1989, National Institute of Infections and Allergic Diseases Director Anthony Fauci, who had by then become an important institutional advocate, announced his support for a "parallel track" in which individuals who were ineligible for clinical trials and unable to take approved medications could have unapproved medications prescribed for them. The idea was actually developed by ACT UP New York member Jim Eigo the previous year who presented it to a federal committee investigating cancer and AIDS drugs (Arno and Feiden, 1992). Fauci's endorsement was an important turning point in the history of treatment activism; it was the beginning of a much stronger alliance between activists and government scientists. Although Fauci had met with representatives of the AIDS community before, the interactions had been adversarial (Dunne, 1987). Fauci recalled, "In the beginning, those people had a blanket disgust with us. And it was mutual. . . . When the smoke cleared we realized that much of their criticism was absolutely valid" (Epstein, 1996: 235).

By the early 1990s, the center of gravity in treatment activism moved from the streets into the corridors of power. AIDS treatment advocacy was becoming dominated by a small core group of people in the Treatment and Data Committee (T & D) of ACT UP–New York (Handleman, 1990), which produced one-page handouts and later, detailed policy papers. Treatment activists became part of the policy process. By 1990, representatives of the AIDS community were attending meetings once closed to them, had gained voting rights comparable to principal investigators, and had seats on all AIDS Clinical Trial group committees including the executive committee (Chambré, 2006).

More of the work of the AIDS community involved alliances with groups and policy actors that were not only diverse in form but also ideology, including former "enemies" including government scientists, political conservatives, civil libertarians, and drug companies. An amfAR-supported conference at Columbia University in July 1989 was sponsored by the CRI and a similar group called the CCC in San Francisco and was described as a "love-in" affirming their common goals. Larry Kramer developed a good working relationship with Tony Fauci whom he had once called a "murderer" (Biddle, 1993). However, treatment activists were careful about these alliances. Despite a concern that drug companies were primarily interested in profits, AIDS advocates came to understand that they had some common interests. A major turning point, which eventually led to the departure of key treatment activists from ACT UP, was a $1 million donation from Burroughs Wellcome to ACT UP for community-based trials (Broder, 1992). Several years earlier, the company's headquarters had been occupied by ACT UP but a company spokesperson announced in 1992, "We as an organization have come to realize that the goals of ACT UP—most notably, the discovery of treatments for HIV disease—are not all that different than ours" (Zonana, 1992). David Barr (1990:7), an ACT UP member doing policy research for GMHC, affirmed, "Working directly with pharmaceutical companies also is a way advocates can ensure that the most promising drugs are researched first."

This alliance led to a split within ACT UP in 1992 and key members of the T & D committee formed the Treatment Action Group (TAG), which operated as a think tank. A journalist writing for *POZ* magazine called the AIDS community's alliance with drug companies "sleeping with the enemy" (Silverstein, 1998). More money from drug companies allowed AIDS organizations to mount conferences and educate patients about treatment, which ensured the demand for the drug companies' products (Morrow, 1999). Drug companies and AIDS advocates also had a mutual interest in lobbying for increased federal funding for the ADAP program, which paid for pharmaceuticals for individuals whose incomes were too high to be eligible for Medicaid.

Thus, a variety of political actors operating in a number of social spheres—the state, civil society, and firms—promoted efforts to find a cure. While demonstrations and other forms of activism were critical in shaping public awareness, the narrative describes how a variety of political actors and strategies influenced the policy process.

## Collaboration and Solidarity in Brazil

Brazil's AIDS policy development is a striking contrast to the United States with a limited number of public protests and a higher level of collaboration between the state and civil society. Brazil is widely recognized to have had a model response to the epidemic (Berkman et al., 2005; Okie, 2006; Rosenberg, 2001). In 1990, the World Bank projected that in the absence of an effective policy, 1.2 million people would be infected with HIV in 2000, considerably larger than the estimated number of cases in 2009, which ranged from 460,000 to 810,000 (Berkman et al., 2005; HIV & AIDS in Brazil). Brazil has developed an integrated model of prevention and treatment providing universal access to medications to all AIDS cases. AZT was given to all registered HIV/AIDS cases in 1991 and anti-retrovirals (ARVs) became universally available one year after they were demonstrated to be effective, starting in 1997.

What accounts for this successful model? Previous observers have pointed to a robust AIDS movement, which contributed to state action and, later, to highly successful collaboration between civil society organizations and an activist state. Biehl (2004) characterizes the politics of AIDS in Brazil as "activism within the state." A second element is cultural. Several features of Brazilian culture strengthened state and civil society commitments and contributed to the fact that the epidemic has not been racialized (Lieberman, 2007). Solidarity and citizenship characterize the response to AIDS. The third element was Brazil's autonomy in terms of its ability to challenge international patent protections and produce a large share of the medications needed by people living with HIV.

The first cases were reported in Brazil in 1982. This was a period of major political transition since Brazil was moving away from many years of dictatorship and was democratizing. It was also a time when several unsuccessful economic strategies, combined with worldwide inflation, contributed to a rise in poverty (Connor, 2000). These factors contributed to an initially slow federal response; the federal government established the National AIDS Program and earmarked funding specifically for AIDS in 1988 (Gauri and Lieberman, 2006). Beginning with the founding of the AIDS Prevention and Support Group, GAPA, in São Paolo in 1985, the number of AIDS NGOs and organizations providing AIDS services or those engaged in advocacy rose sharply. In June 1989, 14 organizations attended the first meeting of NGOs doing AIDS work. Five months later, a second meeting attracted representatives from 38 organizations (Parker, 2003). Four years later, in 1993, there were 120 organizations and 480 in 2003 (Gauri and Lieberman, 2006).

The earliest advocates were part of the country's relatively small gay movement (Parker, 2003) and a small but critical mass of former political exiles who were opponents of the country's military regime. They viewed AIDS as an important political issue but some of them were personally involved because they had AIDS themselves or they had family members with AIDS (Gauri and Lieberman, 2006; Nunn, 2009). Support also came from political parties, labor unions, and a broad range of religious groups including Catholic, Protestant, and Afro-Caribbean (Garcia and Parker, 2011; Parker, 2008).

Of particular importance was an alliance with the sanitary reform movement that was committed to improving health care institutions and altering the underlying social conditions that contributed to poor health. This movement successfully lobbied to incorporate informal sector workers in the national health system in 1990 (Gauri and Lieberman, 2006). In the first six years of the epidemic, the number of cases was relatively small and concentrated in several large cities. Similar to the United States, much of the early advocacy was centered in the gay community, in NGOs, and in local governments (Berkman, Garcia, et al., 2005). These efforts began in São Paolo and in Rio de Janeiro, which are still the nation's epicenters (Teixeira, 2003). By 1984, more than 10 states had established AIDS programs (Connor, 2000). Once federal officials became more committed to AIDS policy, they took a leadership role. Biehl (2004) describes Brazil as an "activist state" in which public officials collaborate with civil society. This is not surprising given the strong public commitment to citizen participation that is integral to some public institutions. For example, the public health system actively engages citizens as elected representatives in Public Health Councils (Berkman et al., 2005).

The Brazilian constitution of 1988 established health care as a right. This made a profound difference in how AIDS advocates operated since they could file class action suits. Rather than needing to engage in protest, the lawsuits were a way to establish the right to free viral-resistance testing and to expand the drug formulary (Berkman et al., 2005; Rios, 2003; Ventura, 2003).

As in the United States, the boundaries between state and civil society actors were highly permeable in Brazil. Some early AIDS advocates became public officials at the local and federal levels. Berkman et al. (2005:1, 168) point out: "The Brazilian response to AIDS thus emerged from the bottom up. It has been characterized by an active collaboration between government and NGOs, as well as by mobilization of activist political support and commitment within the machinery of the state itself, particularly on the part of local service providers in the public health system."

The quality and tone of AIDS activism in Brazil is a striking contrast to the more visible actions in the United States. While policy histories make reference to demonstrations (Nunn, 2009), discussions of Brazilian policy in English do not make reference to very many of them. A review of numerous discussions of AIDS activism in Brazil revealed a small number of public demonstrations. Several, in the fall of 1999 and one year later, led to increased budget allocations to pay for medications. Brazilian AIDS advocates mounted three demonstrations in the spring of 2001: one at the U.S. embassy, part of transnational protests challenging the lawsuit brought by drug companies against South Africa's importation of generics, and a second in Recife, which supported Brazil's introduction of a UN resolution supporting the right of access to medications (Passarelli and Júnior, 2003).

According to Biehl (2004: 108), "AIDS activists left behind antagonism to the state and together, with health technicians, epidemiologists, medical and social scientists, economists, and psychologists constituted a new epistemic community within the state." This was particularly evident in the decision to make access to ARVs universal. Soon after their effectiveness was announced, this epistemic community successfully lobbied for the passage of a federal law that ensured access to ARVs. The decision was framed as having a positive economic impact allowing people to continue to work and reducing the need for disability payments, decreasing the costs of hospital treatment, and preventing HIV transmission (Biehl, 2004). A detailed analysis of the evolution of this policy attributes this law, authored by former president and then-Senator Sarney, to the persuasion by other government officials, like the National AIDS Program director, and the belief that Sarney had family members living with HIV. Sarney himself explained his sponsorship of the bill in the following way: "I never had any direct pressure from political groups; I just went with my instincts about the gravity of the AIDS epidemic. . . . I knew that people wouldn't be able to afford these drugs, so a few days after the Vancouver AIDS Conference, I presented a project saying that the government would provide antiretroviral drugs free to all people living with AIDS" (Nunn, 2009: 88).

Another state official and physician underscored the nature of the collaboration between NGOs and bureaucrats, noting: "NGOs did have a lot of influence. . . . They always participated when we needed them to. When our technical advice wasn't enough to convince politicians to adopt certain policy politicians, they helped. The newspapers helped too because NGOs had a lot of contacts in the media. . . . And I think that this partnership worked well for us . . . the NGOs are our partners. Since we had the same objectives, support from civil society helped. Sure, they threw eggs at us, and we also threw eggs at them. But these partnerships have been, and continue to be, very important" (Nunn, 2009: 66).

Cultural factors have had an important influence on the Brazilian response to the epidemic. In contrast to the United States, where individualism is central, Brazilians stress social solidarity as a key cultural principle (Parker, 2008). Access to treatment is a right of citizenship and the epidemic has not been racialized as it has been in the United States and South Africa.

Gauri and Lieberman (2006: 64) point out that "it is rare to find epidemiological data with racial breakdowns in any government report. Seeing people with AIDS through a lens of solidarity, rather than as the racial other, has contributed to a sharp decline in stigmatization. Relatively few Brazilians are unwilling to have a person with AIDS as a neighbor" (Gauri and Lieberman, 2006). Brazilian culture has contributed to frank public discussion of sexuality and drug use. These have contributed to public policies and programs that communicate clear and direct messages advising people to use condoms. These messages are especially evident in government-sponsored public service announcements and widespread access to sterile syringes (Okie, 2006).

The development of Brazil's AIDS infrastructure has relied heavily on external funding. Several foundations, including Ford and MacArthur, provided financing (1993). Brazil's second NGO, the Brazilian Interdisciplinary AIDS Association, received early funding from the Ford Foundation (Connor, 2000) and, by 2005, from the Centers for Disease Control (CDC), USAID, the German aid agency, and a $1 million Gates Award for Global Health in 2003 (Beyrer, Gauri, and Vaillancourt, 2010; Brier, 2009; World Bank, n.d.). Its most substantial source of external financial support has been from the World Bank, which allocated $430 million in loans by 2002 (de Mattos, Terto, and Parker, 2003; World Bank, n.d.).

While ARV costs have been high in the United States, Brazil addressed the issue directly. It defied international patent protections for pharmaceutical companies and manufactured its own medications through reverse engineering and manufacturing generic versions of existing medications (Biehl, 2004). This had a major impact on the country's ability to contain the epidemic by lowering the cost of ARVs. The cost of ARVs, which were lifesaving, became a global issue and ignited activism in South Africa, the country with the highest number of HIV cases in the world.

## Combating Dissidence and Inaction in South Africa

The emergence of AIDS in South Africa intersects with the final days of the apartheid system, the beginning of democratization, and efforts to promote equality. As in the United States and Brazil, the first AIDS cases in 1985 were among gay white men and the disease was first viewed as a North American problem (Robins, 2004). South Africa is a racially diverse society, like the United States and Brazil, but has far more racial polarization. In addition to the broad social changes taking place at that time, the history of AIDS policy has been complicated by the fact that key government officials, most notably the two-term President Mbecki (1999 to 2008), endorsed a dissident theory that cast doubt on the fact that HIV causes AIDS. In 1999, he declared that AZT was a danger to health and, until the Cabinet overrode him, was unwilling to promote policies to expand access to ARV treatment (Nattrass, 2007).

A definitive timeline of the development of AIDS policy in South Africa begins in 1990—five years after the first cases—with the initiation of ante-natal surveillance surveys and the first AIDS conference (Nattrass, 2007). In addition to the evolution of the South African state, a huge degree of stigma and silence accompanied the epidemic but also brutality with several well-publicized murders of women known to be HIV positive (Power, 2003; Robins, 2004). The issue gained greater urgency in 2001 when a Medical Research Council report estimated that AIDS accounted for one-quarter of deaths in the country (Robins, 2004).

Government policies evolved both belatedly and slowly with a free helpline begun in 1992, the first national AIDS plan in 1994 (Nattrass, 2007), and AIDS-specific funding in 2000 (Gauri and Lieberman, 2006). Civil society activity was limited to the nonpolitical National Association of Persons with AIDS (NAPWA-SA) founded in 1994.

In December 1998, 15 people, some of whom were anti-apartheid veterans and former exiles, formed the Treatment Action Campaign (TAC) in response to the death of gay rights and anti-apartheid activist Simon Nkoli, who was unable to afford ARV treatment (Friedman and Mottiar, 2005). TAC members saw a need for more forceful advocacy since the NAPWA was overtly nonpolitical. The public announcement of this new group, on the steps of St. George's Cathedral in Cape Town, was precisely timed: it was Human Rights Day, not a coincidence since Achmat (2004: 76) describes its work as "a struggle about our constitutional rights to life and dignity and also to equity . . . because without medicine . . . people die," rights that are explicitly mentioned in the South African constitution. Over time, TAC mobilized a young, 90 percent African, mostly female, and rela-tively educated group of people living with AIDS, 80 percent of whom Achmat estimated to be unemployed. While disclosure of HIV status is not stressed as it was in the United States, given the stigma and retribution, most are thought to be living with HIV (Friedman and Mottiar, 2005). Members have been willing to participate in a highly publicized series of campaigns involving civil disobedience. In some cases TAC employed the same rhetoric and strategies used by ACT UP in the United States includ-ing interrupting speeches and accusing drug companies and public offi-cials of being murderers. But beside these highly public strategies were a series of position papers, court cases, and challenges to South African law that together contributed to the South African AIDS community's success in obtaining universal access to ARVs as well as collaborating with the state to challenge international patent law and be able to produce and to import lower cost generic ARVs.

The founding of TAC provided a vehicle for giving political voice to the concerns of people living with HIV and breaking the silence since many of its demonstrations featured people wearing T-shirts with the slogan "HIV positive." This was not meant as a personal disclosure but an expression of solidarity with those who were.

Its first political acts involved close collaboration with the state, which was then challenging international drug patent protections under the TRIPS treaty, which blocked the importation of lower cost generic drugs if they were still under patent protection. South Africa passed the Medicines Act in 1997, which circumvented this treaty and would allow it to import generics. In response, 42 pharmaceutical companies, members of the South African and the U.S. Pharmaceutical Manufacturers Associations, initiated a lawsuit in South Africa challenging the constitutionality of the act and accused it of violating international patent protection under the TRIPS agreement. The United States threatened trade sanctions; and government officials, including Vice President Gore, called for a repeal of the Medicines Act (Grebe, 2011; Power, 2003). In 1999, TAC supported the government's position and mounted protests in Cape Town, Durban, and Pretoria calling for the United States to "stop bullying" South Africa. This effort was reinforced by a series of ACT UP demonstrations during Gore's presidential campaign. TAC joined the government in the case and was admitted as an amicus curiae in 2001. Médicins Sans Frontières (MSF) circulated a petition that requested that the companies drop the suit: close to 300,000 people from more than 130 countries signed the petition (Médicins Sans Frontières, 2001). Eventually, two manufacturers dropped out of the case, the United States ended its pressure, and the remaining drug companies withdrew their lawsuit, thereby freeing South Africa to import and to manufacture generics (Cleary and Ross, 2002).

As the 21st century began, TAC's use of political protests expanded. During the July 2000 International AIDS Conference in Durban, TAC organized a "Global March for HIV/AIDS Treatment" with 5,000 demonstrators, many of them wearing HIV positive T-shirts (Smith and Siplon, 2006). A year later, TAC began to directly challenge the government and had its first march on Parliament calling for a National Treatment Plan in 2000 (Dying for Treatment, 2003). This step was a difficult one due to the leadership's loyalty to the ruling African National Congress party and, according to Achmat (2004: 77–78), "For four and a half years we have negotiated with the government. . . . We have used every instrument that our new democracy gave us. . . . We can no longer put our party loyalty before people's rights to live." In 2000, TAC initiated the Christopher Moraka Defiance Campaign, which directed attention to government responsibility for the death of yet another comrade who was unable to afford AIDS medications (Robins, 2004). Achmat purchased 5,000 doses of fluconazole in Thailand, a treatment for thrush for 28 cents compared to the patented dose, which was sold for as much as $18 (Power, 2003), and TAC imported over 30,000 pills by the end of 2002 using the same strategy as U.S. AIDS activists. These efforts pressured two drug companies to change course. In March 2001, Pfizer offered fluconazole at no cost to state-sponsored clinics and Bristol Myers-Squibb lowered the price of Stavudine from $3.00 (U.S.) per day to $.15 (Nattrass, 2007).

In the winter and spring of 2003, TAC mounted a civil disobedience campaign that ended when the cabinet announced that the state would provide funding for ARV treatment. In February, TAC held a march marking the opening of parliament in Cape Town called "Stand Up for Our Lives" which attracted between 10,000 and 15,000 participants (Health GAP, n.d.; Treatment Action Campaign, 2002). On March 20, demonstrators marched on the Cape Town, Sharpeville, and Durban police stations carrying wanted posters and requesting that police officers arrest the ministers of health and of trade and industry for willful homicide. The goal was to have 600 arrests that day to call attention to the 600 AIDS deaths every day. While many of the demonstrators were charged, there were too few jail cells for them and they were released (Health Gap, n.d.; Power, 2003). In Durban, police sprayed tear gas, used water cannons, and punched some demonstrators (TAC, 2004). A week later, Health GAP and ACT UP initiated a telephone campaign calling the South African embassy in Washington (Health GAP, n.d.). This was followed by a global day of action on April 24, which featured demonstrations and events in Tokyo, Amsterdam, Los Angeles, London, Milan, Boston, and Paris as well as in Durban, East London, Cape Town, Nelspriut, and Tshwane (TAC, 2004).

During the time that TAC was organizing these episodes of contention, President George W. Bush was pressuring the Mbeki government to expand access to ARVs and made a commitment to provide financial support from the newly developed funding stream under the PEPFAR program (Stevenson, 2003). Four months later, the South African government changed course and committed to spending $45 million each year for AIDS treatment.

Edwin Cameron, a Supreme Court of Appeals justice, was the earliest ally within the state. Cameron was the first public figure to disclose his HIV status on television in 1999, nine years after his HIV diagnosis. His disclosure gave the issue a greater sense of urgency and he was the same kind of celebrity patient as Rock Hudson and Magic Johnson in the United States. In addition to his public role, Cameron founded the AIDS Law Project at the University of Witswatersrand in 1993 whose first director was Zackie Achmat (Grebe, 2011). Before TAC, Cameron's individual advocacy had had little impact: He tried to meet with President Mandela in 1996 but instead had an unproductive meeting with the vice president (Power, 2003). TAC later gained support from several members of parliament and former President Mandela who lost several family members including a son to AIDS (Timberg, 2005). In 2002, Mandela was photographed visiting Achmat sporting the HIV-positive T-shirt that Achmat designed (Nattrass, 2007).

TAC's allies, both domestically and internationally, have been critical to its success. TAC itself noted the impact of its allies in its 2002 Annual Report indicating that "TAC's work does not take place in a vacuum. We have developed relationships with organizations who make essential contributions to achieving our common objectives." It has obtained financial support from international NGOs including Bread for the World, Oxfam, international foundations, and European governments (Robins, 2004; Rosenberg, 2006). Elite and grassroots allies from within South Africa include the Congress of South African Trade Unions (COSATU); scientists who criticized the state's reliance on the dissident AIDS paradigm; Anglican Bishop Ndugane who called government inaction on AIDS "as serious as apartheid"; the African National Congress political party; and a host of other NGOs including the Legal Resources Centre and the AIDS Law Project (Grebe, 2011; Nattrass, 2007; TAC Annual Report, 2003).

MSF was also an important ally. In addition to the petition it circulated, it provided significant financial support and established a model clinic. Initially rebuffed by the government, MSF sponsored the first clinic distributing ARVs in a town just outside Cape Town. This clinic demonstrated the feasibility of successfully treating people living with HIV in South Africa (Friedman and Mottiar, 2005). One account of the development of this model clinic notes that its founder, Eric Goemaere, was urged to start the clinic by Achmat (Power, 2003), who had been instrumental in establishing a health clinic in the early 1990s (Grebe, 2011). The clinic also made it clear that more resources were needed since the funding it received from MSF did not allow it to distribute ARVs to all of the patients who needed them (Fox and Goemare, 2006).

TAC and its allies also employed a series of successful administrative complaints and court cases. In one case, initiated at the end of 2001, TAC claimed that the state had an obligation to provide ARV medications to reduce mother-to-child transmission because the constitution established health care as a right. The court ordered the government to supply the ARV nevirapine to prevent transmission (Friedman and Mottiar, 2005). In another case TAC joined with several doctors, COSATU, and several people living with HIV in 2002 to file a complaint with the Competition Commission that GlaxoSmithKline and Boehringer Ingelheim charged excessive prices for several drugs (TAC, 2003).

During a five-year period, TAC had a profound impact on South African AIDS policy. TAC's success can be traced to its charismatic leadership, a broad base of financial support, and its elite and institutional allies and others who supported its positions. In addition to its visible and effective demonstrations, TAC circulated thoughtful policy statements and position papers like U.S. advocates. The organization and its allies contributed to a major change in state policy: a treatment paradigm shift by the government from a dissident position to a commitment to mainstream treatment. It accomplished this by combining a series of outsider political strategies with close collaboration with a host of domestic and global allies. It continues its work with a broad base of global support, serving as an important watchdog, educating people living with HIV, and continuing to promote the evolution of AIDS policy albeit with less public fanfare. Like the two other cases, the evolution of AIDS advocacy in South Africa has important implications for our understanding of the role of civil society organizations in the policy process.

## MOBILIZING AND SUSTAINING A FRAGILE COALITION: FUTURE CHALLENGES

This analysis of the nature of treatment advocacy in these three settings reveals that a diverse set of policy actors coalesced to expand access to ARVs including advocates and activists from all three societal sectors— civil society, the state, and firms—who operate as adversaries and as collaborators, sometimes sequentially and sometimes simultaneously. Activists engaged in demonstrations and civil disobedience have been critical both domestically and globally. Activists provide thoughtful policy blueprints and have initiated successful lawsuits that complemented their publicly visible actions. At the same time, much of the impact of their work has been reinforced if not initiated by various types of institutional advocates including government officials who sometimes promote and encourage activism; staff in nongovernmental organizations (NGOs) who join the activists in political protest; and foundation staff who publish reports, initiate ideas, and fund organizations. Corporate actors, initially targets, have also benefited from the pressure activists have placed on the state and the market to make their products available for sale.

This complex dynamic rests on another contemporary reality: Neoliberal global social policies have contributed to the growth of civil society organizations, both global and domestic. In the modern global economy, advocates and activists target the policies and resource allocations of a diverse set of power centers. In this context, the preferred organizational form for public policies, both domestic and global, is the public-private partnership in which a nongovernmental (NGO) or quasi-nongovernmental organization (QUANGO) is charged with the responsibility of carrying out a social policy drawing on a combination of public, charitable, and corporate resources.

Studies of the impact of social movement and political organizations document rather definitively the complementary role of activism and advocacy and the advantages of a number of organizations collaborating with one another. Professionalized advocacy groups that engage in "routine advocacy tactics" have a large base of participation, and focus on issues that are already of interest to the media tend to gain much more attention in the mass media (Andrews and Caren, 2010). On the other hand, disruptive tactics also garner attention (Amenta, Caren, Olasky, and Stobaugh, 2009) and contribute to political deliberation in the form of public hearings (Olzak and Soule, 2009). The complementary impact of protest and traditional political strategies in focusing attention and promoting deliberation explains a longstanding observation that the actions of a "radical flank" garner public attention and legitimize the efforts of those employing more moderate strategies (Haines, 1984). In addition, the impact of challenger groups is greater when there are a large number of such organizations (Olzak and Ryo, 2007).

This article widens the lens on the nature of AIDS policymaking, noting the broad array of actors and the variety of methods that have shaped AIDS policy in three sites. It focuses on efforts to first find and then expand access to ARVs. While the dynamics of multisector actors in the current neoliberal policymaking environment is not unique to AIDS, there is one feature that is:

The kind of biological citizenship being contested is not merely designed to improve health, but to save lives, what Biehl (2009) calls survival politics. This allows for the application of discursive strategies that render health advocacy especially unique and means that the claims made have a strong and compelling moral tone (Busby, 2010). Human rights is an important claim but saving lives is an even more salient and compelling feature of the discourse. Both individually and in collaboration with a variety of allies, AIDS activists disseminated information, rhetoric, and images about the epidemic; emphasized the moral nature of their claims and the immoral nature of inaction in what American advocates described as a "holocaust; reminded government and drug companies of their responsibility to protect citizens and prolong life; and worked closely with a broad range of political insiders as well as celebrities to forward their cause.

The main future challenge for access to ARVs is the sustainability of the current system of financing and distribution. It is not an exaggeration to describe the current financing arrangement as both insufficient and a "fragile coalition" (Shadlen, 2007). At the end of 2011, 34 million people were HIV positive and at least 8 million in low and middle income countries were being treated with ARVs (Fighting AIDS, n.d.). In 2010, the Global Fund paid for 3 million people and PEPFAR accounted for 3.2 million in 2010 (AmFar, 2010; Fighting AIDS, n.d.). Yet, one in three Africans needing treatment did not receive it (Institute of Medicine, 2010). This shortfall is important because of the lives that may be lost and because treatment reduces the chances that a risky encounter will lead to HIV transmission. Even though the scope of the epidemic has stabilized, the global financing mechanisms are flat and will become even more inadequate in the future, especially in Africa, as the life expectancy of the HIV-positive increases (Institute of Medicine, 2010). Support from U.S. foundations declined by 7 percent between 2009 and 2010 (Funders Concerned About AIDS, n.d.). In the United States, the federal-state–financed ADAP program has a waiting list of over 9,000, which pales in comparison to the shortfall in other societies, but is nonetheless troubling in such a wealthy country (ADAP Waiting List, n.d.). The level of global resources has been greatly affected by the worldwide recession, and some countries committed to the Global Fund have not contributed their "fair share" (Busby, 2010). Toward the end of 2011, the Global Fund announced that it would not make any new grant allocations for two years as a result of funding limitations (Brown, 2011).

Amid this gloomy picture, political leaders and AIDS advocates have begun to reframe the epidemic proclaiming that by 2015, we will have the beginning of the end of AIDS: an AIDS-free generation (Nix, 2011). One person who was cured of AIDS has already survived for several years and the results of a second case are promising (Pollak, 2011). The National Minority AIDS Council in the United States has pointed out the strategy that will result in ending AIDS: a collaboration among people with AIDS, community-based organizations and activists, community health centers, public health departments, health care providers, researchers, public health officials, health insurers, private foundations, pharmacies, and the pharmaceutical industry (National Minority AIDS Council, 2012). These diverse actors have moved policy forward in the past and will hopefully continue to do so in the future as they work together to end the epidemic.

## BIBLIOGRAPHY

Achmat, Z. (2004). The Treatment Action Campaign, HIV/AIDS and the government. *Transformation* 54, 76–84.

ACT UP (1987). Flyer of the First Action, March 24, 1987, Wall Street, New York City. Retrieved from http://www.actupny.org\1stFlyer.htm

ADAP Waiting List (n.d.). Retrieved from http://www.statehealthfacts.org/comparetable.jsp?ind=552&cat=11

Amenta, E., Caren, N., Olasky, S. J., & Stobaugh, J. E. (2009). All the movements fit to print: Who, what, when, where and why SMO families appeared in the *New York Times* in the twentieth century. *American Sociological Review,* 74, 636–656.

Amfar (2010, December). The need for new investments in fiscal year 2012: Assessing the evidence. *Issue Brief.*

Andrews, K. T., & Caren, N. (2010). Making the news: Movement organizations, media attention, and the public agenda. *American Sociological Review,* 75, 6, 841–866.

Annas, G. J. (1992). The changing landscape of human experimentation: Nurenberg, Helsinki and beyond. *Health Matrix,* 2, 119–140.

Armstrong, E. A., & Bernstein, M. (2008). Culture, power, and institutions: A multi-institutional politics approach to social movements. *Sociological Theory,* 26, 2, 74–99.

Arno, P. S., & Feiden, K. L. (1992). *Against the odds: The story of AIDS drug development, politics & profits.* New York: HarperCollins.

Banaszak, L. A. (2005). Inside and outside the state: Movement insider status, tactics, and public policy achievements. In D. S. Meyer, V. Jenness, and H. Ingraham (eds.), *Routing the opposition: Social movements, public policy, and democracy.* Minneapolis: University of Minneapolis Press (pp. 149–176).

Barnett, T., & Whiteside, A. (2002). *AIDS in the twenty-first century: Disease and globalization.* New York: Palgrave Macmillan.

Barr, D. (1990, November/December). Action on AIDS: Shaping the federal AIDS research agenda. *The Volunteer,* 7.

Berkman, A., Garcia, J., Muñoz-Laboy, M., Paiva, V., & Parker, R. (2005). A critical analysis of the Brazilian response to HIV/AIDS: Lessons learned for controlling and mitigating the epidemic in developing countries. *American Journal of Public Health,* 95, 1162–1172.

Beyrer, C., Gauri, V., & Vaillancourt, D. (2010). Evaluation of the World Bank's assistance in responding to the AIDS epidemic: Brazil case study. Retrieved from http://www.oecd.org/dataoecd/28/52/36962873.pdf

Biehl, J. G. (2004). Global pharmaceuticals, AIDS and citizenship in Brazil. *Social Text,* 22, 5, 105–132.

Biehl, J. G. (2009). *Will to live: AIDS therapies and the politics of survival.* Princeton, NJ: Princeton University Press.

Blumenthal, D., & Morone, J. A. *The heart of power: Health and politics in the oval office.* Berkeley: University of California Press.

Boffey, P. (1988a, July 24). F.D.A. will allow AIDS patients to import unapproved medicines. *New York Times,* A1.

Boffey, P. (1988b, July 5). New initiative to speed AIDS drugs is assailed. *New York Times,* C1.

Braun, J. F., Powderly, W. G., Steinberg, C. L., & Torres, G. (1993). A guide to underground AIDS therapies. *Patient Care,* 27, 13, 53.

Brazil's AIDS program wins Gates Award for global health (2003, May 30). *Philanthropy News Digest.* Retrieved from http://foundationcenter.org/pnd/news/story.jhtml?id=34700033

Brier, J. (2009). *Infectious ideas: U.S. political responses to the AIDS crisis.* Chapel Hill: University of North Carolina Press.

Broder, M. (1992, July 12). Wellcome gives $1 million to community research. *QW,* 16.

Brown, D. (2011, November 24). A key group in global AIDS therapy halts new grants. Washington Post, A1.

Brown, L. D., Khagram, S., Moore, M. H., & Frumkin, P. (2000). Globalization, NGOs and multi-sectoral relations. Social Science Research Network. Accessed from papers.ssrn.com/sol3/papers.cfm?abstract_id+253110.

Busby, J. (2010). *Moral movements and foreign policy.* Cambridge, UK: Cambridge University Press.

Carpenter, D. P., & Moore, C. D. (2007). Robust action and the strategic use of ambiguity in a bureaucratic cohort: FDA officers and the evolution of new drug regulations, 1950–1970. In S. Skowronek and M. Glassman (eds.), *Formative acts: American politics in the making.* Philadelphia, PA: University of Pennsylvania Press.

Chambré, S. M. (1995). Uncertainty, diversity, and change: The AIDS community in New York City. In D. A. Chekki (ed.), *Research in Community Sociology,* 6th ed. Westport, CT: JAI Press, 149–190.

Chambré, S. M. (2006). *Fighting for our lives: New York's AIDS community and the politics of disease.* New Brunswick, NJ: Rutgers University Press.

Chase, M. (1985, August 5). Fighting a scourge: Gains against AIDS have come rapidly but a cure is distant. *Wall Street Journal,* 1.

Chase, M. (1987a, October 5). Faster action: FDA rule changes may rush new drugs to very sick patients. *Wall Street Journal,* 1.

Chase, M. (1987b, December 15). Wellcome unit cuts price of AIDS drug 10%: Cites production improvement. *Wall Street Journal,* 1.

Chase, M. (1987c, December 11). AIDS patient advocates, U.S. square off for hearing on drug development suit. *Wall Street Journal,* 52.

Chase, M. (1988, November 23). U.S.-sponsored AIDS drug trials to include private doctors'efforts. *Wall Street Journal,* 1988, 1.

Cimons, M. (1985, November 26). AIDS funds: Tardy but catching up. *Los Angeles Times,* 1.

Cleary, S. & D. Ross (2002). "The 1998-2001 legal struggle between the South African government and the international pharmaceutical Industry: Agame-theoretic analysis. Journal of Social, Political and Economic Studies 27: 445–494.

Clemens, E. S., & Guthrie, D. (2011). Introduction. In E. S. Clemens and D. Guthrie (eds.), *Politics and partnerships: The role of voluntary associations in America's political past and present* (pp. 1–23). Chicago: University of Chicago Press.

Connor, C. (2000). Contracting non-governmental organizations for HIV/AIDS: Brazil case study. Retrieved from http://www.minsa.gob.pe/ogpp/APP/doc_complementarios/Contracting%20Non-organizations%20Brazil%20Case%20Study.pdf

deMattos, R. A., Terto, V., & Parker, R. (2003). World Bank strategies and the response to AIDS in Brazil. *Divulgaçâoem Saùdepara Debate,* 27, 215–227.

Dunne, R. (1987, February 17). Letter to Arnie Kantrowitz and Lawrence Mass. Lawrence Mass papers, Box 7.

Epstein, S. (1996). *Impure science: AIDS, activism, and the politics of knowledge.* Berkeley: University of California Press.

Fighting AIDS (n.d.). Accessed from http://www.theglobalfund.org/en/about/diseases/hivaids/.

Fisher, J. A. (2009). *Medical research for hire: The political economy of pharmaceutical clinical trials.* New Brunswick, NJ: Rutgers University Press.

Fox, R. C., & Goemaere, E. (2006). They call it "patient selection" in Khayelistsha: The experiences of Medecins Sans Frontieres–South Africa in enrolling patients to receive antiretroviral treatment for HIV/AIDS. *Cambridge Quarterly of Healthcare Ethics,* 15 , 3, 313–21.

Friedman, S. (2006). Participatory governance and citizen action in post-apartheid South Africa. International Institute for Labour Studies, Geneva. Retrieved from http://www.ilo.org/public/english/bureau/inst/publications/discussion/dp16406.pdf

Friedman, S., & Mottiar, S. (2005). A rewarding engagement: The treatment action campaign and the politics of HIV/AIDS. *Politics and Society,* 33, 511–565.

Funders Concerned About AIDS. U.S. philanthropic support to address HIV/AIDS in 2010. Retrieved from http://issuu.com/fcaa/docs/final_2011_fcaa_resourcetracking_web/1?viewMode=magazine&mode=embed

Garcia, J., & Parker, R. (2011). Resource mobilization for health advocacy: Afro-Brazilian religious organizations and HIV prevention and control. *Social Science and Medicine,* 72, 1930–1938.

Gauri, V., & Lieberman, E. S. (2006). Boundary institutions and HIV/AIDS policy in Brazil and South Africa. *Studies in Comparative International Development,* 41, 3, 47–73.

Gevisser, M. (1988, December 19). AIDS movement seizes control. *The Nation,* 677.

Global Fund (n.d.). *Fighting AIDS: The global AIDS epidemic.* Retrieved from http://www.theglobalfund.org/en/about/diseases/hivaids/

Goodwin, J., Jasper, J. M., & Polletta, F. (2001). *Passionate politics: Emotions and social movements.* Chicago: University of Chicago Press.

Gould, D. B. (2009). *Moving politics: Emotion and ACT UP's fight against AIDS.* Chicago: University of Chicago Press.

Grebe, E. (2011). Coalition-building through local and transnational networks in the treatment action campaign's AIDS activism. *Journal of South African Studies,* 37, 4, 849–868.

Haines, H. H. (1984). Black radicalization and the funding of civil rights: 1957–1970. *Social Problems,* 32, 1, 31–43.

Handleman, D. (1990, March 8). ACT Up in anger. Rolling Stone, 80–89.

Health GAP (n.d.). *Support the treatment action campaign* (TAC). Retrieved from http://www.healthgap.org/camp/tac.html

Hilts, P. J. (1989a, September 16). Wave of protests developing on profits from AIDS drug. *New York Times,* A1.

Hilts, P. J. (1989b, September 19). AIDS drug's maker cuts price by 20%. *New York Times,* A1.

HIV/AIDS in Brazil (n.d.). Acessed from http://www.avert.org/aids-brazil

Institute of Medicine (2010, November). Preparing for the future of HIV/AIDS in Africa: A shared responsibility. *Report Brief.* Retrieved from http://www.iom.edu/~/media/Files/Report%20Files/2010/Preparing-for-the-Future-of-HIVAIDS-in-Africa-A-Shared-Responsibility/Future%20of%20HIV%20AIDS%202010%20Report%20Brief.pdf

Jasper, J. M. (2012). Introduction: From political opportunity structures to strategic interaction. In J. and J. M. Jasper (eds.), *Contention in context: Political opportunities and the emergence of protest* (pp. 1–36). Stanford: Stanford University Press.

Jordan, A. G. (1981). Iron triangles, wooly corporatism and elastic nets. Journal of Public Policy, 1 (1), 95–123.

Kaiser Family Foundation (n.d.). Globalhealthfacts.org. Retrieved from http://www.globalhealthfacts.org

Kapstein, E., & Busby, J. (2010). Making markets for merit goods: The political economy of antiretrovirals. Global Policy, 1, 75–90.

Karon, T. (2001, April 19). South African AIDS activist Zackie Achmat. *Time.* Retrieved from http://www.time.com/time/nation/article/0,8599,106995,00.html

Kawata, P. (n.d.). NMAC's vision to end the AIDS epidemic in America. National Minority AIDS Council. Retrieved from http://www.nmac.org/component/content/article/63-blog/1294-ending-the-epidemic-nmacs-vision-to-end-it.html

King, B. G., & Soule, S. A. (2007). Social movements as extra-institutional entrepreneurs: The effect of protests on stock price returns. *Administrative Science Quarterly,* 52, 413–442.

Kolbe, M. (1988, August 7). A PWA movement of guerilla clinics. *Gay Community News,* 2.

Kramer, L. (1989, June 27). Read this and live. *Village Voice,* 24.

Leary, W. (1989, July 27). Work on AIDS drugs seen as still too slow. *New York Times,* B4.

Lieberman, E. (2007). Ethnic politics, risk and policy-making: A cross-national statistical analysis of government responses to HIV/AIDS. *Comparative Political Studies,* 40, 1407–1432.

Lugliani, G. (1989, November/December). Medical update: Pressure brings AZT price down. *The Volunteer,* 2.

Marshall, E. (1989, July 28). Quick release of AIDS drugs. *Science,* 4916, 345.

Médicins Sans Frontières (2001). International Activity Report 2001. Retrieved from http://www.doctorswithout borders.org/publications/ar/report.cfm?id1204

McCarthy, J. & Zald, M. (1977). Resource mobilization and social movements: A partial theory. American Journal of Sociology, 82, 1212–1241.

Milner, H. V., & Moravcsik, A. (2009). Power, interdependence and nonstate actors in world politics. Princeton: Princeton University Press.

Mintrom, M. (1997). Policy entrepreneurs and the diffusion of innovation. *American Journal of Political Science,* 41, 738–770.

Morrow, D.J. (1999, September 9). A movable epidemic: Markers of AIDS drugs struggle to keep up with market. New York Times, C1.

Muñoz-Laboy M. A., Murray, L., Wittlin, N., et al. (2011). Beyond faith-based organizations: Using comparative institutional ethnography to understand religious responses to HIV and AIDS in Brazil. *American Journal of Public Health,* 101, 972–978.

Murray, L., Garcia, J., Muñoz-Laboy, M. A., et al. (2011). Strange bedfellows: The Catholic Church and Brazilian national AIDS program in the response to HIV/AIDS in Brazil. *Social Science and Medicine,* 72, 945–952.

National Minority AIDS Council (2012). Ending the epidemic: NMAC's Vision to end it. http://nmac.org/ending-the-epidemic/ending-the-epidemic-nmacs-vision-to-end-it/

Nattrass, N. (2007). *Mortal combat: AIDS denialism and the struggle for antiretrovirals in South Africa.* Scottsville: University of KwaZulu-Natal Press.

Nix, S. (2011, November 9). The beginning of the end of AIDS. *Huffington Post.* Retrieved from http://www.huffingtonpost.com/sheila-nix/hiv-aids-cure_b_1082582.html

Nunn, A. (2009). *The politics and history of AIDS treatment in Brazil.* New York: Springer.

Okie, A. (2006). Fighting HIV—lessons from Brazil. *New England Journal of Medicine,* 354, 19, 1977–1981.

Olzak, S., & Ryo, E. (2007). Organizational diversity, vitality and outcomes in the civil rights movement. *Social Forces* 85, 1561–1591.

Olzak, S., & Soule, S. A. (2009). Cross-cutting influences of environmental protest and legislation. *Social Forces* 88, 1201–1226.

Parker, R. (2003, August). Building the foundations for the response to HIV in Brazil: The development of HIV/AIDS policy, 1982–1996. *Divulgaçãoem Saùdepara Debate,* 27, 143–183.

Parker, R. (2008). AIDS solidarity as policy: Constructing the Brazilian model. NACLA Report on the Americas, 41 (4), 20–24.

Passarelli, C.-A., & Júnior, V. T. R. (2003, August). Nongovernmental organizations and access to anti-retroviral treatments in Brazil. *Divulgaçãoem Saùdepara Debate,* 27, 252–264.

Pear, R. (2001, June 5). AIDS at 20: Advocates for Patients Barged In, and the Federal Government Changed. *New York Times,* A1.

Petryna, A. (2009). When experiments travel: Clinical trials and the global search for human subjects. Princeton, NJ: Princeton University Press.

Pollak, A. (2011, November 29). New hope of a cure for H.I.V. *New York Times,* 1.

Power. S. (2003, May 19). The AIDS Rebel: An activist fights drug companies, the government—and his own illness. *New Yorker.* Retrieved from http://www.newyorker.com/archive/2003/05/19/030519fa_fact_power

Reed, C. (1987, April 14). AIDS patients seek illicit drugs in bid to defy odds. *Toronto Globe and Mail,* A9.

Rios, R. R. (2003, August). Legal responses to the HIV/AIDS epidemic in Brazil. *Divulgaçãoem Saùdepara Debate,* 27, 228–238.

Robins, S. (2004). Long live Zackie, long live: AIDS activism, science and citizenship after apartheid. *Journal of South African Studies,* 30 (3), 1–21.

Rosenberg, T. (2001, January 28). Look at Brazil. *New York Times Magazine,* 26.

Rosenberg, T. (2006, August 30). For people with AIDS, a government with two faces. *New York Times,* 22.

Santoro, W. A., and McGuire, G. A. (1997). Social movement insiders: The impact of institutional activists on affirmative action and comparable worth policies. Social Problems 44, 503–19.

Shadlen, K. C. (2007). The political economy of AIDS treatment: Intellectual property and the transformation of generic supply. *International Studies Quarterly,* 51, 559–581.

Silverstein, K. (1998 June). Sleeping with the enemy. *POZ.* Retrieved from http://www.poz.com/articles/228_1622.shtml

Sirica, J. (1985, October 15). Drugs for AIDS funneled from Mexico to city. Newsday October 15.

Skocpol, T. (2003). *Diminished democracy: From membership to management in American civic life.* Norman: University of Oklahoma Press.

Smith, R. A. & Siplon, P. D. (2006). *Drugs into bodies: Global aids treatment activism.* Westport, CT: Praeger.

Span, P. (1992, April 18). Pharmacy for the desperate. *Washington Post,* D2.

Specter, M. (1989, June 5). AIDS patients insist on treatment role: Researchers report difficulty conducting traditional drug trials. *Washington Post,* A12.

Stevenson, R. W. (2003, July 10). Bush pushes South Africa in fighting AIDS. *New York Times,* A1.

Teixeira, P. R. (2003, August). Universal access to AIDS medicines: the Brazilian experience. *Divulgação em Saùdepara Debate,* 27, 184–191.

Timberg, C. (2005, January 7). Mandela says AIDS led to death of son: Health activists praise ex-president's openness. *Washington Post,* A10.

Treatment Action Campaign (2003). *Treatment Action Campaign (TAC) Annual Report for January 2002—February 2003.* Retrieved from http://www.tac.org.za/Documents/report02to03.pdf

Treatment Action Campaign (2004). *TAC Annual Report for 1 March 2003–29 February 2004.* Retrieved from http://www.tac.org.za/Documents/Annual Report2003.pdf

Ventura, M. (2003). Strategies to promote and guarantee the rights of people living with HIV/AIDS. *Divulgação em Saùdepara Debate,* 27, 239–246.

World Bank (n.d.). AIDS: The World Bank's partnership with Brazil. Retrieved from http://go.Worldbank.org/UNVP29TDE0

Wyrick, B. (1986, July 21). Major test of 6 AIDS drugs near. *Newsday,* 7.

Zonana, V. F. (1992, July 1). AZT Maker Gives $1 Million to Research. *Los Angeles Times,* A20.

# 3

# Discord and Harmony in Biomedical HIV Prevention Technologies: Advancements through Advocacy

*San Patten, Joanne Mantell, and Zena Stein*

The expectation that we would soon see a technological breakthrough against AIDS with an effective and universal vaccine rose with the discovery of the causal agent, but gradually faded as the peculiar properties of HIV emerged. The social and personal changes in many lives required to prevent sexual transmission—celibacy or lifetime mutual monogamy—seemed almost unattainable, with the male condom being the only available alternative in the first decades of the pandemic. With women virtually unable to regard the use of that tool as under their control, active minds turned to other technological possibilities. Currently, several new biomedical approaches to HIV prevention are at various stages in the research and development pipeline, and many have proof-of-concept as viable means of preventing sexual transmission of HIV, but their emergence has taken decades, and the work is not complete.

Not only are the product formulation, laboratory, and clinical testing processes for these products highly complex, but the social processes underlying these technological advances also complicate implementation. Here, we focus on what we call "advocacy," defined as "the functions of an advocate" or "the work of advocating, pleading, or supporting." In the context of HIV, advocates may be concerned with a range of issues: human rights, governmental or legal issues, services (availability, access, affordability), or social inclusion.

In the last 10 years, research around new HIV prevention technologies (NPTs) has accelerated, spurred by a growing advocacy movement

---

### DESCRIPTION OF PREVENTION TECHNOLOGIES

**Microbicide:** Substances still under study that could be used in the vagina and/ or rectum to reduce the risk of HIV transmission during sex. Microbicides could come in the form of creams, gels, films, slow-release vaginal rings, enemas, or suppositories.

**Female Condom:** A thin sheath or pouch that is inserted into the vagina to help prevent pregnancy and sexually transmitted diseases, including HIV.

**PrEP:** A strategy that involves use of antiretroviral medications (ARVs) to reduce the risk of HIV infection via sexual exposure.

---

from communities and researchers and supported by increasing funding opportunities from national governments and international donors. The development, testing, and use of NPTs have been besieged by both tension and optimism, some related to the biomedical approach to HIV prevention, others to the specific technologies, and still others to particular research methods. In this chapter, we will explore how advocacy and political action have been applied to NPTs, since with any new technology, there are advocates and antagonists. We will examine the politics surrounding three categories of prevention technologies: microbicides (rectal and vaginal), female condoms, and oral preexposure prophylaxis (PrEP).

We first note some key successes and pitfalls in the history of HIV prevention advocacy, largely to derive fresh insights for future advocacy efforts. We then look ahead, guided by two main questions: What have been, and will be, the ingredients for successful advocacy and political action on NPTs? What have been, and will be, some key pitfalls for advocacy and political commitment to NPTs? In tackling these questions, the chapter addresses: (1) the history and build-up of advocacy around HIV prevention; (2) key sources of harmony and discord in advocacy and political action around microbicides, female condoms, and oral PrEP; and (3) key lessons learned regarding the conditions that have created harmony and discord around NPT advocacy and political action.

## THE HISTORY OF HIV PREVENTION ADVOCACY

Over the last 30 years, 60 million people around the world have been infected with HIV and nearly 25 million have died of AIDS (UNAIDS, 2010). Early interruption of the HIV pandemic would have required a progressive and truly global response, and would have required national policymakers to address sensitive social issues effectively, such as sexual behavior, drug use, and gender inequities, that drive the epidemic. Unfortunately, the response to the epidemic by most of the world was delayed, inadequate, and inconsistent.

Early prevention successes evolved from collective responses generated by people living with and affected by HIV/AIDS, including family members and community groups. Because of the association of the disease with marginalized populations, sex, intravenous drug use, and death, initial prevention efforts focused on confronting stigma, discrimination, and denial. White gay men, who accounted for 73 percent of AIDS cases in the United States in 1985 (Curran, Morgan, Hardy, Jaffe, Darrow, & Dowdle, 1985), mobilized to fight the strong worldwide stigma that was fueled by moral beliefs and prejudice against homosexuality. The first wave of HIV prevention was a social movement organized and led by people living with HIV (especially gay men in San Francisco and New York City) and their caregivers, with invention of the concept of "safer sex," and with promotion of condom use (Merson, O'Malley, Serwadda, & Apisuk, 2008).

By the mid-1980s, hundreds of community-based groups had been established all over the world to provide care and support, develop and promote prevention strategies, and advocate for more attention from health professionals, scientists, and policymakers. In the face of ongoing and pervasive complacency by governments, activism moved to more aggressive and vocal calls to action targeting governments and pharmaceutical companies (Crimp & Bersani, 1988).

It was not until 1987 that the World Health Organization (WHO) recognized the severity of the pandemic and established the Global Programme on AIDS (GPA), led by the passionate and articulate physician Jonathan Mann. The late Dr. Mann demanded a rights-based response to the pandemic, recognizing and reaching out to activists and community groups to create strong partnerships among the WHO, NGOs, and networks of people living with HIV/AIDS (Fee & Parry, 2008).

Throughout the late 1980s and early 1990s, several foundations, bilateral donor agencies, and international NGOs launched efforts to address HIV/AIDS in developing countries. However, on a global scale, NGO and community responses were uneven and not sufficiently scaled up to match the magnitude of the epidemic. The countries that achieved early success in HIV prevention were those that had strong political leadership that actively encouraged, supported, and expanded civil society responses (Merson, O'Malley, Serwadda, & Apisuk, 2008). The GPA struggled, however, to get governments to address issues that were socially and politically sensitive yet inextricably linked to HIV transmission. In addition, there were some clear tensions even among HIV/AIDS experts over the most effective and cost-efficient levels of intervention: public health approaches that focus on shorter-term and individual behavioral interventions (e.g., condom promotion, social marketing, sexual education of youth, HIV testing, and treatment of sexually transmitted infections) versus longer-term development approaches that address social and structural determinants of HIV vulnerability (e.g., gender, human rights, poverty, and community development).

In 1996, the GPA was replaced by the Joint UN Programme on HIV/AIDS (UNAIDS), which has the mandate to lead an expanded, coordinated, multisectoral global response that includes support for public health interventions as well as programs that address structural determinants of HIV vulnerability. Although the late 1990s were characterized by diminishing programmatic and development assistance from donor countries and financial constraints at UNAIDS, investments and returns in science were experiencing some key successes. Most notably, highly active antiretroviral therapy (HAART) was found to be effective in treating HIV in 1996, and in 1998, the International AIDS Vaccine Initiative (IAVI) was established to encourage the pharmaceutical and biotechnology industry to invest in vaccine development (IAVI, 2006). Research also began to develop and test the safety and efficacy of candidate topical vaginal microbicides. In 1998, a key prevention milestone based on biomedical technology was the finding that a short course of antiretroviral therapy before delivery was highly effective in preventing perinatal HIV transmission to newborn infants (Petra Study Team, 2002).

Advocacy in the late 1990s shifted to treatment access issues. This was a challenging time for activists and communities; the advent of HAART and optimism around vaccine development formed rifts between people living with HIV/AIDS in developing countries and those in wealthy countries.

In 2000, the United Nations Security Council debated the security implications of HIV/AIDS, representing the first time a health issue had ever been discussed on its agenda, and in 2001, Kofi Annan convened a UN General Assembly Special Session on HIV/AIDS (UNGASS) where 180 countries adopted a declaration of commitment that set targets for program delivery and funding levels for donor governments. The Global Fund to Fight AIDS, Tuberculosis and Malaria (GFATM) was formed soon thereafter, and in 2003, the U.S. government announced the President's Emergency Plan for AIDS Relief (PEPFAR). In 2007–2008, the Bill and Melinda Gates Foundation invested significantly in vaccine research, including jointly sponsoring the Canadian HIV Vaccines Initiative along with the Canadian government (Canadian HIV Vaccine Initiative, 2010).

Today, discourse around HIV/AIDS and health systems is prominently featured, with various advocates stressing that the HIV/AIDS response is either essential or detrimental to broader goals of health systems strengthening and health equity. HIV researchers, program planners, and advocates have sometimes created false divides between biomedical approaches and social-structural approaches to HIV prevention, undermining the concept of comprehensive and multifaceted combinations of HIV prevention strategies (LeBlanc et al., 2012). Combination prevention offers the best hope for success in prevention of HIV—a combination of behavioral, structural, and biomedical prevention paradigms and approaches that are adapted and prioritized for local contexts based on scientific evidence and community wisdom (Bertozzi, Laga, Bautista-Arredondo, & Coutinho, 2008).

There is a global consensus that effective HIV prevention is comprised of locally contextualized approaches that are grounded in human rights, and that address individual, dyadic, and societal levels of behaviors, social norms, and structures. HIV responses work in concert with other human rights and development priorities, such as universal access to quality education, economic opportunities for women, an empowered citizenry that can hold governments politically accountable, and human rights for the most marginalized and vulnerable populations (Bertozzi, Laga, Bautista-Arredondo, & Coutinho, 2008).

## BUILDING MOMENTUM FOR NEW HIV PREVENTION TECHNOLOGIES

Without a vaccine, protection of the blood supply, partner selection, and use of the male condom were all that could be advised for HIV prevention. The male condom has been in use for centuries as a method for preventing sexually transmitted infections (STIs) and pregnancies (UNAIDS, 2010; Lewis, 2000). Many initiatives to prevent HIV sexual transmission have focused on reducing the number of sexual partners in addition to promoting condom use. Although abstinence, monogamy and condom use are effective HIV prevention strategies, they require cooperation of the male partner. Such prevention approaches for women are "not only futile but morally bankrupt. Abstinence and condom use may be impossible for women to enforce. Fidelity is of no use unless it is mutual, and men's faithfulness very often lies outside of women's control" (Dunkle & Jewkes, 2007). Many women around the world lack autonomy over their sex lives and are unable to convince their male partners to use male condoms. Structural determinants of health, such as gender inequality, also constrain women's ability for self-protection (Morris & Lacey, 2010) and may deny women's control over procreation (Doyal, 1995).

Effective responses to curb sexual risk of HIV within established intimate relationships have always been the most difficult of prevention challenges. The association of condoms with extramarital sex has stigmatized use and undoubtedly contributes to the hesitance among many men and women to use condoms with their partners (Mantell, Stein, & Susser, 2008). As epidemics mature, a higher proportion of HIV infections occur within marriages or other long-term partnerships (Dunkle, Stephenson, & Karita, 2008), and a key challenge for HIV prevention is to address the challenges within HIV-serodiscordant couples. Many such couples desire to have children, especially with increased availability of ARVs (Cooper et al., 2007; Kaida et al., 2006), and guidance on safer conception options is a critical, unmet need (Matthews & Mukerjee, 2009; Mantell, Smit, & Stein, 2009; Matthews et al., 2010, 2011).

Hence, with the desperate need for alternatives to male condoms, since 1987 advocates have been drawing attention to the need for the development of biomedical HIV prevention technologies to enable women to protect themselves in sexual encounters. The first advocates came from the fields of women's health and contraceptive research and development, and were joined by advocates working on HIV/AIDS, STIs, infectious diseases, and international development. In the early 1990s, as it became apparent that the HIV epidemic in developing countries was driven primarily by heterosexual transmission and that an increasing proportion of global HIV infections occurred in women, women's health activists, such as Dr. Zena Stein (1990), challenged the public health community to develop "women-empowering" methods, giving women greater control over sexual health and fertility.

The trajectory for NPTs began with the development of physical barriers (female condom) and chemical barriers (microbicides, which were initially referred to as virucides). The female condom was the first women-initiated prevention alternative to the male condom. It became available in Europe in 1992, and in 1993, it was approved by the U.S. Food and Drug Administration (Lewis, 2000). In 1996, PATH conceived the Woman's Condom project, dedicated to producing a female condom that would serve women better through a user-driven design. While a female condom has been on the market in several countries for almost 20 years, levels of use have been low. In comparison to the male condom, the female condom is expensive.

In 2008, nearly 35 million female condoms were distributed—still just a fraction of the more than 10 billion male condoms distributed annually worldwide (PATH, 2012).

## ADVOCACY ALONG THE PREVENTION SCIENCE CONTINUUM

Advocacy and institutional support are needed for effective promotion of NPTs. Apart from funding, the NPT advocacy landscape has been challenged by governmental policies and political commitment, disagreements between scientists, communities, and health practitioners as well as between pharmaceutical companies and international nongovernmental organizations.

Advocacy and policy development are key components of prevention science—from identification of prevention needs, to conduct of basic and clinical research, to implementation of findings in public health programs (MacQueen & Cates, 2005). Partnerships among researchers, policymakers, advocates, and affected communities have proven to be vital in this advocacy and policy process and in striving for the greatest societal benefit from prevention research. Advocacy and policy analysis are key, for example, in addressing community-level issues (such as acceptability and access), explicitly considering how research results will be integrated into public health practice, and analyzing new prevention interventions from the perspective of improving health equity.

At the conceptual stage, advocacy is essential in identifying a need for new prevention approaches, creating the demand for research and development, and generating funding and institutional (public and private sector) support. In the experimental stage of prevention research, the advocacy role tends to focus on policy development to ensure protection of vulnerable populations engaged in clinical trials, and engaging communities in the research process such as through Community Advisory Boards (CABs). Partnering with communities may help to increase participant recruitment and retention in trials and help to ensure that access justice and equity issues are addressed in contexts where there is a history of medical- or research-related harm or colonial relationships between research institutions and local communities. Finally, at the applied stage, advocacy and policy guidance are key components in the effort to create consensus guidelines on whether/how to integrate new prevention tools with national and local HIV prevention priorities. Advocacy at this stage of the prevention research process helps build community ownership of the study results and generates demand for the intervention, opening delivery and implementation pathways.

## THE ROLE OF ADVOCACY IN THE PREVENTION RESEARCH CONTINUUM

- In the **conceptual stage,** advocacy is needed to secure the resources to develop effective preventive interventions.
- In the **experimental stage** (clinical research), advocacy centers on acceptability assessments, engaging communities in research processes, and policy development to pave the way for implementation.
- In the **applied stage,** advocacy centers around communities positioning themselves to take ownership of the social dimensions of prevention interventions and ensuring that effective interventions are made available and accessible to those who are most vulnerable.

The effectiveness of integrating advocacy with various research phases has been demonstrated through efforts to make emergency contraception available without a physician's prescription. Organized advocacy became full-fledged in the mid-1990s with the intensive use of media campaigns to increase awareness of emergency contraception (Robinson, Metcalf-Whittaker, & Rivera, 1996). As discussed in more detail in this chapter, women's health advocates have been instrumental in calling for development of topical microbicides and creating greater access for the female condom. Advocacy, raising community awareness, research on hypothetical acceptability, and collaboration between researchers and local communities have been essential in generating support for the potential role of microbicides in preventing HIV infections among women.

## THE ROLE OF THE MEDIA IN ADVOCACY FOR NEW PREVENTION TECHNOLOGIES

HIV advocates have a long history of approaching the media to seed the transformation of public policies in the public interest. Public health advocates for tobacco control and HIV treatment have shared the common achievement of creating a social movement by changing attitudes and behaviors, and exposing corporate greed (Wallack, Dorfman, Jernigan, & Themba, 1993). The social movements around HIV/AIDS issues have been important political forces for improving access and quality of prevention, care, treatment, and support services, as well as creating broader social change.

HIV/AIDS-related advocacy always faces an "image problem" as the people most vulnerable to HIV—gay men and other men who have sex with men, people who use drugs, sex workers, and people from HIV-endemic countries—are not universally seen as worthy of public sympathy or support, and for the most part are on the margins of society. Thus, the social movements stemming from HIV-related advocacy efforts—such as the gay rights movement, harm-reduction movement, and advocacy for access to medicines in resource-poor countries—have had the common goal of raising awareness of and action against inequities based on race, gender, sexuality and sexual orientation, drug use, and class. These social movements would not have been possible without responsive media coverage, and that coverage would not have occurred without effective blending of science, politics, and advocacy.

HIV advocates have been sophisticated in advocacy, grassroots organizing, and using the mass media (and increasingly social media) in innovative ways. Advocates can be a significant force in policymaking and agenda-setting by increasing the visibility of values, people, and issues. In the late 1980s, advocates in the United States employed "disaster relief" and "rapid response" rhetoric to frame their advocacy efforts and mobilize funding for AIDS care services in cities hardest hit by the epidemic. These advocates used demonstrations and aggressive media campaigns, employing a broad coalition and the news media extensively to pressure decision makers to enact the Ryan White CARE Act in 1990.

Several key NPT clinical trials were announced in 2010–2012, and additional new trial results are anticipated over the next few years. With these new advances, it has become apparent that various stakeholders sometimes lack the necessary skills to understand and interpret trial results. This research literacy is particularly important in Africa where HIV rates are the highest, and thus where the majority of research trials take place and where there is ongoing need for participants to enroll in large-scale clinical trials. Media journalists need to be able to understand and in turn report accurately and with sensitivity on NPT research and development efforts, including clinical trial results and ethical concerns.

There have been some egregious examples of sensationalist, biased, incorrect, and inflammatory reporting in the media about NPT trials, some stemming from basic misunderstanding of how clinical trials for NPTs are designed, and others stemming from historical mistrust of Western research institutions and racial tensions (for examples, see Mngxitama, 2010 and Chibulu, 2009). As consumers of media reporting, advocates and community members must be able to see through the "spin"—false hope on one side, outrage/despair on the other. Both extremes are harmful to HIV prevention efforts, as the former can create risk compensation and a false sense of security among individuals, while the latter can hinder efforts to continue NPT research.

## POLITICAL AND COMMUNITY LEADERSHIP IN HIV PREVENTION ADVOCACY

The last 30 years of HIV prevention advocacy have been led by various and evolving dominant discourses and by a wide variety of key players, from grassroots community members most affected by the epidemic, to health equity, women's health, gay rights, and human rights activists, to physicians and specialists. However, there is no clear prevention constituency, and no such constituency has been adequately mobilized to demand scale-up of HIV prevention interventions to the same extent as the treatment movement. It has been a challenge to keep HIV prevention at the forefront of social policy and action, particularly because of the controversies and taboos around sex and drug use, the need to engage many sectors, the long time lag between HIV infection and the appearance of illness, and the pressing need to provide treatment to people living with HIV/AIDS (Piot, Bartos, Larson, Zewdie, & Mane, 2008).

International and country-level leadership on HIV treatment has led to clear results in the rollout of treatment to people living with HIV, but the same kind of leadership for HIV prevention has been inconsistent at best. The lack of explicit and dedicated leadership for HIV prevention can partly be explained by the controversial nature of what works in terms of HIV prevention, such as harm reduction for sex workers and people who inject drugs, sex education for youth, promotion of condom use, and changing homophobic social norms (Piot, Russell, & Larson, 2007). To some extent, the divisive dialogue between treatment and prevention advocates has been neutralized with an increasing recognition of the prevention benefits of scaled-up and early treatment for people living with HIV and a growing discourse of "treatment as prevention."

Such leadership requires a well-designed political strategy with scientific evidence and human rights as its foundation and a broad range of sectors and opinion leaders as its workforce. Great political commitment and courage would be necessary, for example, to change laws that not only present structural barriers to HIV prevention but actually make people more vulnerable to HIV. The political will to decriminalize sex work, drug use, homosexuality, and HIV transmission is necessary but lacking in many parts of the world (Gupta, Parkhurst, Ogden, Aggleton, & Mahal, 2008). Significant advocacy and political commitment are needed, for example, to develop targeted HIV prevention services for gay men, let alone eliminate laws in the 79 countries and territories that criminalize same-sex sexual relations between consenting adults (including six countries retaining the possibility of applying the death penalty for such acts) (UNAIDS, 2010).

Passionate and vocal advocates have played key roles in raising the profile of HIV in the public's and governments' attention. Likewise, individual researchers and physicians have played a key role in advocating and promoting biomedical approaches to HIV prevention. But an HIV prevention constituency must be made up of more than HIV experts. Social mobilization requires political action and advocacy led by a broad-based coalition including youth, women's, gay men's, and faith-based organizations, the media, business leaders, and HIV/AIDS activists (Piot, Bartos, Larson, Zewdie, & Mane, 2008).

Many communities that first generated spontaneous and effective responses combined relative prosperity with traditions of political power or political activism. In many parts of Africa, for example, women of high socioeconomic status (e.g., spouses of financially mobile and successful men) were as likely to become infected with HIV as low-income and low-literacy women. In Western countries, like Canada and the United States, white and relatively prosperous gay men were disproportionately affected by the epidemic. These communities had political skills and access to funding, and used both community self-help, political advocacy, and the media to generate successful responses. At the same time, lower income and more marginalized populations had fewer financial or political resources to organize self-help responses or make claims on governments.

Social mobilization and mass popular demand for HIV prevention has been achieved in various parts of the world through broad civil society reactions to oppressive and divisive states (e.g., in Brazil, Uganda, Thailand, Cambodia, and South Africa); through outreach by faith-based international NGOs and religious leaders; through youth-focused marketing, social networking, and corporate social responsibility; and finally through HIV treatment activist groups that have broadened their mandates to demand HIV prevention (Piot, Russell, & Larson, 2007).

Despite the successes of each of these sectors in generating demand for HIV prevention, these efforts have not yet coalesced as a coherent movement that is able to shift social norms and sexual and drug-use practices. The demands of these sectors have instead been competing or contradictory: "community versus state, religious versus secular, local versus international, private versus public, and medical versus social" (Piot, Bartos, Larson, Zewdie, & Mane, 2008).

## ADVOCACY AND ACTIVISM FOR NPTS: FEMALE CONDOMS, MICROBICIDES, AND ORAL PREP FEMALE CONDOMS

The development of the contraceptive pill in the mid–20th century was gender-transformative (Ehrhardt, 1988). Not only did it reduce the key role the male condom played in pregnancy prevention, but it made it possible for women to control their fertility while circumventing the crucial role of gender power. With the advent of HIV, the inescapable role of gender power came back in full force. However, while the pill gave women power over their fertility, HIV undermined it. Unsurprisingly, then, the widespread instruction for women to use a male condom with their partners was unlikely to appeal to women in the 1990s with emergence of the global HIV pandemic.

In the United States, the FDA permitted the male condom to be "grandfathered" into preventive technology without further tests, a concession not granted to the female condom. The trajectory of the female condom has suffered its ups and downs—from enthusiasm and hope to skepticism and outright negative bias, to resurgence of positive attitudes about its potential contribution in curbing HIV acquisition and transmission. Advocacy for the female condom has been uneven and sometimes plagued by adversities.

Women have long demanded an HIV prevention method that they can initiate and control, not dependent upon male partners or health care providers. More than 100 acceptability studies have shown the female condom (known as FC1, Reality®, or Femidom®) to be acceptable to women and men users, the majority conducted after the female condom was approved by the U.S. Food and Drug Administration in 1993 (Mantell et al., 2005). Consequently, attention to design and packaging features has been inadequate. Health care providers often lack training on female condom use and how to promote the method to clients. The female condom has been marginalized by governments, policymakers, funders, and the media, resulting in it being inaccessible and therefore underutilized by potential users in most countries (CHANGE, 2011; Peters, Jansen & van Driel, 2010). Misconceptions that most women do not like the female condom are often used to rationalize lack of expanded access (McConnell, 2008). Some have argued that treating culture as a barrier to female condom use is a pretext for lack of government advocacy and support, hence limiting method accessibility and uptake (Musoni, 2007; Susser, 2001). Arguments about the high cost of the female condom relative to the male condom and absence of definitive empirical evidence of its HIV prevention efficacy (which is based on pregnancy prevention data, and through extrapolation, efficacy for HIV/STI prevention) have limited universal access to the female condom. The lack of head-to-head testing of the HIV prevention efficacy of the female against the male condom has promulgated little support of the female condom among some implementers, donors, manufacturers, academics, and researchers as well as by some governments in developing countries (FSG Social Impact Advisors, 2008). Such discourse essentially pits the rights of individuals to protection against the costs of protection. The FSG Social Impact Advisors Report cites three challenges to female condom promotion: (1) lack of consistent definition of product success; (2) its cost-effectiveness relative to the male condom; and (3) difficulty in quantifying its female empowerment benefits (FSG Social Impact Advisors, 2008).

The female condom has also been overlooked by policymakers and funders due to "bad press" about its physical properties, especially in North America (Kaler, 2004). The media's negative treatment of the product is also related to skepticism about its feasibility: "Will the female condom ever catch on?" (Tang, 2010); "A tough sell: The female condom" (Clark-Flory, 2010). Most recently, despite new study findings that demonstrate the cost-effectiveness of free female condom distribution in Washington, DC (Holtgrave et al., 2012), a *New York Times* article about this study casts the female condom in a negative way: "Female condoms have never really caught on, either among wealthy women for birth control or among poor women for AIDS protection. In a few counties like Zimbabwe, they are popular among prostitutes" (McNeil Jr., 2012).

In the early years following FDA approval of the female condom, there was little activism and advocacy for it. Negative attitudes toward the female condom have begun to decrease, but a lot more advocacy work is needed. One of the best examples of grassroots advocacy for the female condom was in Zimbabwe where an NGO, the Women and AIDS Support Network, engaged in community mobilization that led to the gathering of more than 30,000 signatures, ultimately persuading the Ministry of Health to approve, procure, and promote the purchase of female condoms for public-sector distribution and social marketing (Kerrigan et al., 2000). Social marketing of the female condom in beauty salons has been an effective strategy for increasing accessibility (Meldrum, 2006). The Brazilian Health Ministry, which has been distributing free female condoms since 1997, recently purchased 20 million female condoms that will be distributed free primarily to women vulnerable to STIs (Joshi, 2012). In the United States, the Center for Health and Gender Equity (CHANGE), an international NGO in Washington, DC, launched a Prevention Now Campaign to expand global access to female (and male) condoms, advocating for policy support and funding for purchase, distribution, and effective programming (Kalkstein, 2012).Through effective advocacy, CHANGE was instrumental in advocating for inclusion of the female condom in PEPFAR reauthorization and has worked internationally with civil society in conducting female condom advocacy workshops. It also coordinated advocacy efforts for the U.S. Food and Drug Administration Advisory Committee hearing for the second-generation female condom, FC2, made of synthetic latex (nitrile), in December 2008. Subsequent FDA approval of FC2 in March 2009 became the catalyst for galvanizing nongovernmental organizations to support FC2, which was not done for the first-generation product. A number of health departments in the United States seized this opportunity to launch FC2 promotion campaigns. Grassroots advocacy efforts have been instrumental in promoting the female condom and microbicides. In Namibia, Susser's ethnographic work documented grassroots advocacy for the female condom and women's desperation to have the method, as they called for "give me the FC!!" (Susser, 2001, 2009).

Another new female condom device, known as Cupid®, has been approved by the World Health Organization (Cupid Ltd., 2012). The Cupid® female condom, made of latex, has an inner sponge used to insert and hold the device in place during sexual intercourse. Other female condoms are currently being developed or are being tested for efficacy. For example, the Women's Condom developed by PATH is being tested in a Phase III clinical trial for contraceptive effectiveness (PATH, 2012), and the V'Amour/Protectiv is in the process of obtaining approval by the World Health Organization (USAID, 2011).

In 2011, the Universal Access to Female Condoms Joint Programme (UAFC), based in the Netherlands, launched a highly innovative paper doll campaign, featuring Zawadi ("gift" in Swahili) Smartlove, to increase local and global advocacy for the female condom (UAFC, 2011). These dolls are sent all over the world and people are asked to write messages on these dolls demanding female condoms. Long chains of these dolls are constructed, reflecting demand for female condoms. The messages are used to garner local and international leadership support. For example, at a Paper Doll Event in the Netherlands, 1,500 messages were displayed at the Dutch Parliament in November 2011. Forty NGOs in 22 countries participated in this campaign and collected more than 6,000 dolls in 2011; another 40 countries will be targeted to participate in the campaign (Universal Access to Female Condoms Joint Programme, 2011).

In Cameroon, which has a UAFC-supported female condom program administered by the Association Camerounaise pour le Marketing Social, a variety of innovative strategies have been used since 2009 to increase method uptake, including advocacy, mass media campaigns with artists, distribution through friendly sales points, training of journalists, and advocacy targeted to decision makers (i.e., government ministries, international organizations, traditional and religious leaders, military high command, media, hairdressing salons, pharmacies, women's groups) (Elat & Kpognon, 2012). Other advocacy strategies included a brochure on female condom programming, establishment of a high-level independent Steering Committee, national launching of the female condom, and presentation of the project at a Parliamentarian session. Another novel marketing strategy developed in Cameroon is a dress constructed of female condoms (Universal Access to Female Condoms Joint Programme, 2011). This dress has been used as an advocacy tool to promote awareness of the need for FCs.

Complementing the UAFC's grassroots initiatives is the Global Female Condom Initiative of the United Nations Population Fund (UNFPA). UNFPA has scaled up its female condom programming and works at the country level with Ministries of Health and other government agencies to develop a country-driven female condom strategy as part of overall condom programming (PATH/UNFPA, 2006).

Within the context of a female condom structural intervention in New York State, Exner and colleagues distributed a policy kit that contained materials (posters, pamphlets, information sheets) to promote female condom policies and practices to directors of agencies funded by the New York State Department of Health's AIDS Institute (Exner et al., 2012). The Tool-Kit and pelvic models were used by sexual risk-reduction counselors to demonstrate correct female condom use with clients. One prominent message promoted in the intervention was that the female condom brought pleasure to both women and men.

In the United States, a Female Condom Access Working Group comprised of researchers, community partners, advocates, program administrators, and health departments (New York City, New York State, Washington, DC, San Francisco, Houston, Atlanta, Baton Rouge) was recently established by the AIDS Foundation of Chicago and CHANGE to develop and implement strategies to increase availability and use of the female condom (FC2). The Chicago Female Condom Campaign works to increase awareness, affordability, access, and use of the female condom through organizing education, training, advocacy, and pooled (bulk) purchasing of the product. Borrowing from Beyoncé , this campaign uses the theme of "Hey Chicagoans: Put a Ring on It" and developed a Campaign Training Corps to enhance outreach (Terlikowski, 2012). The Washington AIDS Partnership in collaboration with the DC Department of Health has implemented an initiative to ensure that female condoms are stocked in CVS pharmacies in the district and ensure distribution of free female condoms in high schools, hair salons, and liquor stores. In addition, the health department has advertisements for the female condom on buses telling people to "Get turned on to it" (Monroe, 2012). A key female condom promotion message centers on women's control over their protection rather than dependence upon men.

More recently, there has been advocacy for anal use of the female condom. Although the female condom has never been approved for anal use (Kelvin et al., 2009, 2011; Mantell et al., 2009), limited empirical evidence suggests that is being used off-label during anal sex (Kelvin et al., 2011). Many health care providers are reluctant to promote it because of the lack of guidelines about use (Mantell et al., 2009). However, several health departments in the United States are promoting anal use of the female condom, despite lack of safety testing and consensus guidelines for use. For example, in 2011, the San Francisco Department of Health launched its "Our Bodies, Our Choices" campaign on Valentine's Day featuring the female condom for women, MSM, and transgender individuals. As part of this initiative, the female condom was promoted for use by the receptive partner during anal sex, as reflected in the poster: "Get Turned On to It" Campaign (SFDoH, 2011; Monroe, 2012). In Africa, increased recognition of the growing numbers of MSM and discourse about heterosexual anal sex suggest there is an untapped market for products that protect against anal STIs (Johnson, 2012).

## Microbicides

Zena Stein's seminal paper in 1990 called for the development of woman-controlled prevention options, specifically microbicides, chemical substances that can potentially kill microorganisms that cause HIV (Stein, 1990). Later that year, her voice was joined by delegates at the U.S. National Conference on Women and HIV Infection. Included among their conference recommendations was the "develop[ment] of better barrier/contraceptive methods and virucides which are effective, safe and acceptable to women," adding that "methods which are woman-controlled and may be used without detection by their sexual partners" are "especially needed" (Global Campaign for Microbicides, n.d.). Vaginal microbicides were seen as the hope for revolutionizing HIV prevention for women, a promising alternative to male and female condoms (Stein, 1990; Elias & Heise, 1994), and for some, a magic bullet.

In the beginning, microbicides faced many challenges. Pharmaceutical companies often resisted developing microbicides not only because of the high research and development costs but also because they anticipated low returns on their investments as the need for such products are greater in low-resource countries. However, well-organized advocacy for microbicides (in contrast to the lack of such advocacy following initial introduction of the female condom) proved to be highly effective in generating positive sentiments about the importance of finding an efficacious microbicide and securing funding for testing these products. This advocacy could be characterized as a quasi-social movement.

In 1991–1992, the United Kingdom's Medical Research Council (MRC) convened a group of experts from the United States, Belgium, and the UK to discuss the challenges and prospects of developing such products. Over three meetings, recommendations from the expert group led to MRC's decision to establish and fund a program of microbicides research. Around the same time, the first consultation on microbicides among women's health and HIV/AIDS professionals was convened by the Population Council in New York, and the International Women's Health Coalition (IWHC) and WHO sponsored a meeting of women's health advocates and scientists in Geneva to discuss contraceptive research priorities. The resulting report, "Creating Common Ground," called for greater attention to user-controlled barrier methods that provide HIV prevention as well as contraception (World Health Organization, 1991).

In 1992, two small but important public funding opportunities for microbicide research were launched, one by the UK's MRC to support the development of an "intravaginal virucide," and one by the U.S. National Institutes of Health (NIH) for studies of vaginal ecology as it relates to disease transmission (as a precursor to consideration of microbicides) (Global Campaign for Microbicides, n.d.).

The first microbicide-specific advocates' coalition, WHAM (Women's Health Advocates on Microbicides), was formed in 1993 by 11 women's health organizations and networks worldwide to shape the Population Council's early microbicide research efforts. WHAM met semiannually for several years and guided the council's microbicide program by helping to design a multicountry study of women's formulation preferences, reviewing draft protocols, exploring ways to better monitor informed consent in clinical trials, and providing recommendations to the council. In 1997, WHAM convened an international symposium called "Practical and Ethical Dilemmas in the Clinical Testing of Microbicides," bringing together 55 participants from 15 countries to build consensus on how best to conduct microbicide trials (Global Campaign for Microbicides, n.d.).

In 1994, also recognizing the need to form a coalition, the scientific community formed the International Working Group on Microbicides (IWGM) with initial support from the WHO Global Programme on AIDS to facilitate collaboration among research institutes working on microbicides. The microbicide field rapidly matured between 1993 and 1997 with new microbicide actors and research focus shifting from the lab to the field as different microbicide candidates began to enter clinical trials. At the XII International AIDS Conference in Geneva (July 1998), the Global Campaign for Microbicides (GCM) replaced WHAM in order to encompass a wider advocacy agenda. GCM was committed to focusing world attention on the critical need for new HIV prevention options, especially for women. With start-up funding from UNAIDS, the GCM aimed to generate political pressure for increased investment in microbicides and to ensure that the public interest was protected and the rights and interests of trial participants, users, and communities were fully represented and respected throughout every phase of scientific process required to develop these new products.

The GCM raised awareness about the need, and created demand, for microbicides through the media, workshops, outreach to policymakers (including launching a major legislative strategy to increase U.S. government investment in microbicide research and development), and supplying grassroots activists with "action kits." By 2001, the GCM had grown into a major global organizing effort with more than 70 partner groups worldwide and hired its first full-time executive director, Lori Heise, a founding member and longtime women's health advocate.

Between July 2000 and February 2002, the Rockefeller Foundation's Microbicides Initiative convened an international group of scientists, research organizations, advocacy groups, pharmaceutical representatives, United Nations organizations, and donors to examine the field and recommend strategies to accelerate microbicides development. A working group on advocacy, public education, and resource mobilization created the report "Microbicides: A Call to Action," offering a blueprint for advocacy action that prioritized capacity-building "for NGOs and their networks to advocate for microbicides and to participate actively in decision-making around research agendas and clinical trial implementation" (Heise, 2002).

The Rockefeller Initiative then gave rise to the European Commission awarding financial support to the International Family Health (IFH) for international networking and advocacy on microbicides over three years. The GCM partnered with IFH to develop a strong presence in key European countries. At the same time, the International Partnership for Microbicides (IPM) was created and also contributed to growing European commitment to microbicides research and development. By this time, the GCM had established a strong grassroots base for microbicides advocacy among allied NGOs and the general public in the United States, Canada, and Europe (Global Campaign for Microbicides, n.d.).

In the global South, in 2002, the GCM launched a clinical trials/community involvement initiative to support community engagement in microbicides research. In 2004, a number of partner groups in Africa formed the Africa Microbicides Advocacy Group (AMAG), a coalition of advocates based in Africa, helping to build capacity in advocacy on the need for prevention methods that women can initiate and a more gendered approach to the epidemic. Today, the GCM has over 300 endorsers from around the world (Global Campaign for Microbicides, n.d.) and continues to advocate for women-controlled prevention options.

The GCM's advocacy efforts largely focused on vaginal microbicides as tools for women's greater autonomy over HIV prevention and sexual and reproductive health. More than a decade ago, activists and public health practitioners began to call for the development of microbicides for anal use. This was especially important given that the risk of an unprotected act of receptive anal sex is 10 to 20 times more likely to result in HIV transmission than an unprotected act of vaginal sex (Gray et al., 2001; Vittinghoff et al., 1999). Interest in rectal microbicides was reflected in the press with article titles such as "Demanding Microbicides: A Chemical Condom in Your Future?" "Beyond Latex: Is There an Invisible Condom in Your Future?" (Forbes, 2011; Straube, 2011). However, there was little support for rectal microbicides at that time, with concerns expressed about diversion of resources for condom promotion (Straube, 2011) and delay in development of vaginal products urgently needed by women (Roehr, 2008). Discomfort in talking about anal sex, common misconceptions that rectal microbicide use would be limited to MSM, and the belief that heterosexual women and men do not engage in anal sex contributed to apathy about rectal microbicide advocacy.

Coordinated efforts to develop a rectal microbicide did not occur until 2004 (IRMA, n.d.). It was not until 2005, after rallying by the advocacy and research communities, that another advocacy group, the International Rectal Microbicides Advocates (IRMA) (under the name of the International Rectal Microbicides Working Group) was established to focus on rectal microbicides that could be used by men or women to prevent HIV transmission during anal sex. IRMA is comprised of over 1,100 advocates, policymakers, and leading scientists from around the world working together to advance a robust rectal microbicide research and development agenda. IRMA focuses its advocacy efforts on creating safe, effective, acceptable, and accessible rectal microbicides for the women, men, and transgender individuals around the world who engage in anal intercourse. IRMA works to confront the institutional, sociocultural, and political stigma around the public health need for rectal microbicide research and to increase funding and commitment within this field of inquiry. Since its creation in 2005, IRMA has acted as a vibrant and reliable central forum for exchange, debate, and networking on not only rectal microbicides, but other new prevention technologies, such as medical male circumcision, vaccines and oral prevention (PrEP), and promotion of existing prevention methods such as male and female condoms as part of a range of prevention options (IRMA).

In 2010, IRMA launched Project ARM—Africa for Rectal Microbicides—to expand community mobilization, enhance capacity of community leaders and advocates, and provide education, engagement, and advocacy around the development of African rectal microbicide research and implementation (IRMA, n.d.). Project ARM is advocating for increased access to lubricants, documenting best practices in anal sexual health and rectal microbicide advocacy, and preparing for the first Phase II rectal microbicide trial (MTN 017), which includes South Africa as a trial site. IRMA-ALC (IRMA–America Latina y el Caribe) was launched in 2008 to advocate for rectal microbicide development and research. A number of rectal microbicide studies were done, including rectal safety and acceptability (RMP-02/MTN-006 and MTN-007) and rectal safety of lubricants (IRMA, 2010a, b). An estimated $25 million was spent on rectal microbicide research between 2007 and 2010 with the U.S. National Institutes of Health as the primary donor (IRMA, 2010a, b). One example demonstrating the relationship between advocacy and research relates to sexual lubricants—IRMA's 2007 global Web-based survey on use, preferences, and acceptability regarding sexual lubricants for anal sex as well as Dr. Charlene Dezzutti's laboratory testing of these products (IRMA, n.d.; 2010a, b). Findings from both of these studies can be used to inform message development. A video, *The Rectal Revolution Is Here—A Video Introduction to Rectal Microbicide Clinical Trials,* has been recently developed by IRMA, the Microbicides Trials Network (MTN), and the Population Council to educate communities and participants about rectal microbicide clinical trials (Pickett, 2012).

## Oral PrEP

Oral PrEP, taking doses of antiretroviral medications on a regular basis *before* being exposed to HIV to reduce the risk of infection, is providing new hope as an NPT for high-risk HIV-negative persons. Several clinical trials have demonstrated the efficacy of daily oral tenofovir (TDF) or Truvada (TDF/emtricitabine), to prevent HIV infection in seronegative persons, including MSM, transgender individuals, and heterosexual men and women (Grant et al., 2010; Thigpen, 2012; Baeten et al., 2012). These studies demonstrate that PrEP is safe and has minimal side effects and no significant risk of drug resistance, and that effectiveness depends upon participants' adherence. The iPrEx trial found an overall 44 percent reduction in HV transmission but more than 90 percent reduction among participants with high adherence (Grant et al., 2010), while the Partners PrEP trial among 4,758 HIV-serdiscordant couples in Kenya and Uganda showed a 75 percent reduction in HIV infections (Baeten et al., 2012). In the TDF2 trial among heterosexual women and men in Botswana, HIV infections were reduced by 62 percent (Thigpen et al., 2012). Concerns about mineral bone density loss and drug resistance to tenofovir and TDF were reported. Also of note are three studies of at-risk women. The first, the CAPRISA 004 trial, showed that use of tenofovir as a topical vagina gel before and after sexual intercourse reduced HIV acquisition by 39 percent (Abdool Karim et al., 2010). The other two women's trials had disappointing results. The Fem-PrEP Phase III trial was stopped early because of lack of efficacy (with 33 new infections in the TDF/FTC arm vs. 35 new infections in the placebo arm (Van Damme et al., 2012). In the VOICE IIB trial of more than 5,000 women in South Africa, Uganda, and Zimbabwe, comparing a daily oral tablet containing tenofovir (PrEP), a daily oral tablet containing tenofovir and emtricitabine (Truvada®), and daily use of a 1 percent vaginal tenofovir gel, none proved to be effective. This result has been attributed to the fact that most trial participants did not use the products as directed. Single women less than 25 years old were least likely to use their assigned products compared to older, married participants (Microbicide Trials Network, 2013; AVAC, 2013). The reasons for the differences in the PrEP studies in women and the other studies is unknown but differences in adherence, penetration of drug in vaginal tissue, degree of HIV exposure, and genital inflammation are possible.

Heated debate about the approval of Truvada to prevent HIV infection in adult men and women flooded the electronic media since publication of the trials' findings. Advocates of PrEP for HIV prevention argue that the drug will provide a new option. However, concerns have been voiced about potential side effects, poor adherence, increased risk behavior, cost of the drug, and accessibility for those already infected. In May 2012, the FDA Antiviral Drug Advisory Committee strongly recommended that Truvada® be approved for use as preexposure prophylaxis among sexually active adult men and women—particularly gay men and other MSM, serodiscordant heterosexual women and men, and other individuals at high risk (FDA Antiviral Products Advisory Committee, 2012). On July 16, 2012—days before the start of the International AIDS Conference in Washington, DC—the FDA approved use of Truvada for HIV prevention by high-risk HIV-negative individuals. But even before FDA approval of PrEP, off-label use of ARVs by seronegative persons to prevent HIV infection had been reported (Kellerman, Hutchinson, Begley et al., 2006; Sandfort, Guidry, Masvawure et al., 2012).

Much of the debate around implementation of PrEP stems from the divergent PrEP trial findings so far regarding effectiveness of ARVs for prevention. A key finding across all of the trials, however, is that the varying effectiveness rates are a product of differences in adherence behavior (van der Straten et al., 2012). PrEP adherence in serodiscordant couples may be understood as a function of the need to reduce HIV risk while preserving a partnered relationship. PrEP use in stable couples may be associated with improved adherence and thus greater effectiveness (van der Straten et al., 2012). Another source of contention relates to equity, justice, and resource allocation; populations who are underserved, or are in under-resourced countries, may have difficulty accessing PrEP, ARVs to HIV-uninfected prior to infected individuals is another controversy (Jay & Gostin, 2012).

From an advocacy perspective, education is needed to ensure that health care providers prescribe PrEP appropriately and that potential users understand their HIV risk and the benefits and disadvantages of PrEP so as to make an informed decision about whether they would benefit from the drug.

## KEY LESSONS LEARNED

The search for promising HIV prevention methods has taken us on a long journey that we are still traveling. Recently, the NPT movement has expanded, embracing the need for disease protection alternatives for all populations, not just women—methods for men, such as medical male circumcision, as well as those for HIV-negative women, men, and trans-gendered people, such as oral PrEP. Short of abstinence, no one method totally eliminates risk and provides 100 percent protection against HIV. This means that a compendium of prevention tools will be required for combination prevention prior to exposure, at the point of HIV transmission, and shortly after exposure.

The sad reality is that despite 25 years of advocacy and political action, global prevention efforts remain woefully insufficient. Key prevention services—those that have been proven to be effective, such as condom distribution, treatment of sexually transmitted infections, and needle exchange programs—currently reach only 9 percent, 20 percent, and 8 percent, respectively, of those who need them (Global HIV Prevention Working Group, 2007). Introduction and widespread use of behavioral interventions and biomedical HIV prevention technologies require extensive political will, government support, and advocacy from both grassroots and research communities. A renewed and revitalized movement for HIV prevention is underway, focusing on scaling up already proven-effective prevention interventions, as well as calling for new biomedical approaches to HIV that would expand prevention options, particularly for those who are unable or unwilling to use condoms. We conclude by highlighting some key lessons from HIV prevention advocacy efforts.

## Avoiding False Divides

In the first decade of the HIV epidemic, a dichotomy of views between levels of interventions impeded the ability of UN agencies, donor organizations, and governments to harmonize their efforts at the country level and served to polarize the HIV/AIDS community. A similar (albeit false) dichotomy has emerged between advocates of social-structural approaches to HIV prevention and those who advocate for new biomedical tools for HIV prevention. Public health specialists, for example, bemoan that individual-level interventions (such as biomedical tools and behavior change initiatives) take up the lion's share of resources and attention over public health and structural interventions (Roberts & Matthews, 2012). However, all biomedical interventions are ultimately social and behavioral interventions; the two approaches are not mutually exclusive, and advocates must be mindful to avoid the creation of false divides between biomedical approaches and social-structural approaches to HIV prevention. As stated by Mitchell Warren: "We need to act on the promise of combination pre-vention—and debate less about the relative merits of one strategy versus another one" (AVAC, 2012).

Although several major speakers at the July 2012 International AIDS Conference in Washington, DC, referred optimistically to the historic goal of ending the epidemic—"of creating an AIDS-free generation" (Clinton, 2012)—it was clear that without major advances at the biological level for an effective vaccine or cure (neither in immediate sight), the sad reality is that a cure for those infected is "way upstream" and depends on future research break-throughs (Fauci, 2012).

## The Prerequisite of Eliminating Stigma and Discrimination

All national-level successes in HIV prevention have been associated with government (often multidepartmental) leadership and community activism, especially in sustaining and renewing responses among populations—such as injecting drug users, sex workers, and men who have sex with men—that continue to face stigma and discrimination and as a result, lack access to prevention services. Removal of discriminatory laws, such as antihomosexuality laws, are vital prerequisites to effective HIV prevention interventions reaching those populations that are most vulnerable.

## Lack of a Global HIV Prevention Constituency

While several sectors have been successful in demanding HIV prevention, a coherent HIV prevention constituency and social movement are still lacking. The need for scale-up of prevention interventions already proven to be effective and investment in research and development of NPTs have not inspired the same international social movement as for HIV treatment. A key challenge will be to build on the vibrant dialogue about, and gradually build consensus on, the value of treatment as prevention, and the value of integrating HIV prevention and treatment interventions from individual to community to national levels.

## The Need for Evidence to Take Precedence over Politics

The synergy between science, political leadership, and public policy has contributed to advancements in public health over the last two centuries, and AIDS (and NPTs) is no exception (Piot et al., 2007). Science can inform policymakers through evidence-driven research—data that needle exchange programs can prevent HIV transmission formed the core of UNAIDS' support for harm-reduction policies (Humphreys & Piot, 2012). Often, policies are driven or swayed by politics that can have negative consequences, as in the many African countries with laws against same-sex relationships, which seriously impede HIV prevention efforts for gay/bisexual men (UNAIDS, 2010).

## Advocates Can Bridge the Gaps

The connections between policy and science are necessarily complex, especially in the context of NPTs because both are driven by advocacy. Both, for example, are dependent upon available funds for further exploration and research. In addition, the politics of global developments in NPTs often assume that funding for these activities will emanate from the United States or United Kingdom, while efficacy trials are likely to be conducted with high HIV incidence populations, often in limited-resource countries. Bridging these cross-national gaps will have to be accomplished by advocates who themselves must overcome differences, not only between governments and communities (geographic, social), but also between politicians, researchers from multiple disciplines, administrative bodies, and funders.

## Hyperbole and False Hope Can Be Detrimental

The development of NPTs has been fraught with disappointments and challenges, but also peppered with overwhelming optimism, sometimes to the point of idealism, fueled by hope and strong desire to prevent HIV acquisition and ultimately reduce new infections. This idealism has also led to hyperbole in the popular press about some of these methods, especially regarding vaginal microbicides, before the first product gel, tenofovir, demonstrated efficacy in the CAPRISA trial. Advocates must seek a careful balance between promotion of NPTs as viable and vital components of the HIV prevention toolkit and avoidance of adverse side effects of their enthusiasm such as risk compensation and a false sense of security.

## Effective Advocacy Is Multipronged and Multilevel

Advocacy for NPTs has taken several forms, including establishment of policies and inclusion of promotion of these methods in country-level national AIDS plans and grassroots community mobilization. Dissemination of research findings on method acceptability, efficacy, and use-effectiveness through social media and publication in professional journals is another platform for advocacy. Promotion of microbicides has reached the level of a social movement with sophisticated media campaigns and grassroots organizing. AVAC now sponsors a fellowship in microbicide advocacy. Other international organizations such as ATHENA and CHANGE have been leading advocates for the female condom and medical male circumcision. Both the GCM and IRMA have engaged civil society in the scientific process of biomedical prevention technologies. These prominent advocacy organizations have effectively cultivated global audiences through the Internet and established regional advocacy groups for NPTs.

The drive for developing safe, acceptable, and efficacious NPTs by the scientific community needs to continue. Civil society must also be a leading force in NPT advocacy efforts, mobilizing creation of demand and establishing and leveraging strategic partnerships with government, international donor agencies, and product manufacturers such as pharmaceutical companies. Since the media can be a potent force in promoting NPTs, advocacy groups need to seek the media to promote their NPT agenda. Advocacy efforts must also be directed at governments and the private sector to commit additional millions of dollars for research and development of new products, efficacy trials of candidate NPTs, as well as postmarketing use-effectiveness trials in real-world settings.

## Clinical Trials of NPTs Must Be Carefully Designed and Conducted

Intervention trials for the prevention of HIV raise special issues and a decade of randomized controlled trials in the field of microbicides and of oral Tenofovir and Truvada have taught the field much. What we might consider its crowning efforts—the success of the trial of the microbicide tenofovir in women in KwaZulu-Natal, and of Truvada in MSM and transgender women internationally—have critically raised the issue of use-effectiveness and efficacy, and the crucial role in trials of the former as opposed to the latter. This was well illustrated in each of the trials that recently followed, as attempts to enhance these results by repetition or by varying the participants, by gender or geography, or by altering the dose. We have learned that to repeat interventions that include both behavior and structure of service (efficacy, for instance) compared to use-effectiveness (does the substance really work against infection) has led to very costly mistakes. If we are searching for consistency, we have to repeat a trial, either by direct transmission or under the very same circumstances, checking the biology and not only the comparison of reported behaviors. We have, moreover, to take extra care that so-called "controls" in a trial— participants who are not to receive the hoped-for benefits of a treatment— will be fully informed, nor is it always agreed that there is no raised risk for controls (Kuhn et al., 2011; Michels & Rothman, 2003).

## CONCLUSION

Since 1987, advocates have been drawing attention to the need for new HIV prevention tools beyond the male condom. The first advocates came from the fields of women's health and contraceptive research and development, and were joined by advocates working on HIV/AIDS, STIs, infectious diseases, and international development. Today, key players in NPT advocacy and political action are women's sexual and reproductive health advocates, the gay men's health movement, HIV clinicians, pharmaceutical companies, private foundations (e.g., Bill and Melinda Gates Foundation), and NGOs and coalitions (e.g., FHI, GCM, PATH, Alliance for Microbicides, IRMA). These key players, through activism, funding support, research, and various forms of political action, have been central to NPT advancements, particularly in response to the failure of the ABC prevention approach, the recognition of the need for women-controlled or at least women-initiated prevention tools, and the continuing incidence of HIV even as treatment was scaled up.

There have been several key sources of discord even among NPT advocates, but most pronouncedly, between NPT advocates and prevention experts who focus on social-structural approaches to HIV prevention. Some other key sources of this discord include, but are not limited to: NPTs being (mis)construed as a "magic bullet," particularly by the media; controversies and ethical concerns around the conduct of clinical trials; and the challenges of scaling up treatment in resource-poor settings, let alone making ARVs available for oral PrEP.

More optimistically, there are also many sources of harmony and unified voices among HIV prevention advocates, including the call for comprehensive prevention, expanding the prevention toolkit, and placing importance on a wider variety of HIV prevention choices; a gender-based analysis of NPTs and their implications for women's sexual and reproductive health; and a growing consensus that HIV prevention and treatment are mutually beneficial.

Overall, advocacy and political action have been central to NPT research and the beginnings of rollout. The HIV movement began with strong advocacy roots, and there are many lessons that can be applied to efforts to expand the HIV prevention toolkit.

## BIBLIOGRAPHY

Abdool Karim, Q., Abdool Karim, S. S., Frolich, J. A., et al. (2010). Effectiveness and safety of tenofovir gel, an antiretroviral microbicide, for the prevention of HIV infection in women. *Science, 329* (5996): 1168–1174.

AVAC (2012). *AVAC Report 2011: The End?* Retrieved from: http://www.avac .org/ht/a/GetDocumentAction/i/40815

AVAC (2013, March 4). VOICE trial changes results underscore need to accelerate development of additional HIV prevention options for women: PrEP strategies remain valuable prevention tool, says AVAC. Retrieved from: http:// www.avac.org/ht/display/ReleaseDetails/i/49160/pid/212

Baeten, J. M., Donnell, D., Ndase, P., & Celum, C. (2012). Antiretroviralprophylaxis for HIV prevention in heterosexual men and women. *The New England Journal of Medicine, 367*: 399–419.

Bertozzi, S. M., Laga, M., Bautista-Arredondo, S., & Coutinho, A. (2008). Making HIV prevention programmes work. *The Lancet, 372* (9641): 831–844.

Canadian HIV Vaccine Initiative (2010). *The Canadian HIV Vaccine Initiative.* Retrieved April 25, 2012, from: http://www.chvi-icvv.gc.ca

Center for Health and Gender Equity [CHANGE] (2011). *Female condoms and U.S. foreign assistance: An unfinished imperative for women's health.* Washington DC: Center for Health and Gender Equity. Retrieved January 15, 2012, from: http://www.genderhealth.org/files/uploads/prevention_now/publications/ unfinishedimperative.pdf

Chibulu, H. (December 23, 2009). Microbicide trials yield disastrous results. *The Post Newspapers Zambia.* Retrieved June 6, 2012, from: http://www .postzambia.com/post-print_article.php?articleId=3510

Clark-Flory, T. (July 29, 2010). *A tough sell: The female condom.* Retrieved March 26, 2012, from: http://www.salon.com/2010/07/29/female_condom_ campaign/

Clinton, H. R. (July 23, 2012). *Remarks at the 2012 International AIDS Conference, Washington, DC.* Retrieved from: http://www.state.gov/secretary/ rm/2012/07/195355.htm

Cooper, D., Harries, J., Myer, L., Orner, P., & Bracken, H. (2007). "Life is still going on": Reproductive intentions among HIV-positive women and men in South Africa. *Social Science and Medicine, 65*(2): 274–283.

Crimp, D., & Bersani, L. (1988). *AIDS: Cultural analysis, cultural activism* (1st ed.). Cambridge, MA: MIT Press.

Cupid Limited. (2012). *Cupid female condom.* Retrieved August 2, 2012, from: http://www.cupidltd.com/

Curran, J. W., Morgan, W. M., Hardy, A. M., Jaffe, H. W., Darrow, W. W., & Dowdle, W. R. (1985). The epidemiology of AIDS: Current status and future prospects. *Science, 229,* 1352–1357.

Doyal, L. (1995). Chapter 4: What makes women sick: Gender and the political economy of health. In *Regulating Reproduction* (93–124). New Brunswick, NJ: Rutgers University Press.

Dunkle, K. L., & Jewkes, R. (2007). Effective HIV prevention requires gender-transformative work with men. *Sexually Transmitted Infections, 83:* 173–174.

Dunkle, K. L., Stephenson, R., & Karita, E. (2008). New heterosexually transmitted HIV infections in married or cohabiting couples in urban Zambia and Rwanda: An analysis of survey and clinical data. *The Lancet, 371:* 2183–2191.

Ehrhardt, A. A. (1988). Preventing and treating AIDS: The expertise of the behavioral sciences. *Bulletin of the New York Academy of Medicine, 64*(6): 513–519.

Elat, J. B., & Kpognon, A. (November 2012). Advocacy for a better uptake of FC programming. Case study: Cameroon. *UAFC Conference on Prevention, Pleasure & Protection.* The Hague, Netherlands.

Elias, C., & Heise, L. (1994). Challenges for the development of female-controlled vaginal microbicides. *AIDS, 8*(1), 1–9.

Exner, T. M., Tesoriero, J. M., Battles, H. B., Hoffman, S., Mantell, J. E., Correale, J., Adams-Skinner, J., Shapiro, D. A., Rowe, K., Cotroneo, R. A., et al. (2012). A randomized controlled trial to evaluate a structural intervention to promote the female condom in New York State. *AIDS and Behavior, 16*(5): 1121–1132.

Fauci, A. (July 23, 2012). Ending the epidemic. From scientific advances to public health implementation. *Remarks at the 2012 International AIDS Conference, Washington, DC. July 23, 2012.* Retrieved August 5, 2012, from: http://www.nytimes.com/2012/07/28/opinion/the-long-uphill-battle-against-aids.html

FDA Antiviral Products Advisory Committee (2012). Background Package for NDA 21–752. Retrieved from: http://www.fda.gov/downloads/Advisory Committees/CommitteesMeetingMaterials/Drugs/AntiviralDrugsAdvisory-Committee/UCM311519.pdf

Fee, E., & Parry, M. (2008). Jonathan Mann, HIV/AIDS and human rights. *Journal of Public Health Policy, 29:* 54–71.

Forbes, A. (June 11, 2011). *Headlines.* IRMA Presentation.

FSG Social Impact Advisors (October 2008). *Smarter programming of the female condom: Increasing its impact on HIV prevention in the developing world.* Retrieved from: http://www.fsg.org/Portals/0/Uploads/Documents/PDF/Female_Condom_Impact.pdf

Global Campaign for Microbicides (n.d.). Retrieved from: http://www.global-campaign.org/mission.htm.

Global HIV Prevention Working Group (2007). *Bringing HIV prevention to scale: An urgent global priority.* Retrieved June 4, 2012, from: http://www.globalhivprevention.org/

Grant, R. M., Lama, J. R., Anderson, P. L., et al. (2010). Pre-exposure chemoprophylaxis for HIV prevention in men who have sex with men. *New England Journal of Medicine, 363*(27): 2587–2599.

Gray, R. H., Wawer, M. J., Brookmeyer, R., Sewankambo, N. K., Serwadda, D., Wabire-Mangen, F., et al. (2001). Probability of HIVv-1 transmission per coital act in monogamous, heterosexual, HIV-1-discordant couples in Rakai, Uganda. *The Lancet, 357*(9263):1149–1153.

Gupta, G. R., Parkhurst, J. O., Ogden, J. A., Aggleton, P., & Mahal, A. (2008). Structural approaches to HIV prevention. *The Lancet, 372*(9640): 764–775.

Heise, L. (2002). *Global advocacy for microbicides: A call to action. A report by the Advocacy Working Group of the Microbicide Initiative.* Advocacy Working Group, Rockefeller Foundation, and the Global Campaign for Microbicides.

Holtgrave, D. R., Maulsby, C., Kharfen, M., Jia, Y., Wu, C., Opoku, J., West, T., & Pappas, G. (2012). Cost–utility analysis of a female condom promotion program in Washington, DC. *AIDS and behavior.* doi: 10.1007/s10461-012-0174-5

Humphreys, K., & Piot, P. (2012). Scientific evidence alone is not sufficient basis for health policy. *British Medical Journal, 344.* doi: 10.1136/bmj.e1316

IAVI (2006). *Imagining a world without AIDS: A history of the International AIDS Vaccine Initiative.* New York, NY: International AIDS Vaccine Initiative, 2006. Retrieved from: http://www.iavi.org/Information-Center/Publications/Pages/Imagining-a-World-Without-AIDS-A-History-of-the-International-AIDS-Vaccine-Initiative.aspx

International Rectal Microbicide Advocates [IRMA] (May 20, 2010a). From promise to product: Advancing rectal microbicide research and advocacy. Retrieved from: http://www.rectalmicrobicides.org/docs/From Product to Promise FINAL English version/FINAL_eng_IRMA_2010.pdf

International Rectal Microbicide Advocates [IRMA] (2010b). Less silence, more science. Advocacy to make rectal microbicides a reality. Retrieved from: http://www.rectalmicrobicides.org/docs/IRMAColorFinalWeb.pdf

International Rectal Microbicide Advocates [IRMA] (n.d.). *Project ARM–Africa for Rectal Microbicides.* Retrieved from: http://www.rectalmicrobicides.org/docs/ProjectARM/fact sheet/FINAL.pdf

Jay, J. S., & Gostin, L. O. (27 July 2012). Ethical challenges of preexposure prophylaxis for HIV. *Journal of the American Medical Association.*

Johnson, T. (February 2012). Universal access to female condoms in South Africa. Regional workshop on HIV prevention among men who have sex with men. PEPFAR meeting, Johannesburg, South Africa.

Joshi, M. (2012). Brazil to distribute 20 mn female condoms. *TopNews.in.* Retrieved March 26, 2012, from: http://www.topnews.in/health/brazil-distribute-20-mn-female-condoms-215316 (Accessed March 26, 2012).

Kaida, A., Andia, I., Maier, M., Strathdee, S. A., Bangsberg, D. R., et al. (2006). The potential impact of antiretroviral therapy on fertility in sub-Saharan Africa. *Current HIV/AIDS Reports, 3*: 187–194.

Kaler, A. (2004). The female condom in North America: Selling the technology of "empowerment." *Journal of Gender Studies, 13* (2): 139–152.

Kalkstein, K. (November 2012). Informed advocacy to expand global access to female condoms. *UAFC Conference on Prevention, Pleasure & Protection.* The Hague, Netherlands.

Kellerman, S. E., Hutchinson, A. B., Begley, E. B., Boyett, B. C., Clark, H. A., & Sullivan, P. (2006). Knowledge and use of HIV pre-exposure prophylaxis among attendees of minority gay pride events. *Journal of Acquired Immune Deficiency Syndromes, 43*(3): 376–377.

Kelvin, E. A., Mantell, J. E., Candelario, N., Hoffman, S., Exner, T. M., Stackhouse, W., & Stein, Z. A. (2011). Off-label use of the female condom for anal intercourse among men in New York City. *American Journal of Public Health, 101* (12): 2241–2242.

Kelvin, E. A., Smith, R., Mantell, J. E., & Stein, Z. A. (2009). Adding the female condom to the public health agenda on prevention of HIV and other sexually transmitted infections among men and women during anal intercourse. *American Journal of Public Health, 99* (6): 985–987.

Kerrigan, D., Mobley, S., Rutenberg, N., Fisher, A., & Weiss, E. (2000). The female condom: Dynamics of use in urban Zimbabwe. Washington, DC: Population Council Ministry of Health (MOH) and Ghana Health Service (GHS). *2001 Annual Report.* Accra: MOH/GHS, 2000.

Kuhn, L., Susser, I., & Stein, Z. (2011). Can further placebo-controlled trials of antiretroviral drugs to prevent sexual transmission of HIV be justified? *The Lancet, 378*: 285–287.

LeBlanc, M. A., Patten, S., Broeckaert, L., Caswell, G., Cazal, S., Haire, B., Ukpong, M., & Webb, R. (2012). A "useless distraction"? Challenges to engaging in new HIV prevention technologies in countries with few/no trials. *2012 International Microbicides Conference (Microbicides 2012).* Sydney, Australia.

Lewis, M. (2000). A brief history of condoms, in A. Mindel, *Condoms.* BMJ Books.

MacQueen, K. M., & Cates, W. (2005).The multiple layers of prevention science research. *American Journal of Preventive Medicine, 28*(5): 491–495.

Mantell, J., Myer, L., Carballo-Diéguez, A., Stein, Z., Ramjee, G., Morar, N., & Harrison, P. (2005). Microbicide acceptability research: Current approaches and future directions. *Social Science & Medicine, 60* (2): 319–330.

Mantell, J. E., et al. (2009). Anal use of the female condom: Does uncertainty justify provider inaction? *AIDS Care, 21*(9): 1185–1194.

Mantell, J. E., Smit, J. A., & Stein, Z. A. (2009). The right to choose parenthood among HIV-infected women and men. *Journal of Public Health Policy, 30*(4): 367–378.

Mantell, J. E., Stein, Z. A., & Susser, I. (2008). Women in the time of AIDS: Barriers, bargains, and benefits. *AIDS Education and Prevention, 20*(2): 91–106.

Matthews, L. T., Baeten, J. M., Celum, C., & Bangsberg, D. (2010). Periconception pre-exposure prophylaxis to prevent HIV transmission: Benefits, risks, and challenges to implementation. *AIDS, 24*: 1975–1982.

Matthews, L. T., Crankshaw, T., Giddy, J., Kaida, A., Smit, J. A., Ware, N. C., & Bangsberg, D. R. (October 29, 2011). Reproductive decision-making and periconception practices among HIV-positive men and women attending HIV services in Durban, South Africa. *AIDS & Behavior.* doi: 10.1007/s10461-011-0068-y

Matthews, L. Y., & Mukherjee, J. S. (2009). Strategies for harm reduction among HIV-affected couples who want to conceive. *AIDS & Behavior, 13*: S5–S11.

McConnell, J. (2008). The female condom: Still an under-used prevention tool. *The Lancet Infectious Diseases, 8*: 343.

McNeil, D. G., Jr. (March 27, 2012). Female condom giveaway is expensive. *The New York Times.*

Meldrum, A. (October 13, 2006). Zimbabwe's hairdressers join HIV fight. *The Guardian.*

Merson, M. H., O'Malley, J., Serwadda, D., & Apisuk, C. (2008). The history and challenge of HIV prevention. *The Lancet, 372*: 475–488.

Michels, K. B., & Rothman, K. J. (2003). Update on unethical use of placebos in randomised trials. *Bioethics, 17* (2): 188–204.

Microbicide Trials Network (2013, March 4). Understanding the results of VOICE. Retrieved from: http://www.mtnstopshiv.org/news/studies/mtn003 (Accessed March 6, 2013).

Mngxitama, A. (July 17, 2010). Research on HIV prevention gel puts black lives at risk. *The Sowetan Newspaper.* Retrieved from: http://www.sowetanlive.co.za/columnists/2010/07/27/research-on-hiv-prevention-gel-put-black-lives-at-risk

Monroe, K. (March/April 2012). National Women's Health Network. The Women's Health Activist. *Put a ring on it.* Retrieved from: http://nwhn.org/newsletter/node/1383.

Morris, G. C., & Lacey, C. J. (2010). Microbicides and HIV prevention: Lessons from the past, looking to the future. *Current Opinion in Infectious Diseases, 23,* 57–63.

Musoni E. Culture Hindering Use of Female Condoms'. The New Times (Rwanda). 2007, June 17. Available at: http://allafrica.com/stories/200706180719.html (Accessed 9 September 2013).

PATH (May 2012). Woman's condom: Technology solutions for global health. Retrieved from: http://www.path.org/publications/files/TS_update_womans_condom.pdf

PATH/UNFPA (2006). *Female condom: A powerful tool for protection.* Seattle: UNFPA, PATH, 2006. Retrieved from: http://www.unfpa.org/upload/lib_pub_file/617_filename_female_condom.pdf

Peters, A., Jansen, W., & van Driel, F. (2010). The female condom: The international denial of a strong potential. *Reproductive Health Matters, 18* (35): 119–128.

The Petra Study Team (2002). Efficacy of three short-course regimens of zidovudine and lamivudine in preventing early and late transmission of HIV-1 from mother to child in Tanzania, South Africa, and Uganda (Petra study): A randomized, double-blind, placebo-controlled trial. *The Lancet, 359*(9313): 1178–1186.

Pickett, J. (March 10, 2012). Beyond condoms: Research and advocacy on new HIV prevention technologies. *Positive Living Conference,* Fort Walton Beach, Florida. Retrieved from www.rectalmicrobicides.org

Piot, P., Russell, S., & Larson, H. (2007). Good politics, bad politics: The experience of AIDS. *American Journal of Public Health, 97* (11): 1934–1936.

Piot, P., Bartos, M., Larson, H., Zewdie, D., & Mane, P. (2008). Coming to terms with complexity: A call to action for HIV prevention. *The Lancet, 372,* 845–859.

Roberts, E. T., & Matthews, D. D. (2012). HIV and chemoprophylaxis, the importance of considering social structures alongside biomedical and behavioral intervention. *Social Science and Medicine.* doi:10.1016/j.socscimed.2012.02.016

Robinson, E. T., Metcalf-Whittaker, M., & Rivera, R. (1996). Introducing emergency contraceptive services: Communications strategies and the role of women's health advocates. *International Family Planning Perspectives, 22*: 71–75.

Roehr, B. (March 6, 2008). Advocating for rectal microbicides. *The Bay Area Reporter.* Retrieved March 26, 2012, from: http://ebar.com/news/article .php?sec=news&article=2773

San Francisco Department of Public Health (2011). Get turned on to it campaign. Retrieved from: http://www.fc2sf.org/

Sandfort, T., Guidry, J., Masvawure, T. B., et al. (July 22–27, 2012). Knowledge of and attitudes toward PrEP in a New York City sample of sexually active MSM (A-452-0193-16254). *XIX International AIDS Conference (AIDS 2012).* Washington, D.C.

Stein, Z. A. (1990). HIV prevention: The need for methods women can use. *American Journal of Public Health, 80*: 460–462.

Straube, T. (July/August 2011). The anal dialogues. *POZ.* Retrieved from: http:// www.poz.com/articles/Microbicides_Anal_HIV_2634_20673.shtml

Susser, I. (2001). Sexual negotiations in relation to political mobilization: The prevention of HIV in comparative context. *AIDS and Behavior, 5*(2): 163–172.

Susser, I. (2009). AIDS, sex, and culture. In *Global politics and survival in Southern Africa.* Chichester: Wiley-Blackwell.

Tang, J. C. (April 10, 2010). Will the female condom ever catch on? *The Daily Beast.* Retrieved from: http://www.thedailybeast.com/articles/2010/04/10/will-the-female-condom-ever-catch-on.html

Terlikowski, J. (November 2012). Chicago female condom campaign. Put a ring on it. AIDS Foundation of Chicago. *UAFC Conference on Prevention, Pleasure & Protection.* The Hague, Netherlands.

Thigpen, M. C., Kebaabetswe, P. M., Paxton, L. A., et al. (2012). Antiretroviral preexposure prophylaxis for heterosexual HIV transmission in Botswana. *New England Journal of Medicine, 367:* 423–443.

UNAIDS (2010). Human rights and gender equality. Chapter 5. In *Global Report: UNAIDS Report on the Global AIDS Epidemic.* Retrieved from: http:// www.unaids.org/globalreport/Global_report.htm

Universal Access to Female Condoms Joint Programme (UAFC 2011). Retrieved November 16, 2011, from: http://www.condoms4all.org/newsarticle/589/Paper_Doll_Campaign_continues_in_2012

USAID. (November 18, 2011). *The female condom.* Retrieved from: http://transition.usaid.gov/our_work/global_health/aids/TechAreas/prevention/femalecondom.html (Accessed July 24, 2012).

Van Damme, L., Corneli, A., & Ahmed, K. (2012). Pre-exposure prophylaxis for HV infection among African women. *New England Journal of Medicine, 367*: 411–422.

van der Straten, A., van Damme, L., Haberer, J. E., & Bangsberg, D. R. (July 22–27, 2012). How well does PREP work? Unraveling the divergent results of PrEP trials for HIV prevention. *XIX International AIDS Conference (AIDS 2012).*Washington, D.C.

Vittinghoff, E., Douglas, J., Judson, F., McKirnan, D., MacQueen, K., & Buchbinder, S. P. (1999). Per-contact risk of human immunodeficiency virus transmission between male sexual partners. *American Journal of Epidemiology, 150*(3): 306–311.

Wallack, L., Dorfman, L., Jernigan, D., & Themba, M. (1993). *Media advocacy and public health: Power for prevention.* Newbury Park: Sage.

World Health Organization (1991). *Creating common ground: Women's perspectives on the selection and introduction of fertility regulation technologies.* Geneva: World Health Organization.

# 4

# Building "HIV/AIDS-Competent Communities" in Resource-Poor Settings: Creating Contexts That Enable Effective Community Mobilization

*Catherine Campbell and Morten Skovdal*

Community participation is widely accepted as a vital component of effective HIV/AIDS management, especially in many of the marginalized settings in which HIV/AIDS flourishes. However, successful community mobilization is extraordinarily difficult to bring about. Historically heavy emphasis has been placed on the challenge of building community skills and capacity in the areas of HIV prevention, care, treatment, and impact mitigation. There has been too little parallel attention to the challenges of building social environments that enable and support effective community empowerment. This is particularly the case in relation to ensuring that communities are supported by enabling partnerships with the public sector, NGOs, and donors, and by social policies that institutionalize the need for community engagement.

We present our model of "community HIV/AIDS competence" as a frame for greater context-friendly analysis and action, illustrating it with two very different rural African case studies. Both of these externally funded programs sought to support the development of community HIV/AIDS competence (in relation to the provision of home-based care to the sick and dying, and the support of HIV-affected children, respectively) through empowering local communities with HIV/AIDS-related capacity and skills and building social environments that supported their effective implementation. We explore the obstacles and opportunities each project faced along the way, linking our argument to wider debates about the extent to which externally designed and funded projects open up or close down opportunities for agency by marginalized communities in resource-poor settings.

## THREE GENERATIONS OF APPROACHES TO HIV/AIDS MANAGEMENT

Community mobilization has emerged as part of the "third generation" of approaches to HIV/AIDS management (Campbell & Cornish, 2010). The first generation, which dominated in early prevention efforts, focused on providing individuals with information about health risks, on the assumption that people engaged in unprotected sex due to lack of knowledge about HIV/AIDS, the fact that they themselves might be at risk, and how to prevent infection. This second generation of approaches targeted the peer group rather than the individual, on the assumption that peer norms were the most significant determinant of health-related behaviors, related both to prevention and care. As the emphasis in the response shifted from a primary emphasis on prevention and care to include greater attention to treatment and impact mitigation, a third generation of approaches targeted not only the individual and peer groups, but also the community, in order to create local community contexts that were most likely to support effective local responses to HIV/AIDS.

Such approaches focus on building HIV-competent community contexts. Because public health interventions most commonly target their efforts at geographically defined communities, we use a place-based definition of community in our work. We characterize HIV-competent communities in terms of the psychosocial features of a community in which local people are most likely to collaborate with one another and outside support agencies to develop effective local responses to the challenges of prevention, care, treatment, and impact mitigation (Campbell, Nair, & Maimane, 2007a; Nhamo, Campbell, & Gregson, 2010). The concept of community HIV/AIDS competence serves as a framework for the design, implementation, and evaluation of community-led approaches to HIV/AIDS seeking to facilitate safer sexual behavior, stigma reduction, service access, treatment adherence, and impact mitigation.

Community involvement is a pillar of international HIV/AIDS intervention and policy rhetoric. It is considered vital for three reasons (Campbell & Cornish, 2010). The first relates to the need to "translate" externally conceived HIV/AIDS management approaches into locally and culturally appropriate discourses and practices in real-world settings. People's experiences of, and responses to, HIV/AIDS may be embedded in local worldviews and survival strategies that have a poor fit with the biomedical and behavioral frames of reference that tend to dominate globally conceived programs. Second, community mobilization is deemed necessary for building local capacity to "sustain" externally funded programs once their funded period is over. The participation of local people in HIV/AIDS management and impact mitigation efforts is also central to the "task shifting" agenda that is increasingly emphasized in global responses to health (WHO, 2008), with its emphasis on the need to strengthen health systems in affected settings.

The third reason for community participation, most relevant to this chapter, relates to the social psychology of health-related behavior change. People are most likely to behave in ways that optimize effective HIV/AIDS management if they live in social environments that enable and support health-enhancing behavior (Tawil, Annette, & O'Reilly, 1995). To date, efforts to mobilize communities tend to be pursued in an ad hoc way in the absence of clear underlying models of the psychosocial processes that mediate between participation and health. In our work, we draw on the "social psychology of participation" (Campbell & Jovchelovitch, 2000) to conceptualize the social environments in which people are most likely to work together to facilitate effective community responses to HIV/AIDS.

## Promoting HIV/AIDS-Competent Communities

Opportunities for positive social participation are core to creating HIV/AIDS competence. There is growing evidence for the direct and indirect health-enhancing impacts of positive local participation (in informal or formal networks related to friendship, leisure, spiritual faith, community activism, and so on, as well as health-oriented projects) (Gregson, 2012). Directly, social participation can lead to benefits such as increased access to information about health problems and how best to avoid or respond to them; better access to practical, emotional, and material support for the ill; and the confidence to cope with or challenge social stigma. Indirectly social participation may be associated with various forms of empowerment (e.g., increased income-generation opportunities, enhanced social recognition, opportunities for community activism), which may also increase opportunities for health, both at the individual and the collective levels (Blane et al., 1996; Gregson, 2012).

An HIV-competent community has six psychosocial characteristics (Campbell et al., 2007a; Campbell, Nair, Maimane, & Sibiya, 2008; Nhamo et al., 2010): knowledge, social spaces for dialogue, a sense of community ownership of the problem and responsibility for tackling it, recognition of individual and local strengths for doing this, a sense of local solidarity around developing more effective community responses to HIV/AIDS, and partnerships with relevant support agencies outside of the community. Each of these is discussed in turn below.

First, as stated above, programs should seek to ensure that community members have the knowledge and skills necessary to respond effectively to HIV/AIDS. Second, they should work with local people to create safe social spaces for critical thinking about the causes of HIV/AIDS, obstacles to more effective responses, and how to avoid these. Here we are informed by Paulo Freire's (1973) notion of "critical thinking," which suggests that people are more likely to change their behavior as individuals when working collectively with others (at best) to tackle the social circumstances that place their health at risk, or (at least) to develop strategies for alleviating their negative impacts. Freire argues that in conditions of deprivation and social injustice people commonly respond by viewing their negative life situations as the result of individual failings or bad luck. He argues that the development of understandings of the shared social causes of problems is a vital first step to the formulation of collective plans to begin to recognize and alleviate these.

Dialogue among liked and trusted peers may occur spontaneously in the course of indigenous forms of social participation—in local faith-based organizations or women's groups, or in daily peer networks of various sorts. It may also be purposively facilitated by health programs using methods such as "community conversations" (UNDP, 2004) or peer education (Campbell & MacPhail, 2002) with a carefully selected range of local groups representing different local interests. Community interventions have also used initiatives such as sport and microfinance as arenas for promoting critical thinking about health. Such approaches train local community health workers to facilitate discussions where local people air reservations about new health programs, "translate" unfamiliar medical information about health problems or services into concepts and practices that make sense to them, brainstorm locally appropriate responses to health problems, and begin to put these into practice (Campbell & Scott, 2010).

Such collective debate and action is seen to support the third characteristic of an HIV-competent community, namely a sense of community ownership and responsibility for tackling HIV/AIDS, rather than the more fatalistic style of waiting passively for outsiders to come to the community and solve the problem. It would also be essential for facilitating the fourth characteristic, recognition of individual and collective strengths to tackle the problem. Small-scale acts of kindness to the AIDS-affected will be invaluable in tackling stigma, for example, and there is much that local community groups (e.g., church groups, patient self-help groups) can do to promote collective action to support more effective responses by local people. The fifth characteristic, a sense of local solidarity around tackling HIV/AIDS, also potentially results from ongoing community dialogue about local obstacles and how to respond to and avoid them, as well as building on preexisting local solidarity.

The concept of social spaces rests on the conceptualization of dialogue developed by authors such as Billig (1987), Freire (1973) and Jovchelovitch (2007), who emphasize the key role of debate and dialogue in the processes through which people's sense of their possibilities for action are reproduced or transformed. Such spaces provide contexts where people can collectively work through doubts and uncertainties about taboo topics. Through a process of dialogue they can make this information relevant to their own lives—processing it in ways compatible with their preexisting frames of reference, vocabularies, and social practices. Dialogue among liked and trusted peers may occur spontaneously in the course of indigenous forms of social participation—in local faith-based organizations or women's groups, or in daily peer networks of various sorts. It may also be purposively facilitated through approaches such as the "community conversations" approach, where trained local facilitators work with local groups to further understandings of, for example, local cultural obstacles to change and to brainstorm locally appropriate ways of tackling these (Moulton, Miller, Offutt, & Gibbens, 2007; UNDP, 2004); HIV support groups where patients encourage one another to adhere to treatment and support one another in responding to stigma (Campbell et al., 2011); participatory peer education (Campbell & MacPhail, 2002; Vaughan, 2010); interventions such as "PhotoVoice" (Skovdal, 2011b; Wang, Yi, Tao, & Carovano, 1998); and the use of activities such as microfinance groups (Kim et al., 2007) and sports (Jeanes, 2011) as the basis for opening up spaces for discussions about responding to HIV/AIDS. Such social spaces provide people with safe opportunities where they can talk about AIDS—still a taboo topic in many contexts—working with liked and trusted peers to develop critical understandings of obstacles to effective prevention and care, brainstorm ways they could respond more effectively, both as individuals and in groups, and generate awareness of the types of outside support they would need to optimize the effectiveness of their responses.

The latter point takes us to the sixth component of an HIV-competent community, namely the need for communities to develop partnerships with outside organizations and agencies that are willing to support their efforts to improve their opportunities for health. Positive changes in the lives of the most marginalized are unlikely without significant support by powerful social actors and groups from both within and outside of communities, as well as their "political will" to assist the most marginalized in improving their opportunities for well-being (Campbell, Cornish, Gibbs, & Scott, 2010).

The issue of partnerships has been relatively neglected in the theory and practice of HIV/AIDS-related community mobilization. Efforts have usually focused at the level of small-group activism and empowerment through small, bottom-up projects, usually involving narrowly defined marginalized groups. Such projects are often successful in building the skills and capacities of the poor, but less successful in building "receptive social environments." Projects often assume that poor people themselves will be able to capture the attention of the powerful once they have been empowered (Jones, 2001). Yet this is often not the case. The field of community mobilization still has much to learn about how best to supplement their "bottom-up" work with marginalized communities with appropriate parallel efforts to create receptive social environments in which powerful social actors are willing to heed the demands of the marginalized and work with them to improve their opportunities for health and well-being.

This latter aspect of community competence is informed by the work of Bourdieu (1986), who argues that social inequalities are caused by the unequal distribution of access to empowering social networks. We extend this to argue that poor health in marginalized communities is closely related to poor people's lack of access to health-enabling social networks, presenting community health programs with the challenge of not only mobilizing community capacity and consciousness, but also facilitating the development of social networks that enable effective community mobilization, which Putnam (2000) and Woolcock & Narayan (2000) would refer to as bridging and linking social capital.

## Case Studies

It is against this background that we discuss two case studies of community mobilization. Both sought to promote HIV/AIDS competence through building capacity, skills, and confidence in a marginalized community, as well as developing "receptive social environments" where more powerful groupings would be willing and able to support the community in working for better health. In many ways the projects are very different, but both have sought to empower very poor local people to cope with HIV/AIDS in rural African contexts. Both projects have been extensively written up elsewhere, and we draw on this literature to construct our argument in this chapter.

## BUILDING COMMUNITY HIV/AIDS COMPETENCE: HOME-BASED CARE IN RURAL SOUTH AFRICA

### Nature and Context of Problem

Entabeni is a rural community in KwaZulu-Natal, South Africa, about 30 km from the nearest towns or hospitals. The first author was part of the Center for HIV/AIDS Networking (HIVAN), a university-based NGO located about two hours' drive away. HIVAN's Community Responses to AIDS program had a particular interest in developing approaches to HIV/AIDS management that sought to identify and facilitate indigenous community responses rather than imposing externally designed interventions. In 2003, HIVAN was invited to conduct research in Entabeni by a local resident's grandson, who was employed at the university and deeply concerned about levels of HIV (36 percent of pregnant women were HIV-positive at that time). He introduced the researcher to the local *Inkosi* (traditional leader), who agreed that the research could take place, and introduced HIVAN members to local volunteer health workers. The project had three phases: research (2003), dissemination and intervention design (2004), followed by a three-year intervention (2005–2008) (Campbell, Nair, Maimane, & Gibbs, 2009). In 2012, HIVAN researchers returned to the community to explore the long-term impact of the intervention on the community.

Entabeni is an isolated area with no electricity or running water and few tarred roads. Homesteads are dotted about a hilly and rocky landscape. Droughts in recent years have made it hard for people to make a living from subsistence farming, and opportunities for formal employment are scarce. Many inhabitants are illiterate and not able to speak English. Access to television and radio is limited, and aside from HIV, residents suffer from high levels of tuberculosis and periodical cholera outbreaks. The *Inkosi* has an authoritarian leadership style, and local power relations are strictly dominated by adult males. Thus for example, women are expected to go down on their hands and knees when talking to the leader and his local representatives. Polygamy is common. Husbands pay *lobola* (bride-wealth) to their wives' parents in exchange for their domestic and sexual services and as a result, women have relatively little power in intimate relationships.

HIVAN's baseline research in Entabeni (Campbell et al., 2007a; 2008) found that the only support available to people dying of HIV/AIDS was offered by a group of about 80 volunteer home-based carers, local women, usually unemployed, with low levels of literacy and English language skills. This group had arisen over a number of years with very patchy and temporary inputs from various short-term NGO and public-sector community development initiatives. Their work involved walking from one homestead to another, often one or two hours apart up and down hills in intense heat, to assist the families and households of AIDS sufferers with rudimentary nursing, housework, and prayer. They had a male leader who was paid a small salary by the regional Primary Health Care services to lead the group, but the women themselves worked with no financial support, little training, and little recognition or input from local community leaders or the regional health and welfare services. They felt that their ability to perform their role was heavily constrained by their lack of even a basic stipend to cover their expenses, and by lack of recognition of the value of their work by other community members, in a context of high levels of denial of HIV/AIDS in the face of the terrible stigma that prevailed at the time (Campbell, Nair, and Maimane, 2007b).

HIVAN researchers fed back their findings to a series of workshops with community leaders and organizations using a "dissemination as intervention" approach, in which researchers reported back their findings to communities in workshops designed to facilitate local debate about how the community might put the findings into action in community-led initiatives (Campbell, Nair, Maimane, Sibiya, & Gibbs, 2012). At these workshops there was general agreement that the health volunteers played a vital role in assisting the AIDS-affected, and that this should be strengthened. The volunteers themselves said they were willing to take on an expanded role, but that they would require training and support to do this, as well as a stipend. They suggested that HIVAN members might assist them in expanding their work, and HIVAN agreed to play the role of "external change agent" over the three-year period—putting the community in touch with potential training networks and supporting them in setting up a project management committee that would include local public-sector and NGO agencies in the health and welfare sectors. HIVAN members were able to raise funding from a large U.S. funder for a project that centered on a fairly standard "empowerment via participation" approach to community development. Using the model of HIV/AIDS competence as its guiding frame, the project aimed to empower volunteer workers to lead an expanded community response to HIV/AIDS, supported by HIVAN in the first instance for a three-year period and thereafter run by the volunteers themselves. The proposal outlined three core activities aimed toward the development of a sustainable and community-led response:

1. Empowering volunteer health workers to lead an expanded local response.
2. Assisting volunteers in mobilizing support for their role from local people, particularly traditional leaders and men (who had traditionally given them little support) as well as young people. The project anticipated that the latter group would play a key role in helping in the delivery of an expanded response, given high levels of youth unemployment and the desire, expressed by many young people in the project's baseline research, for opportunities for skills building, viewed as a bridge to formal employment.
3. Building partnerships between the community and outside support groups of various sorts. Each of these challenges is discussed below.

## Empowering Local Volunteers to Lead an Expanded Response

This aspect of the project's goals was relatively straightforward to achieve. The project was easily able to link the volunteer group to various NGOs offering training in the topics they asked for: home-based nursing, bereavement counseling, how to set up and run a small organization, primary health care liaison, peer education to share these skills. NGOs appreciated the opportunity to engage with such a remote and hence "hard-to-reach" community. The volunteers eagerly attended courses and set up a cascade peer education system to share their new skills with other community members. The courses were backed up with high-profile formal "graduation ceremonies," where trainees received certificates followed by celebrations with food, singing, and dancing. A local leader donated an unused building, which the volunteers set up as an outreach center, where community members could come with HIV/AIDS-related questions. As a result of this enhancement of their skills and profile, the volunteers felt a surge of joyful confidence and a renewed commitment to their work.

## Building Local Support for the Volunteers' Work

This was a slightly more complex challenge. While the local *Inkosi* made every effort to facilitate the research and the intervention, his support raised a series of complex dilemmas (Campbell, 2010). Thus, for example, he instructed his six wives to attend an HIV awareness course run by the volunteers and attended their graduation ceremony at the end of their training. His attendance at this event was a fantastic coup for the project, which sought to raise its profile in the community, and it was particularly well attended. However, at the ceremony he gave a long speech eulogising the virtues of masculine sexual potency and female chastity, saying that while he had five girlfriends in addition to his six wives and did not want to interrupt his God-given obligation to father children by using condoms, he knew that he was not in danger of contracting HIV/AIDS because his wives and girlfriends were virtuous and faithful. He drew approving cheers from men in the audience when he rejected the claim that polygamy caused AIDS, arguing that neither of the two groups most vulnerable to AIDS, gay men and youth, practised polygamy. Aside from this, the *Inkosi's* highly authoritarian leadership style, involving complete obedience by women and youth to adult men, also undermined the project's anticipated strengthening of the confidence of women and young people to provide strong community leadership of the local struggle against AIDS and to protect their own sexual health (Campbell, Nair, Maimane & Gibbs, 2009).

Efforts to mobilize male support for the project were largely unsuccessful. There were at least three ways in which the project failed to resonate with macho masculinities. Men viewed caring for the sick and promoting health as women's work. They were extremely contemptuous of the activity of volunteering, arguing that unpaid work held no dignity for men, and sneering even at women who were prepared to work hard for no material gain. Finally, the project's emphasis on partner reduction and condom use contradicted associations of manhood with sexual insatiability and willingness to take risks (Campbell et al., 2009). Similarly, young people—who had expressed strong interest in project participation at the dissemination phase—were equally hard to mobilize. Detailed investigation suggested that they too did not see any dignity in unpaid work. Furthermore, they said they had had their fingers burned in the past in projects that had persuaded youth to engage in volunteer work with false promises that volunteering would open up opportunities for paid work. It also emerged that rural youth had a dim view of their local surroundings, seeing that the route to advancement lay in opportunities outside the community and saving their energy for plans to get away rather than stay and strengthen their rural base (Gibbs, Campbell, Maimane, & Nair, 2010).

Across the community there was little support for women taking over leadership from the project from the older man originally appointed by the *Inkosi* to run the volunteer team. When HIVAN periodically urged him to gradually delegate leadership responsibilities to women, he always agreed politely, but simply did not do so. HIVAN's one attempt to organize a confidential meeting of volunteers to develop a strategy for asserting themselves backfired when one of the volunteers broke ranks and told the male leader of the "secret" meeting. His resulting fury terrified the women into continued submission. This led to great bitterness among the team, who felt that their hard work was not being rewarded by increased involvement in project decision making.

## Mobilizing Partnerships between Community Volunteers and Outside Agencies

The project had strong support from two small local one-woman NGOs (run by a Norwegian missionary and a retired British businesswoman, respectively) that ran on shoestring budgets and were able to be immediately responsive to community needs. They provided the bulk of the training of volunteers, served tirelessly on the project's management committee, and were able to provide small sums of money to fund core activities (e.g., provision of furniture for the outreach center, and meat and cold drinks for graduation ceremonies). They, together with HIVAN staff, also provided a sense of support and solidarity for the volunteers, with the NGOs, HIVAN, and the volunteers serving as invaluable sources of recognition of the importance and value of their intensive efforts. Without the NGOs' assistance the project would simply not have survived. However, these were small groups with insecure funding, run by older women, so they were not sustainable long-term project resources.

The project's greatest disappointment lay in its failure to get buy-in from public-sector partners (Nair & Campbell, 2008). A key pillar of the project's rationale had been that over a three-year period, formal involvement in the project's activities would become formally institutionalized into the job descriptions of health and welfare department officials in the region. This was a key element of the proposed long-term sustainability of the project. Prior to the project's start, senior public-sector officials in the region had enthusiastically pledged commitment, viewing the project as a potential pilot study for the development of "best practice" models that would create frameworks for them to implement high-level national health and welfare policy commitments to increased community outreach in all aspects of their work. However, over time, this initial commitment did not translate into practice by the less senior public servants who should have been the ones to turn this commitment into action. Health and welfare department officials had no formal training in community outreach, so they simply lacked the expertise to take this mandate forward. While HIVAN was well qualified and more than ready to assist them in developing these skills, they appeared to be overwhelmed by the immense challenges of tackling health and welfare in under-resourced departments. They had little motivation to see poor community members as equal partners in their work in a highly status-conscious environment. Moreover, government departments were mired in red tape and a very rigid hierarchy, in which lower-level civil servants were precluded from suggesting new or interesting action plans to their superiors. Yet they were the ones that had face-to-face contact with communities. Thus there were no mechanisms for "bottom-up" communication of community needs and views to the supervisors who controlled the daily activities of public-sector workers.

The second and possibly most key reason for public-sector support of the project lay in the volunteers' very strong motivation to secure some small payment of their expenses and a small stipend for their work. The government had made vague promises that local home-based carers would receive small payments, and one of the key aims of the project was that HIVAN would assist volunteers in securing these. However, the state repeatedly changed the goal posts for such payment. Initially announcements were made that volunteers would be paid. After some time this was clarified further: namely, that only volunteers with a school certificate would get payments. This excluded the majority of the Entabeni volunteers. However, even then when the small handful with school certificates attempted to access the stipend, they were told that they would need to register as a formal NGO, which involved many preconditions they could not meet. Some of the volunteers were older women supported by employed husbands and strong Christian convictions who saw the virtue of unpaid community service. However, many others were desperately poor with children to support, and they had been motivated to volunteer by the prospect of eventual payment. In such a context the dropout rates of volunteers were very high. These two failures dented the project's prospects of long-term sustainability beyond its three-year life.

Another challenge facing the project was the withdrawal of its U.S. government funding sooner than expected. Initially the funder had been very supportive of the project's slow community empowerment approach. However, halfway through the project's life a new funding controller was appointed in Washington, DC, who decided that women's empowerment was "not a deliverable of value to the U.S. government" and thus no longer appropriately funded by the agency (Campbell et al., 2009). Moving forward, programs would be evaluated strictly in terms of "numbers reached" and the production of context-free approaches and manuals that could be used in countries across the world. The project was able to reduce its activities and string the funding out for longer than originally anticipated. Furthermore, the community was extremely appreciative of the funding they did receive, which was put to good use in supporting local HIV/AIDS management activities over a three-year period. However, in the face of the project's agenda to increase local people's HIV-related agency, this situation sent the community very clear messages that (1) the funders' primary accountability was to their own controllers, who had no interest in the community's own views of how best to proceed, and (2) their hard work was controlled by far-flung figures in another country with complete power to give money or take it away. This experience highlighted the strong contradiction inherent in the "bottom-up" policy rhetoric of community consultation and the "top-down" reality of absolute funder power over activities.

## Lessons and Outstanding Challenges

At the end of a three-year period when HIVAN withdrew from the project, morale was low and volunteers doubted if they had the confidence or commitment to continue alone. When HIVAN members returned to the community three years later, only a small handful of women were conducting home-based care, and the organizational support structure HIVAN had worked with them to establish was no longer in existence (Campbell, Maimane, & Gibbs, 2012). There is no doubt that the HIVAN-supported Entabeni Project was extremely successful in mobilizing a confident and enthusiastic group of volunteers during its three-year life. It provided them with a range of new and highly relevant skills, including home nursing, bereavement counseling, and peer education, all of which enhanced their ability to provide an expanded home-based care service, as well as an active community outreach center over the project's three-year life (Mqadi, 2007). However, it was less successful in creating a sustainable and community-led service beyond its funded life. Various resistances and obstacles—at the local, national, and global levels—may have contributed to this. In summary, while the project had some success in building the skills and capacity of a small marginalized group of women to offer a valuable local welfare service, it was less successful in creating a social environment that supported them in using this new capacity to create a sustainable locally led response. Before discussing this further, we turn to look at a very different and arguably more successful community project in Kenya.

## BUILDING COMMUNITY HIV/AIDS COMPETENCE: SUPPORTING HIV-AFFECTED CHILDREN IN WESTERN KENYA

### Nature and Context of Problem

Bondo District lies along the shore of Lake Victoria in the Nyanza Province of Western Kenya. The second author has played an active role in the district for several years, both as a researcher and as a consultant for a local NGO (WVP Kenya) and the Ministry of Gender, Children and Social Services. WVP Kenya is a youth-focused NGO that reaches some of the most vulnerable and HIV-affected children in Bondo District through partnerships with local community-based organizations (CBOs). Bondo has the highest prevalence of orphanhood in Kenya. Staff from WVP Kenya are from Bondo, have experienced poverty and disease firsthand, and speak the local language. They see vulnerable children best supported through local structures and knowledge systems, albeit in partnership with respectful and more resourceful organizations.

Bondo District is among the poorest districts in Kenya, with 68 percent living in poverty, the majority surviving through subsistence farming and fishing. Homesteads are scattered across a varied landscape. Disease, particularly HIV and AIDS, is rife. Estimates of HIV prevalence in Bondo vary from 13.7 percent, which is twice the national average (NACC, 2006), to double the figure. One in three children have lost one or both parents and one in nine have lost at least one parent (Nyambedha, Wandibba, & Aagaard-Hansen, 2003).

Many children in Bondo have to deal with hardship on a scale that is unimaginable to most people. As parents fall ill, children take on a caregiving role, which may include nursing (e.g., administering drugs, washing the parents, and taking them to the toilet), household chores (e.g., cleaning, cooking, and washing), and income and food generation (e.g., paid work for neighbors, farming) (Skovdal, 2011a). Locally, engaging in such activities is often regarded as part of a child's socialization in the community. However, in contexts of limited social support, caring duties can compromise a child's health, education, and psychosocial well-being (Skovdal & Ogutu, 2009).

WVP Kenya is committed to seeing children as social actors and learning from their coping strategies, as a springboard for activities that seek to strengthen traditional support mechanisms that can further facilitate their resilience. This framework informed the second author's baseline research into the coping strategies of HIV-affected children caring for their sick or elderly guardians. Using participatory research methods like PhotoVoice, the study found that caregiving children cope through income-generating activities, mobilizing social support, and constructing positive social identities (Skovdal, Ogutu, Aoro, & Campbell, 2009). However, the extent to which a child is able to cope depends on: (1) the ongoing negotiation between a child and its community in shaping social identities; (2) access to local support networks and resources; and (3) the quality of the community and its ability to share resources (ibid.).

To ensure that children are in a better to position to successfully negotiate access for support from their social environment in this context, WVP Kenya programs and activities aim to support HIV-affected children in three ways: (1) empowering local children (through scholarships and microfinance activities); (2) strengthening local capacity to support children (through community-based capital cash transfers); and (3) mobilizing partnerships and supportive policy environments. These three foci will now be discussed.

## Empowering Local Children

WVP Kenya empowers local children through three programs. First, through combining sports activities and health education, it seeks to provide children and youth with a social space to discuss HIV and health-enabling behaviors. Second, a scholarship program identifies out-of-school children in partnership with local community groups and provides them full school scholarships, including elements of household support where identified as necessary. A third program works with HIV-affected and caregiving children and engages them in group-based income-generation activities. This program arose as a result of the study on their coping strategies. Reflecting on the themes from the PhotoVoice exercise, the children, grouped into two youth clubs, were supported to collectively plan and implement activities to strengthen their coping capabilities and address some of their problems (Skovdal, 2011b). With social action funds made available from WVP Kenya, 14 children from one club started a maize-selling business and 15 children in another club began rearing chicken and growing kale (Skovdal, 2010). Not only did the children gain access to food and small amounts of income, they also gained entrepreneurial skills and respect and recognition of their capabilities among local community members and guardians. WVP Kenya continues to support groups of caregiving children with social action funds.

## Strengthening Local Capacity to Support Children

WVP Kenya recognizes that even highly marginalized communities in Bondo have social resources that can support HIV-affected children. To utilize these, the program builds children's and communities' participation into all their activities and emphasizes the need for agencies to support local communities. Therefore, in addition to the above activities, which target children directly, WVP Kenya also provides local CBOs with community-based capital cash transfers (CCCTs) to capitalize on their resources and strengthen wider community ability to support vulnerable children.

One community in Bondo, for example, after having reflected on local skills, resources, and viable business opportunities, decided that they wanted to set up a social enterprise to provide services for events, like funerals, with the revenue supporting some of the most vulnerable children in their community. The social enterprise was set up over a three-year-period and involved intensive training of community members on orphan care and support, children's rights and responsibilities, project management, bookkeeping, as well as project-specific training (e.g., catering). The first social action plan devised by the community asked for funds to buy a large marquee and plastic chairs to rent out during local events. This business required relatively little time and was cash-generative. A year later WVP Kenya asked the community if their social enterprise could be expanded to increase their profit margin. The community developed yet another action plan, asking for funds to train as caterers, to buy catering uniforms and cookery utensils, to offer their catering services, either together or separately from their marquee/chair business. Eight months later, WVP Kenya, with a remaining pot of money, asked the community for a last time if they could think of ways to expand their social enterprise. The community decided to buy a sound system complete with speakers and a microphone, which they could also rent out, either separately or together in a package with their catering and marquee/chairs services. This social enterprise was set up with $6,000 and has transformed the capacity of this particular community to provide for the needs of vulnerable children in their area.

Experiences from Bondo and beyond have found that this type of community mobilization program not only provides community members with the power and control to address the hardships experienced by children in their local area, but also offers recognition of, and confidence in, local knowledge, strengths, and resources (Skovdal, Mwasiaji, Morrison, & Tomkins, 2008; Skovdal, Mwasiaji, Webale, & Tomkins, 2011). The programme helps sensitize the community to the needs and circumstances of HIV-affected children, placing a focus on their marginalization, which in turn helps foster a sense of wider solidarity and unity for HIV-affected children, supported by their capacity to help them (ibid.).

Although CCCT has worked reasonably well in Bondo, it is by no means a magic bullet. Both WVP Kenya and the Ministry of Gender, Children and Social Services have experienced numerous difficulties in implementing CCCT, primarily relating to the notion of community. Community dynamics are complex and characterized by competing agendas, interests, and motivations. To minimize the risk of such dynamics undermining the success of CCCT, it has proved important to target communities that have a shared objective and members committed to implementing it, such as CBO members committed to assisting children in difficult circumstances. This is not the case in many communities.

In Bondo, the Ministry of Gender, Children and Social Services used project staff that had traveled the country to help with the facilitation of social action plans. With the best of intentions they facilitated workshops using participatory learning and action tools (see Rifkin & Pridmore, 2001), encouraging the communities to brainstorm ideas for their social enterprise. In the process they were giving examples of activities they could implement. Despite their intention to engage with communities as equals, their demeanor, dress code, level of education, and experience represented authority and power to the community members. When communities had to decide which projects to implement, rather than putting forward their own ideas linked to particular local strengths, they tended to "decide" to engage in activities that were perceived to be prescribed "from above." They interpreted examples provided by the project staff as instructions, which they dutifully incorporated into their social action plans. This misunderstanding unwittingly undermined the role of the project in creating opportunities for local self-determination and local experiences of control over project design and planning (Skovdal et al., 2008).

## MOBILIZING PARTNERSHIPS AND SUPPORTIVE POLICY ENVIRONMENTS

### Alliances between Communities, NGOs, and Donors

WVP Kenya has developed long-lasting and synergetic partnerships with a small number of European NGOs who provide the bulk of their funding. Their donors are committed to a long-term partnership with WVP Kenya that evolves in relation to the multiple and changing needs of vulnerable children in Western Kenya. It is only because WVP Kenya has donors who understand and share their interest in sustaining a long-term relationship with their target communities that they have been able to stay involved with their partner communities, supporting local efforts in their care of children and youth on an ongoing basis.

WVP Kenya serves as a bridge between global donors and local beneficiaries, mediating between their very different realities. Although both the local and global actors share the same objectives (i.e., to improve the welfare of children and youth), their value systems differ significantly and they are accountable to very different stakeholders. This presents significant challenges for WVP Kenya, which needs to juggle donor reporting and expectations on one hand and local realities and values on the other. Being a local NGO, WVP Kenya tends to prioritize local values and therefore happily engages in a critical dialogue with its donors if they make recommendations for program changes that are not aligned with local values and are likely to come with unintended consequences. Not all global donors appreciate being challenged, let alone take the time to listen to local perspectives and make changes accordingly (Kelly & Birdsall, 2010). The donors who support WVP Kenya not only listen to what they have to say, but actively encourage ongoing three-way dialogue between the donors, the NGOs, and their target community about how best to "do development."

One recommendation that WVP Kenya contested with its primary scholarships donor came about after representatives from the donor agency came to Kenya and met some of the primary school girls they supported through WVP Kenya. To the donors' dismay they discovered that WVP Kenya had not given all their scholars a pair of shoes as part of their uniform. They were also unhappy about meeting scholars they had sponsored whose uniforms were torn and dirty. Unhappy about what they saw, they immediately recommended that WVP Kenya buy shoes for all their scholars and make sure the scholars always wear neat uniforms. While WVP Kenya did indeed have money available to buy shoes and replacement uniforms for its scholars, in deciding not to purchase these items they were in fact being sensitive to the local context.

The children seen by the donor representatives went to schools in areas with extreme levels of poverty, where few parents can afford uniforms and shoes for their children. WVP Kenya felt that new shoes and uniforms would mark the scholars out as "supported kids," which opened them to possible HIV-related stigma—given that most NGOs supporting children in Bondo focus on the impacts of HIV. Rather than just accepting the recommendation, WVP Kenya disagreed with the donor, who accepted their guidance on this issue. This example highlights not only the importance of partnerships in enabling local organizations and communities to respond to the needs of vulnerable children, but also the need for such partnerships to be rooted in mutual respect and learning, where communities are respected as having expertise of equal value to that of donors and NGOs (Apfell-Marglin, 1990).

## Putting Young Caregiving on the Policy Agenda

Although young caregiving is a phenomenon known to practitioners and policy actors, little has been done practically to include caregiving children in existing programmatic responses and to include this particularly vulnerable group on the national or international policy agendas. In the interests of promoting awareness of the situation of children caring for their AIDS-sick parents and influencing wider institutional networks, WVP Kenya teamed with the London School of Economics (LSE) and the Kenyan national Ministry of Gender, Children and Social Services in a project that sought to influence policy actors and practitioners at local, national, and international levels by transmitting community perspectives to more powerful policy actors (see Skovdal & Campbell, 2013).

This process started with WVP Kenya feeding back its research findings to local community organizations in Bondo, getting their own perspectives on the types of assistance that would best enable them to offer support to caregiving children. These community perspectives and recommendations were in turn fed to a meeting of national policy actors and practitioners in Nairobi. The outcomes of the Nairobi meeting were fed to a forum of international policy actors in London. This multilevel engagement generated new levels of awareness of the need to include caregiving children in policy and practice, framed by community perspectives on how best to do this.

Two key concerns emerged in these discussions, highlighting the potentially different value and knowledge systems characterizing local-global encounters. The first was the view expressed by some that efforts should focus on abolishing young caregiving, and that efforts to support children in caring for their parents might unwittingly constitute support for child labor. The second was the concern that the earmarking of caregiving children for special support might make them vulnerable to HIV-stigma (Skovdal & Campbell, 2013). These debates highlight the wider challenges that arise from seemingly straightforward efforts to promote multilevel dialogue on what initially seemed a fairly uncontroversial issue.

### Reasons for Success, Outstanding Challenges

WVP Kenya does not aim to create social change, but targets children's welfare directly (e.g., through scholarships, sports, and health education) and indirectly (e.g., through community-based capital cash transfer). Either way, children are identified and supported through long-term partnerships with local community groups and organizations.

The head office of WVP Kenya is located in Bondo and not Nairobi. Their staff are young, from the local area, and speak the local language. They have experienced disease and poverty firsthand and can relate to community members and children in ways that nobody from the outside can. They appreciate the importance of providing local community groups with access to valued resources, participation, and self-determination in ways that optimize the agency and competence of community members, enabling them to support vulnerable children (Prilleltensky, Nelson, & Peirson, 2001). This, however, does not only apply to the NGO-community partnership, but also holds true for the donor-NGO partnership.

The work done by WVP Kenya is only possible because of the synergistic donor-NGO-community partnership. It allows WVP Kenya to stay involved with its partner communities and support them in a slow and incremental manner that strengthens their competence to care for HIV-affected children.

WVP Kenya faces two key challenges to their approach. First, providing welfare to children does not come cheap and requires a steady source of income. Although they work carefully to ensure that none of their beneficiaries become dependent on them and would like to see the community-run social enterprises as sustainable, in the provision of child welfare they are not striving for sustainability. Second, their reliance on the donor-NGO-community synergy presents a limit to what they do. Few donors are willing to give local NGOs the kind of flexibility and control that WVP Kenya asks. Similarly, few community groups show the level of compassion and commitment to support HIV-affected children that WVP Kenya is looking for in their partner— excluding children who live in areas with no or poorly organized community groups. Despite successes, WVP Kenya faces many outstanding challenges for the future as they seek to work with less coherent community groups and attract funds from more prescriptive donors.

### DISCUSSION

What are the social determinants of effective community mobilization? We began this chapter by referring to three generations of HIV/AIDS strategies seeking to empower people to respond more effectively: information-based approaches, peer education, and community mobilization, targeting the individual, peer group, and community, respectively, as the primary focus of change. We criticized community mobilization approaches for their narrow focus on empowering small marginalized groups with inadequate attention to creating wider contexts that support small groups in putting their newly acquired skills and confidence into action. Against this background we have reported on two very different case studies that have sought not only to empower marginalized groups but also to create social contexts that are supportive of their empowerment.

The Entabeni Project was ambitious, setting goals that would have required two sorts of fairly significant political changes in the social relations of a deeply conservative and neglected community. First, it sought to strengthen women's ability to lead and sustain a strengthened local response to HIV/AIDS in a highly patriarchal setting, in the context of a project focused primarily on supporting the highly stigmatized victims of an epidemic shrouded in fear and denial. Second, it sought to implement an ambitious model of public sector–community liaison through promoting partnerships between health and welfare officials and highly marginalized community members with no political or economic influence, in the context of a community so remote that many officials were initially not even aware of its existence, in an under-resourced public sector overwhelmed by the twin challenges of HIV/AIDS and poverty, with many public servants keen to distance themselves from settings of marginalization that they themselves might have had to battle against in their own lives (Jewkes, 1998).

While the Entabeni Project arose from a consultation exercise between community and NGO, its form was significantly influenced by Western feminist ideals of "empowerment via participation." In order to attract funding, its plans were "massaged" into a standard three-year plan characteristic of many international donor funding cycles. Initially supportive of its social change approach, the project donor changed tack in midstream, withdrawing funding because the project did not conform to its increasingly strict emphasis on quantifiable "deliverables" (numbers reached, the development of context-independent training manuals, and so on).

WVP Kenya has implemented a far more successful project. To a certain extent, the degree of blame and shame attached to AIDS-affected children might be slightly less than that attached to "sinful" and "diseased" adults (Campbell et al., 2007b), leaving a child-focused community project with slightly more room to maneuver. However, this observation teaches us fewer actionable lessons than attention to WVP's style of response, which differed from Entabeni's in at least three significant ways. First, WVP has never had any kind of social change agenda. Its aim has always been very clearly a small-scale welfare one: to assist a finite number of children to cope with the burdens of nursing sick parents in conditions of desperate poverty, and to enable them to access the education that will make a very significant difference to their future life chances. Second, the project developed from more realistic expectations, guided by an ethos to provide children and youth with opportunities to fulfill their potential in an organic and very cautious way, which did not involve any kind of "grand vision" beyond what could be achieved by particular children from one day to the next. Third, the project has been blessed with funders who were completely willing to respond to the needs of the project and the community as they arose, with definitions of success continually negotiated between funders, NGOs, and community, with such negotiations focusing on concrete achievements on a case-by-case basis rather than any preconceptions of what would constitute an acceptable outcome.

WVP Kenya seems also to have operated with an intuitive understanding of Wieck's (1984) principle of "small wins." Wieck argues that community programs should focus on achieving small wins as early stepping-stones to long-term and more ambitious changes. He would urge caution to those seeking to define problems (e.g., lack of home-based care in Entabeni) in terms that are too wide for a small NGO-funded community project to achieve realistically in a short time span (e.g., the empowerment of women to lead a local AIDS response in a strongly conservative and male-dominated setting). From Wieck's perspective, it is most helpful for projects to start by identifying relatively quick, tangible first steps as WVP did (e.g., helping 100 children buy school uniforms)—goals that are only modestly related to grander political outcomes (e.g., challenging the social marginalization of children in conditions of poverty). Small-scale successes then provide a material and experiential basis for more ambitious future action over time (Alinsky, 1973). Ironically, in retrospect, Entabeni did indeed achieve many small wins, providing effective home-based care and support to AIDS-affected households and so on over a three-year period. However, the project rhetoric excluded the inclusion of these achievements as significant successes, no doubt contributing to a disappointed sense (both in the community and in the NGO) that the project had not been as successful in achieving its goals as it might have been. Furthermore, the project simply wasn't conceptualized in the gradual and long-term evolutionary way that framed WVP Kenya.

The comparisons above support our growing calls for the need to rethink how best to use concepts such as "critical thinking," "empowerment," and "gender" in the social development context (Campbell and Cornish, in preparation). While we are fully sympathetic with the spirit of 20th-century critical theory, which framed the development of these terms, in many ways they have outlived their usefulness and require dramatic reformulation. Thus, for example, critical gender theorists are increasingly referring to the poor resonances between Western liberal notions of gender and women's empowerment, and the experiences and aspirations of marginalized African women—citing these as partial explanations for the dismal failure of many "gender mainstreaming" efforts to improve the lives of oppressed women in the HIV/AIDS and other contexts (Amede Obiora, 2003; Bates et al., 2009; Mannell, 2010). Critical human rights thinkers (e.g., Englund, 2006) highlight ways in which concepts such as empowerment and participation often serve as blunt tools for critical political analysis and action because of an emphasis on the civil or political rights of the excluded—an emphasis that completely neglects the fact that economic inequalities and poverty often make it extremely unlikely that new civic and political entitlements would increase people's capabilities to lead the lives they would choose to lead (Seckinelgin, 2012).

In many ways, the WVP project was not shackled by these conceptual framings in the way that Entabeni was. Neither was it imprisoned by the constraints of accepting money from large external funding bodies whose primary loyalties, sense of accountability, and shifting agendas over time are determined by Western decision makers who prioritize the interests of their own countries and constituencies over the communities that they claim to serve. To date, WVP funders have been particularly sensitive to the need for local-global partnerships in which communities and outsiders are seen as equal partners, bringing different forms of local and technical expertise in program design, implementation, and evaluation. They also acknowledge their responsibility to long-term engagement in ongoing "relationships for aid" (Eyben, 2006), where community, NGO, and funder are locked into ongoing dialogue about how best to proceed to optimize community opportunities for well-being.

## CONCLUSION

There is an urgent need for a "fourth generation" of approaches in HIV/ AIDS research, one that pays greater attention to those dimensions of wider social context that support or undermine efforts to empower poor communities to respond more effectively to HIV/AIDS (Campbell & Cornish, 2010). There is a need for increased documentation of factors that enable or limit efforts to build community HIV/AIDS competence through more case studies of particular interventions in particular settings. In-depth case studies of projects in real settings potentially provide fertile spaces for critical activists to pay closer attention to the contexts of programs, with particular emphasis on the "spaces of engagement" opened up by externally funded interventions in highly marginalized communities (Campbell, Cornish, & Skovdal, 2012), accumulating more detailed examples of real projects to examine the contexts that best open up or close down opportunities for the development of community HIV/AIDS competence in marginalized groups.

## BIBLIOGRAPHY

Alinsky, S. (1973). *Rules for radicals.* Random House.

Amede Obiora, L. (2003). "Supri, Supri, Supri, Oyibo?" An interrogation of gender mainstreaming deficits. *Journal of Women in Culture and Society,* 29 (2), 49–63.

Apfell-Marglin, F., & Marglin, S. (eds.) (1990). *Dominating knowledge: Development, culture and resistance.* Oxford: Clarendon Press.

Bates, L., Hankivsky, O., & Springer, K. (2009). Gender and health inequities. *Social Science and Medicine,* 69, 1002–1004.

Billig, M. (1987). *Arguing and thinking: A rhetorical approach to social psychology.* Cambridge: Cambridge University Press.

Blane, D., Brunner, E., & Wilkinson, R. (eds.) (1996). *Health and social organisation: Towards a health policy for the twenty-first century.* London: Routledge.

Bourdieu, P. (1986). The forms of capital. In J. G. Richardson (ed.), *Handbook of theory and research for the sociology of education* (pp. 241–258). New York: Greenwood Press.

Campbell, C. (2010). Political will, traditional leaders and the fight against HIV/AIDS: A South African case study. *AIDS Care,* 22 Suppl 2, 1637–1643. doi: 10.1080/09540121.2010.516343

Campbell, C., & Cornish, F. (2010). Towards a "fourth generation" of approaches to HIV/AIDS management: Creating contexts for effective community mobilisation. *AIDS Care,* 22 Suppl 2, 1569–1579. doi: 10.1080/09540121.2010.525812

Campbell, C., & Cornish, F. (in preparation) (guest editors). Beyond empowerment: New directions for community health psychology in the 21st century. *Journal of Health Psychology.*

Campbell, C., Cornish, F., Gibbs, A., & Scott, K. (2010). Heeding the push from below: How do social movements persuade the rich to listen to the poor? *Journal of Health Psychology,* in press.

Campbell, C., Cornish, C., & Skovdal, M. (2012). Local pain, global prescriptions? Using scale to analyse the globalisation of the HIV/AIDS response. *Health and Place.*

Campbell, C., Gibbs, A., Nair, Y., & Maimane, S. (2009). Frustrated potential, false promise or complicated possibilities? Empowerment and participation amongst female health volunteers in South Africa. *Journal of Health Management,* 11(2), 315–336. doi: 10.1177/097206340901100204

Campbell, C., & Jovchelovitch, S. (2000). Health, community and development: towards a social psychology of participation. *Journal of Community and Applied Social Psychology,* 10(4), 255–270.

Campbell, C., & MacPhail, C. (2002). Peer education, gender and the development of critical consciousness: Participatory HIV prevention by South African youth. *Social Science and Medicine,* 55, 331–345.

Campbell, C., Maimane, S., & Gibbs, A. (2012, in prep.). Sustainability of a three-year "empowerment via participation" programme for HIV/AIDS management: Going back to a rural community four years later. Manuscript in preparation.

Campbell, C., Nair, Y., & Maimane, S. (2007a). Building contexts that support effective community responses to HIV/AIDS: A South African case study. *American Journal of Community Psychology,* 39(3–4), 347–363.

Campbell, C, Nair, Y., & Maimane, S. (2007b). "Dying twice": Towards an actionable multi-level model of the roots of AIDS stigma in a South African community. *Journal of Health Psychology.* May 2007, 12:3. http://eprints.lse.ac.uk/2794/

Campbell, C., Nair, Y., Maimane, S., & Gibbs, A. (2009). Strengthening community responses to AIDS: Possibilities and challenges. In P. Rohleder, L. Swartz, & S. Kalichman (eds.), *HIV/AIDS in South Africa 25 years on.* London: Springer.

Campbell, C., Nair, Y., Maimane, S., & Sibiya, Z. (2008). Supporting people with aids and their carers in rural South Africa: Possibilities and challenges. *Health and Place,* 14(3), 507–518.

Campbell, C., Nair, Y., Maimane, S., Sibiya, Z., & Gibbs, A. (2012). Dissemination as intervention: Building local AIDS competence through the report-back of research findings to a South African rural community. *Antipode,* in press.

Campbell, C., & Scott, K. (2010). Rhetoric and the challenges of HIV/AIDS management: Promoting health-enabling dialogue through mediated communication. *African Journal of Rhetoric,* 1(2):10–37. http://eprints.lse.ac.uk/32173/

Campbell, C., Skovdal, M., Madanhire, C., Mugurungi, O., Gregson, S., & Nyamukapa, C. (2011). "We, the AIDS people . . .": Through what mechanisms has antiretroviral therapy created a context for ARV users to resist stigma and construct positive identities? *American Journal of Public Health,* 101(6), 1004–1010.

Englund, H. (2006). *Prisoners of freedom: Human rights and the African poor.* London: UCLA Press.

Eyben, R. (2006). *Relationships for aid.* London: Earthscan.

Freire, P. (1973). *Education for critical consciousness.* New York: Seabury Press.

Gibbs, A., Campbell, C., Maimane, S., & Nair, Y. (2010). Mismatches between youth aspirations and participatory HIV/AIDS programmes in South Africa. *African Journal of AIDS Research*, 9(2), 153–163. doi: 10.2989/16085906. 2010.517482

Gregson, S. (2012, forthcoming). Evaluation of community responses to HIV/AIDS. *AIDS Care.*

Jeanes, R. (2011). Educating through sport? Examining HIV/AIDS education and sport-for-development through the perspectives of Zambian young people. *Sport, Education and Society*, 1–19. doi: 10.1080/13573322.2011.579093

Jewkes, R. (1998). Why do nurses abuse patients? Reflections from South African obstetric services. *Social Science and Medicine*, 47 (11), 1781–1795.

Jones, E. (2001). *Of other spaces. Situating participatory practices—a case study from South India.* Sussex: IDS Working Paper 137.

Jovchelovitch, S. (2007). *Knowledge in context: Representations, community, and culture.* New York: Routledge.

Kelly, K. J., & Birdsall, K. (2010). The effects of national and international HIV/AIDS funding and governance mechanisms on the development of civil-society responses to HIV/AIDS in East and Southern Africa. *AIDS Care, 22*(sup2), 1580–1587. doi: 10.1080/09540121.2010.524191

Kim, J. C., Watts, C. H., Hargreaves, J. R., Ndhlovu, L. X., Phetla, G., Morison, L. A., . . . Pronyk, P. (2007). Understanding the impact of a microfinance-based intervention on women's empowerment and the reduction of intimate partner violence in South Africa. *Am J Public Health, 97*(10), 1794–1802. doi: 10.2105/ajph.2006.095521

Mannell, J. (2010). Gender mainstreaming in practice: Considerations for HIV/AIDS community organisations. *AIDS Care* 22 (Suppl. 2), 1613–1619.

Moulton, P. L., Miller, M. E., Offutt, S. M., & Gibbens, B. P. (2007). Identifying rural health care needs using community conversations. *The Journal of Rural Health*, 23(1), 92–96. doi: 10.1111/j.1748-0361.2006.00074.x

Mqadi, N. (2007). *External evaluation of the community responses to HIV/AIDS project.* Durban, South Africa: HIVAN.

NACC (2006). *Kenya HIV/AIDS data booklet 2006.* Republic of Kenya: National AIDS Control Council.

Nair, Y., & Campbell, C. (2008). Building partnerships to support community-led HIV/AIDS management: A case study from rural South Africa. *African Journal of AIDS Research* 7(1), pp. 45–53.

Nhamo, M., Campbell, C., & Gregson, S. (2010). Obstacles to local-level AIDS competence in rural Zimbabwe: Putting HIV prevention in context. [Research Support, Non-U.S. Gov't.] *AIDS Care*, 22 Suppl 2, 1662–1669. doi: 10.1080/09540121.2010.521544

Nyambedha, E., Wandibba, S., & Aagaard-Hansen, J. (2003). Changing patterns of orphan care due to the HIV epidemic in Western Kenya. *Social Science & Medicine*, 57(2), 301–311.

Prilleltensky, I., Nelson, G., & Peirson, L. (2001). The role of power and control in children's lives: An ecological analysis of pathways toward wellness, resilience and problems. *Journal of Community and Applied Social Psychology,* 11, 143–158.

Putnam, R. D. (2000). *Bowling alone: The collapse and revival of American community.* New York: Simon & Schuster.

Rifkin, S., & Pridmore, P. (2001). *Partners in planning. Information, participation and empowerment.* London: TALC/Macmillan Education.

Seckinelgin, H. (2012, forthcoming). The global governance of success in HIV/AIDS policy: Emergency action, everyday lives and Sen's capabilities. *Health and Place.*

Skovdal, M. (2010). Community relations and child-led microfinance: A case study of caregiving children in Kenya. *AIDS Care,* 22 Suppl 2, 1652–1661. doi: 10.1080/09540121.2010.498876

Skovdal, M. (2011a). Examining the trajectories of children providing care for adults in rural Kenya: Implications for service delivery. *Children and Youth Services Review,* 33(7), 1262–1269.

Skovdal, M. (2011b). Picturing the coping strategies of caregiving children in Western Kenya: From images to action. *American Journal of Public Health.*

Skovdal, M., & Campbell, C. (2013). Public engagement and policymaking for HIV-affected children in sub-Saharan Africa. In R. Smith (ed.), *HIV Public Policy and Policymaking.* Westport, CT: Praeger.

Skovdal, M., Mwasiaji, W., Morrison, J., & Tomkins, A. (2008). Community-based capital cash transfer to support orphans in Western Kenya: A consumer perspective. *Vulnerable Children and Youth Studies,* 3(1), 1–15.

Skovdal, M., Mwasiaji, W., Webale, A., & Tomkins, A. (2011). Building orphan competent communities: Experiences from a community-based capital cash transfer initiative in Kenya. [Research Support, Non-U.S. Gov't.] *Health Policy and Planning,* 26(3), 233–241. doi: 10.1093/heapol/czq039

Skovdal, M., & Ogutu, V. (2009). "I washed and fed my mother before going to school": Understanding the psychosocial well-being of children providing chronic care for adults affected by HIV/AIDS in Western Kenya. *Globalisation and Health,* 5:8, doi:10.1186/1744-8603-5-8

Skovdal, M., Ogutu, V., Aoro, C., & Campbell, C. (2009). Young carers as social actors: Coping strategies of children caring for ailing or ageing guardians in Western Kenya. *Social Science and Medicine,* 69(4), 587–595.

Tawil, O., Annette, V., & O'Reilly, K. (1995). Enabling approaches for HIV/AIDS promotion: Can we modify the environment and minimise the risk? *AIDS,* 9, 1299–1306.

UNDP (2004). *Upscaling community conversations in Ethiopia 2004: Unleashing capacities of communities for the HIV/AIDS response.* Addis Ababa: UNDP.

Vaughan, C. (2010). "When the road is full of potholes, I wonder why they are bringing condoms?" Social spaces for understanding young Papua New Guineans' health-related knowledge and health-promoting action. *AIDS Care, 22* (supp 2), 1644–1651. doi: 10.1080/09540121.2010.525610

Wang, C., Yi, W., Tao, Z., & Carovano, K. (1998). Photovoice as a participatory health promotion strategy. *Health Promotion International,* 13(1), 75–86.

WHO (2008). *Task shifting: Global recommendations and guidelines.* Geneva: World Health Organisation.

Wieck, K. (1984). Small wins. Defining the scale of social problems. *American Psychologist,* 39 (1), 40–49.

Woolcock, M., & Narayan, D. (2000). Social capital: Implications for development theory, research, and policy. *The World Bank Research Observer,* 15(2), 225–249.

# 5
# Citizen Scientists and Activist Researchers: Building and Sustaining HIV Prevention Research Advocacy in the "Era of Evidence"

*Emily Bass, Julien Burns, Mitchell Warren, and Deirdre Grant*

The history of the AIDS epidemic is, in part, the history of laypeople claiming the right to act as experts in the often highly technical fields of study that contribute to understanding of the virus and strategies to treat and prevent infection. Immunology, virology, pathogenesis, clinical trial protocol review, drug development, regulatory processes were just some of the arenas in which nonscientists asserted their right to informed participation. Groups like ACT UP, Treatment Action Group, Project Inform, and the AIDS Treatment and Data Network are just some of the civil society organizations in the United States that were hubs for gathering, analyzing, and disseminating information, formulating scientific agendas, and generating highly specific critiques of decisions and plans put forward by major research and policy entities such as the National Institutes of Health, the Food and Drug Administration, the office of the U.S. Trade Representative, the World Bank, and others (Hilts, 1990; *Washington Post*, 2001). There were parallel efforts in Europe, South Africa, Brazil, Thailand, and many other countries around the world (Bass, Gonsalves, & Katana, 2008).

In the early years of the epidemic, the focus of the majority of these efforts was on identifying effective treatments for opportunistic infections and antiretroviral agents that would block viral activity directly. With the syndrome of opportunistic infections that defined acquired immune deficiency syndrome, health professionals at this time were confronted with not one but many diseases that they had never seen and for which treatments were scarce, nonexistent, or poorly defined (Bayer and Oppenheimer, 2002; Shilts, 2007). The terrible reality of facing a pathogen that neither doctors nor laypeople understood, and which political leaders and federal and municipal health authorities were shockingly slow to address, was the environment in which AIDS activists became citizen scientists, fighting for their lives and the lives of the people they loved.

What exactly is a citizen scientist? In this chapter, and focusing specifically on the AIDS epidemic, we use the term to describe individuals who did not have formal training in a relevant field but nonetheless engaged in meaningful analysis of the content, goals, and strategies of one or more scientific arenas—HIV immunology, drug development, tuberculosis, clinical trials in women, and so on—fighting for and, often, securing "a place at the table" with the scientists, policymakers, and donors whose academic and professional credentials vouchsafed their presence.

Many authors, including activists themselves, have documented the tactics and remarkable successes of the AIDS activist movement and its formidable cadre of citizen scientists who learned what they had to in an effort to save their own lives and the lives of their communities (Epstein, 1998; ACT UP, 2012; Smith & Siplon, 2006). Many, if not most, of these studies have described the activism that focused on identifying and securing access to antiretrovirals (ARVs) to effectively treat HIV and opportunistic infections. The work of individuals and groups working on biomedical HIV prevention research has also been documented, though to a lesser extent (Cohen, 2001; Thomas, 2001), and largely in the context of the years when various trials were being planned and there was no proof of concept for an AIDS vaccine, a microbicide, preexposure prophylaxis (PrEP), or voluntary medical male circumcision (VMMC). The term *microbicide* is used to refer to a range of products (gels, suppositories, rings) that could be used vaginally or rectally to reduce the risk of HIV infection. PrEP is a strategy that uses antiretrovirals to reduce the risk of HIV infection in HIV-negative individuals.

This chapter seeks to establish the contours, challenges, and priorities of a new era for citizen scientists and activists working on HIV. Since 2006, there have been scientific breakthroughs in the form of positive results in efficacy trials of VMMC, an AIDS vaccine (a "prime-boost" combination of two vaccines called ALVAC and AIDSVAX), a vaginal microbicide candidate (1 percent tenofovir gel), and daily oral PrEP using the combination antiretroviral TDF/FTC (Gray et al., 2007; Bailey et al., 2007; Auvert et al., 2005; Karim & Karim, 2011; Rerks-Ngarm et al.,

2009; Grant et al., 2010; Baeten et al., 2012). These developments raise novel issues and priorities in play for advocates and activists working in this arena; new alliances and antagonisms as citizen scientists make the case for various approaches in the context of scarce resources; and unprecedented decisions about the level of benefit that warrants introduction of new strategies, even in the hardest-hit populations in the world.

The previous two decades of biomedical prevention advocacy and activism provided limited preparation for the world as it is today. In hindsight, this is not surprising. The type of advocacy needed to raise awareness about yet-to-be-identified strategies, and to engage in the conduct of ethical clinical trials that leave communities better off, involves a specific vocabulary and stakeholder array, which only partially overlaps with the language and coalitions needed to track and ensure access to strategies for which there is evidence of benefit. Moving from research to rollout, or from bench to the bush, is a complex and multilayered process. While prevention research advocates discussed and anticipated the challenges that would be involved, prior to 2006, some of the most immediately relevant experience came from research on use of ARVs in HIV-positive pregnant women during pregnancy and/or labor and/or breastfeeding to reduce the risk of passing the virus to the infant (strategies collectively known as prevention of vertical transmission) and the female condom. Trials of strategies to prevent vertical transmission provoked early controversies about the ethics of placebo-control trial design in prevention studies, when short-course regimens such as single-dose nevirapine were evaluated in placebo-controlled trials in developing countries after a longer, AZT-based regimen showed efficacy and was adopted as standard of care in the United States and Europe. Impassioned debates about the appropriate standard of prevention and care for participants in prevention trials have continued since then. On the implementation side, both the female condom and programs to prevent vertical transmission have been introduced as public health interventions (albeit very different ones), and the experiences associated with program design, financing, messaging, staffing and evaluation provide salutary lessons in the challenges of bringing interventions with known benefit to scale.

However, while lessons from the experiences are important, neither of these interventions is a direct analogy for the current context. What has emerged and is still in process is a new set of advocacy tools and tactics, deployed by citizen scientists with questions and demands that were impossible to frame until very recently. The necessity of creating advocacy strategies in the context of mixed and positive evidence has caused important shifts—several of which are discussed below—whose significance and effectiveness will be judged in years to come.

## "MIND THE GAPS": CHALLENGES IN THE NEW ERA OF BIOMEDICAL PREVENTION RESEARCH ADVOCACY

Broadly speaking, advocates and activists working in biomedical prevention research focused on three broad types of activity prior to 2005. First: tracking the plans, priorities, and funding levels of biomedical prevention research efforts (AVAC, 1998–2004). Second: critiquing trial designs (McGrory, Irvin, & Heise, 2009; Forbes & Mudaliar, 2009: Burton et al., 2004). Third: raising awareness of and community demand for new prevention strategies.

So, for example, the AIDS Vaccine Advocacy Coalition (AVAC) began its activities in 1995 with a report tracking industry involvement in AIDS vaccine research, and a subsequent campaign demanding that the National Institutes of Health set transparent milestones for its AIDS vaccine research program (AVAC, 1998). In terms of critiquing trial design, some of the earliest biomedical prevention research engagement in Africa focused on the ethical implications of conducting placebo-controlled trials of PMTCT regimens, including short-course nevirapine, given the evidence that extended AZT was highly effective (NIAID, 2005; HPTN, 2011). Other trials that received intense focus and often criticism include proposed trials of an AIDS vaccine in Thailand; preexposure prophylaxis in Cambodia, Cameroon, Ghana, Nigeria, and Thailand (McGrory, Irvin, & Heise, 2009; Forbes & Mudaliar, 2009; Peterson et al., 2007); and a planned microbicide trial in Zambia (*Lusaka Times*, 2009). These controversies, while not the focus of this chapter, have been described in a number of publications and were the impetus behind the development of the Good Participatory Practice Guidelines for Biomedical Prevention Research (AVAC & UNAIDS, 2011), a guidance document that maps best practice for stakeholder engagement before, during, and after a trial, and which has been recognized by U.S. President Barack Obama as being a foundational tool for all clinical research (AVAC, 2011).

The third area of activity—raising awareness of new strategies—involves educating various constituencies, including potential users, policymakers, service providers, and others about the possibility of and pipeline for new strategies such as a microbicide, PrEP, or an AIDS vaccine. Such activities are ongoing and obviously essential to mobilizing any additional steps—what has changed, as is described in this chapter, is some of the content and much of the context for these discussions.

Prior to 2005, all of the efforts described above took place in a "data-free" zone. Simply put: nothing worked. There were no clues or findings that could definitively point scientists down one path and close off others for these new prevention options. There was no proof of concept—for example, evidence of effectiveness in a human clinical trial—for a candidate microbicide, PrEP, or a vaccine. While great strides were made in treating HIV infection and opportunistic infections, the prevention "tool box" in 2005 was almost identical to what it had been 10 years earlier.

All of this began to change in 2005 with the data from the randomized controlled trial of male circumcision for HIV prevention in Orange Farm, South Africa (Auvert et al., 2005). In 2006, trials of male circumcision in Uganda and Kenya confirmed this result (Gray et al., 2007; Bailey et al., 2007). In 2009, the trial known as RV144, which enrolled 16,000 people in Thailand, became the first vaccine trial to find evidence that a vaccine regimen had protected against HIV infection (Rerks-Ngarm et al., 2009). In 2010, the CAPRISA 004 trial of the microbicide candidate 1 percent tenofovir gel found evidence of protection among 889 South African women (Abdool Karim et al., 2010). Later that year, the iPrEx trial of oral preexposure prophylaxis using tenofovir-emtricitabine (TDF-FTC) found efficacy among gay men and transgender women (Grant et al., 2010). In 2011, HPTN 052 reported that treating an HIV-infected individual who had a CD4 cell count between 350 and 550 nearly eliminated his or her chances of transmitting the virus to an uninfected stable partner, when compared to HIV-infected individuals who delayed treatment initiation until they met the criteria set by their national guidelines (Cohen et al., 2011).

Thus in half a decade, there have been more positive results from biomedical HIV prevention trials than there were in the previous two decades of the epidemic. Some of these results, like CAPRISA 004, have been followed by trials of identical or similar strategies, which showed no effect in different populations or using different dosing strategies. Others, like the Orange Farm trial of VMMC, were followed in quick succession by two other trials in Rakai, Uganda, and Kisumu, Kenya, which found highly comparable levels of effectiveness. The concordance of these three trials, in different populations, age ranges, and using different surgical techniques, has been called an epidemiological grand slam—but as is discussed in the next section, even this level of evidence has eliminated skepticism and opposition to the new intervention.

As the results—positive, confounding, negative—have flowed in since 2005, the data-free zone has given way to a complex, even congested territory in which advocates, activists, and scientists compare and contrast the evidence for multiple strategies that have shown proof of concept, with vociferous debates about feasibility, timing, and necessity of implementation, future research agendas, and resource allocation as funds grow increasingly scarce.

The most immediate challenge in the context of the "data-full" zone has been parsing what a positive trial result means, particularly in practical terms to the communities who have been recruited as advocates for research into new strategies—a major thrust of biomedical prevention research advocacy until 2005 and through the present. The work that had been done to raise awareness of and demand for new tools did not prepare communities for the nuances of a trial result showing modest evidence of benefit.

In the pre-2005 world, biomedical HIV prevention research advocates worked in a theoretical space. No one could predict what a product would look like, or what level of effectiveness it would achieve, and though there were a range of publications and curricula that focused on the concept of "partial efficacy," these all dwelt in the intangible realm of future possibility (Bass, 2005). At the most basic level, the message to stakeholders was: If a product moves through Phase I, II, and III trials with positive safety and/or efficacy findings at the conclusion of each trial—then it will become available. The numbered phases of clinical trials refer to a general progression from trials in relatively small numbers of people to establish safety and, sometimes, define optimal dosing strategies and gather other relevant information (Phase I), to larger trials that gather additional safety information in a broader range of individuals (Phase II), to trials measuring the product's efficacy or effectiveness in reducing HIV risk (Phase III). There are nuances and caveats, such as the need for confirmatory trials and for studies to establish efficacy in other populations (e.g., adolescents), but for many years, the overall message was seemingly simple: Support the research, and the product will come.

The truth, as evidenced by the past six years, is far more complicated. As one trial after another has yielded evidence of modest or moderate efficacy, advocates have confronted the reality that evidence from a single trial does not lead to immediate implementation. For some trials (PrEP, microbicide, vaccine), this is because the initial proof of concept needs to be followed up with confirmatory trials and a regulatory approval process. For others (e.g., VMMC), even with relatively swift activity on the part of normative agencies—the WHO and UNAIDS issued guidance recommending VMMC as a new HIV prevention tool within four months of the initial data from the Ugandan and Kenyan trials—the pace of implementation has been uneven and often slow in the countries that stand to benefit most (WHO & UNAIDS, 2007).

None of these scenarios has conformed to a "Phase 1, 2, 3—then access" model, where a new intervention progresses smoothly through safety, dosing, and efficacy trials with unambiguous results and then is made immediately available to those who need it. Nor have theoretical conversations about partially effective products prepared communities and individuals for consensus on "how good is good enough" when it comes to a new strategy. The concepts that were the foundation of affirmative, product development–oriented advocacy prior to 2005 were simply not sophisticated enough for the conversations that needed to happen in the era of positive results.

Hence, the first challenge for biomedical prevention advocates working since 2005 has been to expand and refine their vocabulary for describing trial results and the various sequences of events that can be expected after an initial proof of concept. CAPRISA 004 reduced participants' risk of acquiring HIV by approximately 39 percent with a 95 percent confidence interval of 6 to 60 percent. (In this example, 39 percent is the "point estimate" for the product's efficacy. In any trial, this estimate is situated within a range of possible values—in this instance, 6 to 60 percent. The 95 percent confidence interval reflects that there is at most a 5 percent chance that the positive result occurred by chance.) In the iPrEx trial of oral TDF/FTC as PrEP among gay men and transgender women, the benefit was around 44 percent with a confidence interval of 15–63 percent; and in the case of the Thai RV144 trial, the benefit was 31 percent with a confidence interval of 1–51 percent (Karim & Karim, 2011). Are these results positive, disappointing, modest, or meaningful? What types of confidence intervals are communities comfortable with? Should every positive signal from a trial trigger another randomized controlled trial to confirm the result—common practice in drug development—or are there cases where the initial strategy has drawbacks that make it more prudent to take the "proof of concept" (the first positive evidence associated with a new strategy—e.g., the positive result from RV144 provided the proof of concept that an AIDS vaccine is possible) as a green light for refining and accelerating testing of second-generation products?

Between 2005 and 2012, much biomedical prevention research advocacy and education/outreach has been concerned with how to react to, understand, and advocate around—or across—the gap between the completion of a trial with a positive result and the launch of the next step—be it a follow-on confirmatory trial, demonstration project, development of a national guideline, or other policy. The latter scenario is affected by a range of variables—many quite technical—which can hinder advocacy engagement.

Paradoxically, it can be harder to formulate an advocacy demand after a positive research result than it is in the absence of such data. One of the most vivid recent examples of this concerned the aftermath of the CAPRISA 004 microbicide trial, which showed an overall HIV prevention benefit of 39 percent (see previous explanation of the statistical finding). Following this initial result, some advocates argued that additional placebo-controlled trials were unnecessary and even unethical and that open-label access programs should be used to gather additional data on safety and effectiveness. Other advocates supported follow-on research, which included the ongoing VOICE trial that was testing the same product in a different dosing strategy (Stein & Susser, 2010). Here the argument was that gathering more precise data on the strategy would lead to stronger programs and social marketing efforts, as well as a more robust regulatory dossier for licensure.

Other advocates who were aware of the initial positive result but less engaged with the debate on what follow-on trials, if any, should look like, expressed confusion and consternation about the apparent delay in the next steps—summed up succinctly as, "Where the hell's the gel?" (Coulterman, 2011).

The era of evidence has also brought the field of biomedical prevention research into immediate dialogue with a far broader array of stakeholders than followed this arena prior to 2005. With the prospect of new prevention strategies competing for scant resources and potentially representing the hope to turn the tide of the epidemic—or consume resources desperately needed for basic services—advocates, activists and other stakeholders traditionally focused on treatment and prevention have begun to weigh in on the appropriateness of new prevention options. With complete justification, individuals and communities who paid little or no attention to the hypothetical interventions prior to the first proof of concept in the form of positive evidence from an efficacy trial are now concerned, interested, enthusiastic, or wary of the potential that a new tool could be on the horizon. Thus the first challenge—refining the vocabulary—is firmly linked to a second one: developing a common language and/or advocacy agenda with an expanded array of stakeholders.

A third, interconnected challenge is developing a coherent advocacy agenda for biomedical prevention research that spans interventions, rather than focusing on one or more specific strategies. At the precise moment when it is necessary to parse the development pathways for a microbicide versus oral PrEP using TDF/FTC versus an AIDS vaccine based on ALVAC-gp120, it is also necessary to develop an agenda and outlook that brings all of these interventions and others, such as earlier treatment of HIV to reduce infectiousness in HIV-positive people, together into a single, coherent advocacy—and action—platform. Maintaining specificity while forging linkages between various interventions—this challenge, which is only possible when the previously described issues have been addressed, may be the most important of all.

## EMERGING SOLUTIONS: THE NEW ERA OF IMPLEMENTATION ADVOCACY

The previous section outlines three core challenges in the new era of biomedical prevention research and implementation advocacy: revising the vocabulary for discussing trial results and follow-on scenarios for specific products or interventions including PrEP, microbicides, vaccines, and VMMC; creating and executing a common agenda with a broader array of stakeholders; and building an advocacy movement that persuasively and effectively articulates the need for a range of new strategies—a comprehensive approach—while keeping the focus on the critical next steps for specific interventions. This section seeks to identify some of the tactics and approaches that have emerged as potential solutions to these defining conditions of the new era of biomedical prevention advocacy and activism.

### Revising the Vocabulary

Adding nuance to the vocabulary used to describe trial results and follow-on scenarios is both critical and persistently challenging. Starting in early 2009 with the release of data from the MDP 301 microbicide trial that showed a nonstatistically significant trend toward efficacy among women who received a topical gel candidate known as PRO 2000, there has been an uptick in efforts to (self-) educate about statistical analysis, with particular focus on the confidence intervals surrounding a point estimate, the $p$ value, and the point estimate itself (Karim, 2010). Advocacy groups began stressing that the point estimate—the single value that is the "best guess" for the efficacy of an intervention, and that is often the only piece of data to make it into media coverage—is not the full picture of a trial result (AVAC, 2009). Prespecified and post-hoc analyses also became increasingly relevant. A prespecified analysis is one that is planned for as part of the trial's original design—comparing rate of infections in the experimental and placebo arms of HIV prevention trials is an example of a prespecified analysis for an HIV prevention trial. Post-hoc analysis is one that is undertaken after the data are available. It can reveal a trend, but because it was not part of the trial's original design, post-hoc analysis is not as powerful in terms of drawing conclusions about the data. In the case of the RV144 AIDS vaccine trial, post-hoc analysis of infection rates at 12 months after immunization showed that the vaccine strategy reduced infection risk by about 60 percent. This waned over time to the 31.2 percent reported in the final, prespecified analysis. Still, the post-hoc analysis finding at 12 months led to efforts focused on sustaining that level of efficacy with an improved regimen.

This is not entirely new territory: The statistical skill set required to analyze the results from data on prevention trials is not dissimilar from that required to analyze the results of treatment trials, with the critical difference being that HIV treatment trials have historically focused on delay in disease progression, control of viral load, or CD4 cell decline, and the majority of HIV prevention trials focus on new infections averted. But if the broad parameters are similar, the framework for interpretation is quite different. A marginal improvement in quality of life or risk of death is quite different from a marginal improvement in prevention. If a new drug has 30 percent less toxicity or reduces morbidity from tuberculosis, for example, by 30 percent compared to existing interventions, this will likely be considered a clear-cut success. But it is not as clear that an HIV prevention strategy that reduces risk by 30 percent should be adopted as a public health intervention. This is especially true given continuing concerns that male and female condoms, harm reduction, and other highly effective prevention tools remain underfunded and underutilized.

The greatest successes in this arena have been due, in part, to trial teams developing clear roadmaps for how they would react on the basis of a given result—prior to the results being released. One exemplary instance is the Thailand-based RV144 trial, which had a multi-component plan for next steps in the instance of results of low, moderate, or high efficacy (Hankins, Macklin, Michael, & Stablein, 2010). The clarity provided by the trial team framed the discussion for advocates and largely dissipated debates about whether placebo recipients should be given access to the vaccine, whether the vaccine warranted further study, and so on.

Other strategies include providing forums—both in-person and virtual—for researchers to explain their findings and their implications immediately after the release of trial results. Global teleconferences, stakeholder engagement meetings, and community-focused sessions at scientific conferences have all been used to speed and streamline the process of disseminating new results. Such "real-time" responses to emerging data provide the opportunity for stakeholders to work together to revise the vocabulary based on the results of a specific trial.

The challenge, which is further explored in the following section, is that adjusting expectations after a positive result so that advocates no longer expect immediate or even imminent access can also result in a loss of advocacy momentum or enthusiasm. The question "Where the hell's the gel?" raised by women advocates at an AIDS conference in 2011 is both an activist-oriented demand and a genuine question reflecting confusion about what appropriate next steps might be given the modest efficacy seen in CAPRISA 004 and the flat result seen in the VOICE trial in late 2011.

In the preresults era, the focus of advocacy and activism was on mobilizing demand and research activity focused on new strategies. This work is ongoing, but the new vocabulary is much more focused on managing expectations so that a positive result is not seen as triggering immediate access. Success is, in some ways, measured by demands that do not get made. Informed advocates understand that a product showing modest effect in a single Phase IIb trial (an intermediate-sized trial, usually smaller than a full-scale Phase III efficacy trial, which can provide an initial indication of efficacy but is generally not designed to meet the requirements for seeking product licensure by a regulatory authority such as the U.S. Food and Drug Administration; Phase IIb trials are often followed by Phase III confirmatory trials) with wide confidence intervals should be evaluated in an additional trial. But silence is not the sought-after condition of successful advocacy and activism. Rather, as the following section explores, the key is to develop a cadre committed to advocating for incremental next steps over the long haul.

## Broadening the Coalition

If the prevention research advocate's challenge is to manage expectations and work in increments, it is also to garner allies among the activists, implementers, donors, and policymakers who will be needed to ensure eventual access, even if it is many years down the road. Securing theoretical good will—"sure, I will support a microbicide if one becomes available"—is much easier than securing support for an emerging strategy with initial proof-of-concept in the context of many other real-time priorities and issues.

Responses to VMMC represent one of the more striking examples of the friction between prevention research–oriented advocates and potential allies around a new biomedical prevention strategy. VMMC is the most rigorously validated new biomedical prevention strategy. It is the only one that has been implemented on a broad scale; unlike strategies currently under investigation, its effectiveness is lifelong and based on a one-time intervention. For all of these positive aspects—and comparisons to a 60 percent effective vaccine—many advocates were hesitant to embrace VMMC as a "campaign" issue or focus for sustained pressure on governments or donors to set and meet targets, as has been the case for ARV treatment, PMTCT, condom distribution, and many other interventions.

Where did the resistance come from? There are no simple answers, but rather a multiplicity of factors. Women's groups raised strong concerns that a male-targeted strategy would divert resources away from women-controlled prevention and would embolden men to refuse condoms, coerce women into sex, and increase their number of sexual partners (AVAC, 2010; AVAC, 2008). There was a fear that the public health or individual HIV prevention benefit from the intervention would be overwhelmed by other effects unrelated to the inherent effectiveness of the strategy. The advent of the VMMC results also coincided with a vigorous advocacy movement around health care human resources. While there was no formal opposition to VMMC as such, advocates and activists focused on the health care worker issue were initially more likely to raise concerns about feasibility of the intervention than to add it to the list of strategies to be implemented by already overtaxed health care systems.

Perhaps the biggest hurdle was low awareness among the groups and individuals in African countries who would make natural allies and champions of new interventions. In 2006 and 2007, when the data were emerging, these groups were largely focused on tracking other interventions, particularly ART rollout. Knowledge of VMMC was low and, in countries such as Uganda or South Africa where the government did not take a supportive position immediately, there was a general sense of not being convinced that the findings were relevant to the current context.

The strategies that have emerged in response to these conditions of wariness, overt opposition, and passive disinterest are: (1) validating concerns—using them as the basis for engagement; (2) strategic use of epidemiological modeling with a focus on country-specific data; and (3) identifying principles and expectations of policymakers—that is, that positive findings should prompt a government reaction—and mobilizing around those expectations and principles, even as support for the intervention itself was being consolidated.

So, for example, a civil society coalition worked in conjunction with the World Health Organization and UNAIDS to hold joint discussions about VMMC and implications for women, and then followed up with a series of small grants designed for women to document the experiences with VMMC introduction in their communities. In some settings, women realized that the slow pace was the issue—not the potential implications for women, as no one male or female was being impacted by the service—and shifted gears. Four years later, many of these women's groups are now forerunners of informed, focused advocacy campaigns for VMMC (AVAC, 2008; AVAC, 2010).

Another key tool for advocacy has been increasingly specific epidemiological impact modeling, which projects the effect on HIV incidence if countries achieve their VMMC targets. As the rhetoric and reality around the epidemic have moved into a discussion of "an AIDS-free generation" or "ending AIDS in our lifetime," the rationale for dramatic scale-up of new strategies has become more compelling (Clinton, 2011; Obama, 2011). Models showing the impact of VMMC or accelerated treatment initiation for people with HIV also show that immediate investment can lead to long-term savings in funds, new infections, and lives (Hankins et al., 2011). This type of impact projection is a powerful mobilizer. In particular, it has helped to dissipate some, though not all, of the concern from many stakeholders that it's not possible to spend more on the AIDS response when existing resources are stretched thin and coverage of needed interventions is still far from universal. Current models suggest that spending more now will actually save money in the long term, shifting the argument from "we cannot afford to scale up evidence-based strategies" to "we cannot afford not to scale up evidence-based strategies." One of the most immediate tensions in biomedical prevention research today involves the role of preexposure prophylaxis (PrEP) versus "treatment as prevention" or earlier treatment initiation (at CD4 cell counts >350) to both preserve health and reduce infectiousness in people living with HIV. The iPrEx, Partners PrEP, and TDF2 trials all evaluated daily oral PrEP using TDF or TDF/FTC in HIV-negative people. All of these trials found moderate to high levels of risk reduction compared to the trial participants in the placebo arm (Baeten et al., 2012). These trials also have found that risk reduction is directly linked to adherence—PrEP only works if it is taken as prescribed. They have also found that when people take the drug, their risk of HIV is reduced—often quite dramatically. The benefit has been seen in heterosexual men and women, men who have sex with men, and transgender women.

The PrEP results came in the same 12-month period as results from HPTN 052, which found earlier treatment dramatically reduced risk of transmission to the HIV-negative partner in a serodiscordant couple (Cohen et al., 2011) and also provided clinical benefit to the HIV-positive partner, specifically in terms of reduction in morbidity associated with extrapulmonary tuberculosis. "Treatment as prevention" is the first new biomedical prevention tool for HIV-positive individuals and has the added benefit of being a "double" or even "triple-whammy" in that it also preserves health and life, and, in preliminary results from the trial, reduced risk of extrapulmonary tuberculosis.

Tension—sometimes creative, frequently uncomfortable—is inevitable in a world where there is the potential to use ARVs as prevention in both HIV-negative and -positive individuals. The drugs tested in the first generation of PrEP trials are well tolerated, have simple dosing regimens, and have unique resistance profiles. (As it replicates, HIV makes errors in its genetic code and some of these mutations can give rise to viral strains that are not susceptible to antiretrovirals. The specific mutations that make HIV resistant to particular drugs are known as the resistance profile. TDF and TDF/FTC-resistant HIV are still susceptible to many other antiretrovirals.) Because of these characteristics, the drugs are highly sought after as first-line treatment for HIV-positive people. The possibility of introducing PrEP using TDF or TDF/FTC at a time when people with HIV still need the drug is unacceptable to many, if not all, stakeholders engaged in the discussion. At the same time, it is difficult for many prevention advocates to accept complete foreclosure of a tool (daily oral PrEP) that could reduce HIV risk for many individuals—including married women who often cannot negotiate condom use, even with partners of known HIV-positive status. While the debate often takes more nuanced forms, these "zero-sum" terms have been made explicit and are part of the divide that has to be bridged if biomedical prevention research advocacy is to remain relevant in the era of positive results.

Here, one essential step is refining goals and expectations for new interventions. A broad-reaching skepticism about the feasibility of PrEP—summed up, frequently, by statements like "we can't put tenofovir in the drinking water"—is reasonable as long as the presumption is that antiretrovirals would be given to all HIV-negative sexually active adults, as condoms presently are. The conversation shifts when advocates identify the specific populations who might benefit from the intervention: for example, women who cannot successfully or consistently negotiate condom use and seek a method that lends itself to discrete or covert use; women or men in serodiscordant relationships whose partner may not be willing or able to initiate highly effective antiretroviral therapy. Once the discourse moves away from a presumption of universal access—the foundation of the AIDS treatment movement—and to definition of specific niche approaches, stakeholders who may have been staunchly opposed to the intervention become cautiously neutral—and may even become allies.

Successful advocacy also depends in many instances on holding repeated consultations and smaller one-on-one briefings with key stakeholders, in order to build awareness of and familiarity with an intervention well before trial results are available. As an example, Kenyan and Ugandan stakeholder engagement on PrEP began three years before there were data from the trials taking place in those countries. In these two countries, a loose coalition of allies including research teams, civil society groups, and international partners organized one to two meetings per year, as well as follow-up briefings with key individuals such as members of drug regulatory authorities and members of national AIDS control programs.

As research results were published, the leadership for some of these convenings was shifted from the trial sponsors—who could be perceived to have a stake in the outcome of the conversation—to neutral parties and then to national-level actors. In mid-2011, the Ugandan UNAIDS country office helped to convene a dialogue on PrEP; later in that same year, the Ministry of Health AIDS Control Program took the lead in convening a follow-up dialogue.

The progression in leadership on an issue from research sponsors to normative agency to national health policy entities is not a given. It can stall at multiple points and/or result in meetings with no tangible outcomes. In the most successful processes, civil society advocates have both tracked and participated in every stage of the consultations. They have often been the individuals to raise the need for an additional meeting, identify the ideal convener, highlight key issues, and push for such a meeting to happen. In other words, advocates have helped to map the processes by which research results can be turned into policy. In the many instances where no map existed, they have helped to create one by assigning responsibility and demanding accountability.

The need for multiple meetings to build stakeholder commitment and consensus is not, in and of itself, a novelty in the AIDS response overall. But within the arena of biomedical prevention research, the first 20 years were largely defined by stakeholder engagement initiated by research sponsors. While civil society worked on raising awareness of and, in most cases, support for research on new options, the research sponsors and in-country teams engaged policymakers, regulatory authorities, and key decision makers in support of the proposed research. Some civil society efforts focused on country-level planning for or investment in research, but the most detailed engagement was between national authorities and research entities.

In this new era, civil society demand for, and leadership on, dialogues that are not led by research entities has been essential to advancing conversations on potential implementation. These dialogues might have faltered if research entities were perceived to be pushing their own agenda. In today's context, there is increasing trust by research entities that civil society stakeholders acting independently of research groups will realize outcomes that synergize with the goals of the research process. This is a significant evolution from earlier days of biomedical prevention research advocacy in which affirmative civil society engagement with specific trials at a national level was relatively uncommon outside of formal community advisory mechanisms.

Today, trials *and* interventions have civil society champions and, while there is still anxiety about representation and accuracy, research teams are increasingly aware of the potential benefits of advocacy allies seeking to catalyze action based on their findings.

## Creating a Comprehensive Agenda

If advocacy in the "era of evidence" is concerned with defining expectations and niches for emerging products and mapping research-to-rollout pathways, it is also deeply engaged with dismantling the intervention-specific "silos" (advocacy and activity focused specifically and exclusively on development of a microbicide or a vaccine or PrEP instead of work across common issues) that have been a historical reality, and replacing them with an agenda framed around "combination prevention" (Clinton, 2011; Tutu, 2011). Combination prevention, a phrase that is gaining increased popularity, is understood in various ways. In terms of public health strategy, it refers to coordinated use of multiple evidence-based prevention options (VMMC, ARVs for treatment, prevention of vertical transmission) to efficiently stop the spread of the virus. In practice, this translates into agendas that push for increased expenditures and strategic planning on both treatment-as-prevention *and* voluntary medical male circumcision, while also keeping a focus on the potential impact of tenofovir-based PrEP in the near- to mid-term, other ARV-based topical and oral prevention in the mid-to-long-term, and a preventive vaccine and a cure in our lifetimes. This is a busy and even cacophonous agenda, especially at the country level, where a PrEP trial or microbicide trial may be concluding or launching even as a dialogue about ending AIDS using VMMC and TasP is getting underway.

Here, the most successful advocacy strategy has hinged on the argument that a combination of interventions implemented rapidly, strategically, and efficiently can help to end the AIDS epidemic in our lifetimes. The success of this tactic depends on carefully marshaled evidence, particularly modeling of the course of HIV with and without scale-up of key interventions and funding streams (Schwartländer et al., 2011; Hankins et al., 2011; Blandford, 2012).

In Kenya, a coalition of advocates shared PEPFAR modeling projections on the trajectory of the epidemic with and without accelerated rollout of ARVs to people living with HIV. The difference in impact is striking—as is the projection that maintaining current spending levels will result in a relatively flat slope for rates of new infections. As a result of this "teach-in" on impact modeling, civil society launched a successful campaign to secure expanded AIDS spending commitments from the Kenyan national government. These commitments, in turn, were leveraged to secure an increased investment in ARV treatment from the PEPFAR country program.

The use of data on population-level prevention impacts is not unheard of—though many arguments for expansion of ARV programs have been made on the basis of benefit to individual health and cost savings to employers, health, and formal and informal social welfare systems. What is new and profoundly energizing is an advocacy argument that predicts an end to the AIDS epidemic if specific goals are met in the near- and midterm. Also exciting is the degree to which prevention outcomes are at the heart of this argument—without coming at the expense of treatment for people living with HIV. Looking ahead, the most successful and, arguably, impactful advocacy for the coming five to 10 years will almost certainly be generated by coalitions of prevention and treatment advocates combining their agendas, tactics, and skill sets to work toward a single ambitious but utterly necessary goal.

## THE SEARCH CONTINUES: FAMILIAR CHALLENGES AND UNCHARTED TERRITORY FOR CLINICAL TRIALS–RELATED ADVOCACY

Perhaps the greatest challenge facing biomedical prevention research advocacy is the need to capitalize on the momentum of the movement to begin to end AIDS using existing tools more efficiently and at the level of population coverage that is projected to have the optimal impact—while also sustaining support for ongoing trials of emerging strategies including PrEP, microbicides, and a vaccine. *Why* do more clinical trials need to happen if we already have the tools we need today? A closely related question is: *How* can we do clinical trials—which must, by definition, take place in the context of some measurable HIV incidence—when we have tools to bring incidence down to negligible levels?

In developing countries, some of the most passionate advocacy regarding the "why" question has come from individuals and communities who have historically been underserved by existing prevention strategies. Paradoxically, or perhaps inevitably, communities that have received limited attention from HIV prevention programming and/or have been unable to utilize the strategies that have been offered to them have become passionate advocates for emerging technologies. So, for example, gay men and other men who have sex with men, along with transgender women, have become outspoken PrEP and rectal microbicide advocates—even as they affirm and eloquently describe the structural barriers of criminalizing legislation and rampant homophobia, along with the lack of basic prevention: lube, condoms, stigma-free clinics, and service providers (Project ARM, 2012; Amfar et al., 2011).

Women, including women living with HIV, also remain mobilized around the need for sustained research. There is a vibrant history of grassroots awareness-raising and advocacy for women-controlled HIV prevention focused primarily on female condoms and microbicides. More recently, both PrEP and TasP have been configured as potentially female-controlled prevention strategies, with HIV-positive women vocalizing the need for PrEP for both men and women. As one participant at a community consultation said, "I want PrEP because I am HIV-positive and I don't want the burden of prevention to be on me as an HIV-positive woman."

Women have been vocal in calling for further research, including continued investigation of specific interventions such as a slow-release, microbicide-infused ring or long-acting injectable PrEP agent. They have also been clear that biomedical research has to take place in the context of sociobehavioral research and consultation to understand what women's needs, priorities, and questions are regarding emerging interventions.

If there is consensus on the fact that research must continue, there is far less clarity about what these future trials might look like in terms of their design and the standard of prevention offered to participants and communities. This debate has been active over the course of biomedical prevention research with notable discussions about whether or not to incorporate ARV treatment for HIV-infected participants into vaccine trials between 2000 and 2004 (prior to the introduction of free or low-cost antiretroviral therapy for people with HIV in developing countries), or what to provide for participants who became infected in a proposed PrEP trial in

Cambodia and Cameroon. The issue emerged again in the context of the Phambili AIDS vaccine trial in South Africa, which launched in 2007 just after data showed that VMMC was highly effective in that country, but before the national government had developed a VMMC policy (AVAC, 2007; SAAVI, 2007). And it is almost certainly going to emerge when planned vaccine trials, second-generation PrEP trials, and other clinical research are proposed in communities that have validated PrEP treatment as prevention, and possibly a microbicide.

If the territory is familiar, the solutions are not. Now that evidence has emerged about which tools work well—and which may work in the future—the argument is to implement the most effective tools we have at the scale that is needed to truly alter the course of the epidemic. It's possible, and highly desirable, to imagine a context in which VMMC, treatment as prevention, targeted PrEP, and a range of other offerings are in place such that incidence slows dramatically—and even stops. This audacious vision of an end to the epidemic of new infections is years from coming to fruition. But the creative tensions and frictions at play in the world of biomedical prevention research today are the growing pains of a movement seeking to ensure that it does.

## BIBLIOGRAPHY

Abdool Karim, Q., Abdool Karim, S. S., Frohlich, J. A., Grobler, A. C., Baxter, C., Mansoor, L. E., Kharsany, A. B. M., et al. (2010). Effectiveness and Safety of Tenofovir Gel, an Antiretroviral Microbicide, for the Prevention of HIV Infection in Women. *Science, 329*(5996), 1168–1174. doi:10.1126/science.1193748

ACT UP (2012). *ACT UP Oral History Project.* Retrieved April 2, 2012, from http://www.actuporalhistory.org/

Amfar, Foundation for AIDS Research, Johns Hopkins University–Center for Public Health and Human Rights, UNDP, & IAVI (2011). *Respect, Protect, Fulfill: Best Practices Guidance in Conducting HIV Research with Gay, Bisexual, and Other Men Who Have Sex with Men (MSM) in Rights-Constrained Environments.*

Auvert, B., Taljaard, D., Lagarde, E., Sobngwi-Tambekou, J., Sitta, R., & Puren, A. (2005). Randomized, Controlled Intervention Trial of Male Circumcision for Reduction of HIV Infection Risk: The ANRS 1265 Trial. *PLoS Med, 2*(11), e298. doi:10.1371/journal.pmed.0020298

AVAC (1998). *AVAC Report: 9 Years and Counting: Will We Have an HIV Vaccine by 2007?* (1). New York: AVAC.

AVAC (1998–2004). *AVAC Report* (1–7). New York: AVAC.

AVAC (2007). *AVAC Report: Resetting the Clock* (10). New York: AVAC.

AVAC (2008). *Meeting Report: Civil Society Dialogue on Male Circumcision for HIV Prevention: Implications for Women.* Mombasa, Kenya: AVAC. Retrieved from http://www.malecircumcision.org/publications/documents/Mombasa_civil_society_meeting_MC_implications_women.pdf

AVAC (2009). *AVAC Guide to Statistical Terms.* AVAC. Retrieved from http://www.avac.org/ht/a/GetDocumentAction/i/4255

AVAC (2010). *Making Medical Male Circumcision Work for Women: Report of the Women's HIV Prevention Tracking Project (WHiPT).* New York: AVAC.

AVAC (2011, December 20). Commission for Bioethics Cites GPP as Essential for Community Engagement. *Advocate's Network.* New York.

AVAC & UNAIDS (2011). *Good Participatory Practices for Biomedical Prevention Research.* Geneva, Switzerland.

Baeten, J., Donald, D., Ndase, P., Mugo, N., Mujugira, A., & Celum, C. (2012, March 6). *ARV PrEP for HIV-1 Prevention among Heterosexual Men and Women.* Presented at the Conference on Retroviruses and Opportunistic Infections, Seattle, Washington.

Bailey, R. C., Moses, S., Parker, C. B., Agot, K., Maclean, I., Krieger, J. N., Williams, C. F., et al. (2007). Male Circumcision for HIV Prevention in Young Men in Kisumu, Kenya: A Randomised Controlled Trial. *The Lancet, 369*(9562), 643–656. doi:10.1016/S0140-6736(07)60312-2

Bass, E. (2005). Partially Effective Vaccines. In P. Kahn (ed.), *AIDS Vaccine Handbook.* New York: AVAC.

Bass, E., Gonsalves, G., & Katana, M. (2008). Advocacy, Activism, Community and the AIDS Response in Africa. In D. Celentano & C. Beyrer (eds.), *Public Health Aspects of HIV/AIDS in Low and Middle Income Countries: Epidemiology, Prevention and Care* (pp. 151–170). New York: Springer.

Bayer, R., & Oppenheimer, G. M. (2002). *AIDS Doctors: Voices from the Epidemic: An Oral History.* Oxford University Press.

Blandford, J. (2012, January 26). *Global Webinar: The Impact of Treatment as Prevention—Models to Guide Ending the Epidemic.* Presented at the AVAC. Retrieved from http://www.avac.org/ht/d/ContentDetails/i/41812

Boyle, G. J., & Hill, G. (2011). Sub-Saharan African Randomised Clinical Trials into Male Circumcision and HIV Transmission: Methodological, Ethical and Legal Concerns. *Journal of Law and Medicine, 19*(2), 316–334.

Burton, D. R., Desrosiers, R. C., Doms, R. W., Feinberg, M. B., Gallo, R. C., Hahn, B., Hoxie, J. A., et al. (2004). A Sound Rationale Needed for Phase III HIV-1 Vaccine Trials. *Science, 303*(5656), 316–316. doi:10.1126/science.1094620

Clinton, H. R. (2011, November 8). Remarks on "Creating an AIDS-Free Generation." Retrieved from http://www.state.gov/secretary/rm/2011/11/176810.htm

Cohen, J. (2001). *Shots in the Dark: The Wayward Search for an AIDS Vaccine.* W. W. Norton.

Cohen, M. S., Chen, Y. Q., McCauley, M., Gamble, T., Hosseinipour, M. C., Kumarasamy, N., Hakim, J. G., et al. (2011). Prevention of HIV-1 Infection with Early Antiretroviral Therapy. *New England Journal of Medicine, 365*(6), 493–505. doi:10.1056/NEJMoa1105243

Coulterman, A. (2011, December 1). *Where the Hell Is the Gel? NGO Delegation to the UNAIDS PCB.* Retrieved from http://unaidspcbngo.org/?p=15682

Epstein, S. (1998). *Impure Science: AIDS, Activism, and the Politics of Knowledge.* University of California Press.

Forbes, A., & Mudaliar, S. (2009). *Preventing Prevention Trial Failures: A Case Study and Lessons for Future Trials from the 2004 Tenofovir Trial in Cambodia.* Washington, DC: PATH.

Grant, R. M., Lama, J. R., Anderson, P. L., McMahan, V., Liu, A. Y., Vargas, L., Goicochea, P., et al. (2010). Preexposure Chemoprophylaxis for HIV Prevention in Men Who Have Sex with Men. *New England Journal of Medicine, 363*(27), 2587–2599. doi:10.1056/NEJMoa1011205

Gray, R. H., Kigozi, G., Serwadda, D., Makumbi, F., Watya, S., Nalugoda, F., Kiwanuka, N., et al. (2007). Male circumcision for HIV prevention in men in Rakai, Uganda: A randomised trial. *The Lancet, 369*(9562), 657–666. doi:10.1016/S0140-6736(07)60313-4

Hankins, C., Forsythe, S., & Njeuhmeli, E. (2011). Voluntary Medical Male Circumcision: An Introduction to the Cost, Impact, and Challenges of Accelerated Scaling Up (S. L. Sansom, ed.). *PLoS Medicine, 8*(11), e1001127. doi:10.1371/journal.pmed.1001127

Hankins, C., Macklin, R., Michael, N., & Stablein, D. (2010). *Recommendations for the Future Utility of the RV144 Vaccines to the Thai Ministry of Health Report on Meeting in Bangkok, Thailand, March 16–18, 2010.* New York: Global HIV Vaccine Enterprise.

Hilts P. J. (1990, May 22). 82 Held in Protest on Pace of AIDS Research—New York Times. *New York Times.* New York. Retrieved from http://www.nytimes.com/1990/05/22/science/82-held-in-protest-on-pace-of-aids-research.html

HPTN (2011). HIVNET 012: A Phase IIB Trial to Determine the Efficacy of Oral AZT and the Efficacy of Oral Nevirapine for the Prevention of Vertical Transmission of HIV-1 Infection in Pregnant Ugandan Women and Their Neonates. Retrieved from http://www.hptn.org/research_studies/hivnet012.asp

Karim, A. (2010). Results of Effectiveness Trials of PRO 2000 Gel: Lessons for Future Microbicide Trials. *Future Microbiol, 5*(4), 527–529.

Karim, S. S. A., & Karim, Q. A. (2011). Antiretroviral Prophylaxis: A Defining Moment in HIV Control. *Lancet, 378*(9809), e23–25. doi:10.1016/S0140-6736(11)61136-7

*Lusaka Times* (2009). No More Microbicide Clinical Trials on Women—Mazabuka Central MP (n.d.). *LusakaTimes.com—Keeping You Informed for Free.* Retrieved from http://www.lusakatimes.com/2009/12/29/no-more-microbicide-clinical-trials-on-women-mazabuka-central-mp/

McGrory, E., Irvin, A., & Heise, L. (2009). *Research Rashomon Lessons from the Cameroon Pre-exposure Prophylaxis Trial Site.* Washington, DC: PATH.

Morris, B. J., Bailey, R. C., Klausner, J. D., Leibowitz, A., Wamai, R. G., Waskett, J. H., Banerjee, J., et al. (2012). Review: A Critical Evaluation of Arguments

Opposing Male Circumcision for HIV Prevention in Developed Countries. *AIDS Care*. doi:10.1080/09540121.2012.661836

NIAID (2005, April 7). *Questions and Answers: The HIVNET 012 Study and the Safety and Effectiveness of Nevirapine in Preventing Mother-to-Infant Transmission of HIV.* NIAID. Retrieved from http://www.niaid.nih.gov/news/newsreleases/2005/pages/hivnet012qa.aspx

Obama, B. (2011, December 1). Remarks by the President on World AIDS Day. Retrieved from http://www.whitehouse.gov/the-press-office/2011/12/01/remarks-president-world-aids-day

Peterson L., Taylor D., Roddy R., Belai G., Phillips P., et al. (2007). Tenofovir disoproxil fumarate for prevention of HIV infection in women: a phase 2, double-blind, randomized, placebo-controlled trial. PLoS Clinical Trials 2(5): e27. doi: 10.1371/journal.pctr.0020027.

Project ARM (2012). *On the Map: Ensuring Africa's Place in Rectal Microbicide Research and Advocacy.* Chicago, IL: IRMA.

Rees Helen (2010). *Recommendations Arising from the Expert Consultation on the Future Utility of the RV144 Vaccine Regimen.* Bangkok, Thailand: WHO.

Rerks-Ngarm, S., Pitisuttithum, P., Nitayaphan, S., Kaewkungwal, J., Chiu, J., Paris, R., Premsri, N., et al. (2009). Vaccination with ALVAC and AIDSVAX to prevent HIV-1 infection in Thailand. *The New England Journal of Medicine, 361*(23), 2209–2220. doi:10.1056/NEJMoa0908492

SAAVI (2007). *First Large-Scale Study of HIV Vaccine Starts in South Africa.* Cape Town, South Africa: South African AIDS Vaccine Initiative.

Schwartländer, B., Stover, J., Hallett, T., Atun, R., Avila, C., Gouws, E., Bartos, M., et al. (2011). Towards an Improved Investment Approach for an Effective Response to HIV/AIDS. *The Lancet, 377*(9782), 2031–2041. doi:10.1016/S0140-6736(11)60702-2

Shilts, R. (2007). *And the Band Played On: Politics, People, and the AIDS Epidemic.* New York: Macmillan.

Smith, R. A., & Siplon, P. D. (2006). *Drugs into Bodies: Global AIDS Treatment Activism.* Greenwood.

Stein, Z., & Susser, I. (2010). *Transparency, Accountability and Feminist Science— What Next for Microbicide Trials?* Athena Network & AIDS Legal Network.

Thomas, P. (2001). *Big Shot: Passion, Politics, and the Struggle for an AIDS Vaccine.* Public Affairs.

Tutu, D. (2011, September 20). An End to AIDS Is within Our Reach. *The Washington Post.* Retrieved from http://www.washingtonpost.com/opinions/an-end-to-aids-is-within-our-reach/2011/09/18/gIQABAbGjK_story.html

*Washington Post* (2001, November 2). *US Stance on Patents Decried.* Washington, DC.

WHO & UNAIDS (2007). *WHO / New data on male circumcision and HIV prevention: Policy and programme implications.* Retrieved from http://www.who.int/hiv/pub/malecircumcision/research_implications/en/index.html

# 6

# Contesting Conspiracies: Science, Activism, and the Ongoing Battle against AIDS Denialism

*Nicoli Nattrass*

AIDS conspiracy theories pose a challenge for the international AIDS response because they promote distrust in the science of HIV prevention and treatment. AIDS conspiracy theories range from the claim that HIV is a manmade bio-weapon to the "AIDS denialist" assertions that HIV is harmless and antiretroviral drugs themselves cause AIDS. All make what I term a "conspiratorial move" against HIV science by implying that scientists and clinicians have either been duped by, or are part of, a broader conspiracy to inflict harm (Nattrass, 2012). This, in turn, reduces the credibility of HIV prevention and treatment messages. A growing body of research shows that AIDS conspiracy beliefs in the United States (where the struggle for HIV treatment started) and South Africa (home to the greatest number of HIV-positive people on earth) are linked with risky sex (Bogart & Thorburn, 2003; Bogart & Thorburn, 2005; Ross et al., 2006; Bogart et al., 2010; Grebe & Nattrass, 2011), not adhering to antiretroviral treatment (Bogart, Wagner et al., 2010), and not testing for HIV (Bogart & Latkin, 2009; Bogart et al., 2010; Tun et al., 2010).

AIDS conspiracy theories about HIV being invented as a genocidal bio-weapon have been blamed for diverting the attention of leaders and community media away from the risk behaviors underpinning the epidemic among African Americans (Cohen, 1999). AIDS denialism has also undermined the AIDS response by encouraging HIV-positive people to deny their deadly disease and to reject antiretrovirals either for mother-to-child transmission prevention or AIDS treatment (Kalichman, 2009).

AIDS denialism started as a set of "dissident" claims by Berkeley virologist Peter Duesberg that AIDS was caused by a host of environmental and sexually transmitted co-factors (Epstein, 1996; Mass, 2011). As the evidence mounted showing that HIV causes AIDS and that antiretroviral drugs help treat it, most dissidents changed their stance. But Duesberg and a small group of supporters (mainly journalists and alternative therapists) continued to assert that HIV was harmless (despite never having done any research on it) and that HIV science rested on rotten and corrupt foundations (Kalichman, 2009). As HIV scientists became increasingly frustrated with Duesberg's refusal to accept evidence running counter to his beliefs, he relied more and more on the media to construct a rival social basis of authority outside of the scientific community (Epstein, 1996, pp.105–178).

The growing gulf between HIV science and AIDS denialism had major implications for AIDS activism. Notably, ACTUP in the San Francisco Bay Area fractured into rival (and at times hostile) pro-science and AIDS denialist factions (Smith & Siplon, 2006, p. 36) with correspondingly different approaches to treating AIDS. In South Africa, pro-science AIDS activists fighting for the introduction of antiretroviral drugs into the public health sector had to contend with a much more powerful obstacle: a state president (Thabo Mbeki) who was deeply suspicious of the science of HIV pathogenesis and treatment.

We know that HIV is not a biological weapon because it originated a long time ago from the cross-species transmission of the simian immunodeficiency virus (SIV) from primates to humans (see Worobey et al., 2008). There is also a substantial body of scientific and clinical evidence showing that HIV causes AIDS and that antiretrovirals help treat it (see reviews in Chigwedere & Essex, 2010; Volberding & Deeks, 2010). But pointing to the scientific evidence alone does not convince the skeptics because HIV science is all too easily dismissed as "part of the conspiracy." Issues of credibility—whose voice to believe—thus loom large in the contestation. For example, David Gilbert had some success contesting AIDS conspiracy theories among prisoners precisely because he was in jail himself for revolutionary activities linked to the Black Panthers and thus could not easily be dismissed as part of the conspiracy (Nattrass, 2012). Credibility battles against AIDS denialists, by contrast, seek to expose flaws such as the involvement of AIDS denialists in the alternative medicine industry and the deaths of HIV-positive people who refuse to take antiretrovirals.

This chapter examines different ways in which HIV scientists and AIDS activists have mobilized scientific evidence and engaged in credibility battles with AIDS denialists. It highlights the AIDS policy debacle in South Africa under President Mbeki and how the fight against longstanding AIDS denialist Peter Duesberg has involved both scientific rebuttals and credibility battles, including attempts by scientists and AIDS activists to deny his work the imprimatur of science. It concludes with a discussion of how credibility battles against AIDS denialism have extended in new ways in the Internet era, for example, publicizing the deaths of iconic AIDS denialists. Precisely because AIDS denialists claim that you can live healthily as an HIV-positive person without antiretroviral treatment, their deaths are especially symbolically important. Accordingly, the actions of pro-science activists who post news of the deaths of AIDS denialists may well be more effective in combating AIDS denialism than scientific rebuttals. The chapter thus shows that the struggle for science and reason is alive and well in the Internet era.

## AIDS DENIALISM AND THE FIGHT FOR HIV TREATMENT IN SOUTH AFRICA

When Mbeki succeeded Mandela as president in 1999, almost one in five South African adults was infected with HIV. About 300,000 people had already died of AIDS, but during Mbeki's presidency the death toll skyrocketed to include another 2.7 million more. Two independent estimates have concluded that of these, over a third of a million people died unnecessarily because Mbeki and his health minister, MantoThsabalala-Msimang, delayed the introduction of antiretroviral drugs in the public sector (Chigwedere et al., 2008; Nattrass, 2008).

The South African AIDS policy debacle has been told in more detail elsewhere (Fourie, 2006; Nattrass, 2007; Cullinan & Anso, 2009; Geffen, 2010), but to highlight the key issue, it was that rather than basing AIDS policy on the scientific consensus, Mbeki took seriously the claims of self-styled "dissidents" that HIV science was fundamentally flawed and corrupted by the pharmaceutical industry and that antiretroviral drugs were unacceptably toxic. There are many theories as to why Mbeki did this, ranging from his personality (arrogant, "prophet in the wilderness" image), his political socialization, desire to find "African solutions," rejection of Western stereotyping of the sexually driven AIDS epidemic, economic considerations (to limit government liability for AIDS-related health services), postcolonial suspicions of Western biomedicine, and so on (see review in Nattrass, 2012, pp. 96–103). But none of this satisfactorily explains why he accepted Western science in all other respects, or why he rejected the views of South African HIV specialists, many of whom were black, opting instead to support the views of a small group of white, foreign fringe scientists and alternative therapists. South Africa's tragedy is simply that he did convert to AIDS denialism, for whatever reason, and with terrible consequences for the AIDS response.

Soon after taking power, Mbeki convened a "Presidential AIDS Advisory Panel" with half the seats allocated to AIDS denialists and half to HIV scientists and clinicians. This effectively elevated a fringe set of unsupported claims to the same status as the scientific consensus on HIV, resulting in widespread confusion about the pathogenesis and treatment of HIV. Meanwhile, his health minister, Tshabalala-Msimang, rejected reports from South Africa's Medicines Control Council (MCC) that antiretrovirals were safe and effective—describing them instead as "poison" (Garrett, 2002). As medical professionals and AIDS activists started mobilizing for evidence-based AIDS policy, she starved the MCC of resources and obstructed donor funding for antiretrovirals. She hired Roberto Giraldo, a leading AIDS denialist, to promote nutritional alternatives, and she invited him to a meeting of southern African health ministers where he told the audience that "the transmission of AIDS from person to person is a myth" and that "malnourishment is at the center of its progression" (Nattrass, 2007, p. 107). Tshabalala-Msimang also supported Mattias Rath, a vitamin magnate who ran clinical "trials" in Khayelitsha in which patients were encouraged to go off antiretroviral treatment and onto his therapies instead—with predictably dire consequences (Geffen, 2010).

In 2002 Mbeki and Tshabalala-Msimang were forced to concede ground over the use of antiretroviral drugs to prevent mother-to-child transmission after the constitutional court ruled in favor of a coalition of AIDS clinicians, legal activists, and the Treatment Action Campaign (TAC). Civil society activism then concentrated on demanding access to antiretroviral treatment for people living with AIDS. This and a related civil disobedience campaign paid political dividends, and the following year the cabinet overruled Mbeki and announced that antiretroviral treatment would be provided through the public sector. Even so, precisely because Tshabalala-Msimang remained health minister, the rollout of antiretroviral drugs for both HIV prevention and AIDS treatment was plagued by inefficiencies and poor leadership at the national level.

Another problem was that Mbeki and Tshabalala-Msimang sowed suspicion about antiretrovirals by promoting conspiracy theories about HIV science. Mbeki alleged that the CIA, working with the large pharmaceutical companies, was part of a conspiracy seeking to promote the view that HIV was the sole cause of AIDS and that toxic antiretrovirals were the only treatment (Barrell, 2000; Feinstein, 2007, p. 124). He later withdrew from public discussion on AIDS in the face of resistance from within the

ANC and from civil society, but some of his supporters continued to voice suspicions about the origins of HIV. As late as 2006, the political executive in charge of health in KwaZulu-Natal Province, Peggy Nkonyeni, drew connections between "this thing called bioterrorism or biological warfare" and HIV (Geffen & Cameron, 2009, pp. 1–2).

Tshabalala-Msimang sparked controversy in 2000 by circulating extracts from *Behold a Pale Horse* by the American conspiracy theorist William Cooper (1991). Cooper believed that AIDS is part of a gigantic historical conspiracy involving the U.S. government working in cahoots with aliens from outer space, Jews, and ancient secret societies. According to Cooper, HIV was created by the U.S. military/CIA and injected into the African population during the 1970s through a smallpox eradication campaign, and into the African American and homosexual population through hepatitis-B vaccinations. He argued that this was part of a Club of Rome plot to address global overpopulation and that only "the elite" had (secretly) been provided with a prophylaxis. He also asserted that a cure for AIDS existed, but would only be released when enough people had died. Already influential for being "much read in both UFO and militia circles" (Barkun, 2003, p. 60), *Behold a Pale Horse* was, through Tshabalala-Msimang, now provided an influential airing in the highest reaches of the South African government and was widely discussed in the media and on the radio.

It is impossible to measure precisely the impact of the promotion of AIDS conspiracy theories by national political figures such as the health minister. However, analysis of a representative survey of young South Africans in Cape Town in 2009 revealed that people who said they trusted Tshabalala-Msimang more than her successor as health minister were less likely to use condoms—and that this relationship holds after controlling for a large set of other potential determinants of condom use (Grebe & Nattrass, 2011). The study also points to the importance of the role of civil society resistance to Mbeki and Tshabalala-Msimang's policies: Controlling for whether respondents said they kept up with the news, those who had never heard of the TAC were half as likely to use condoms as those who had (Grebe & Nattrass, 2011).

TAC had an impact directly, via court cases against the South African government, and indirectly through its organized protests (to raise public awareness and put pressure on the government) and its "treatment literacy program," which promoted scientific understandings of HIV and AIDS treatment at the local (branch) level. Indeed, it was TAC's commitment to treatment literacy that encouraged Médecins Sans Frontières (MSF) to come to South Africa and set up a pilot antiretroviral treatment program in the Western Cape. The resulting partnership with local and provincial governments illustrated how pro-science activism was able to mobilize and draw on support from the medical profession and government structures despite state-sponsored AIDS denialism at the national level (Hodes & Holm-Naimak, 2011; Grebe, 2011).

TAC's Treatment Literacy Program was, and remains, South Africa's most important mass cultural project in support of science. It started in 2002 when Sipho Mthathi (subsequently the TAC general secretary) was tasked with formalizing and expanding the treatment literacy initiatives she had initiated as a grassroots organizer. The program produces fact sheets and posters about HIV disease, antiretrovirals, and CD4 count monitoring, which are distributed at national, regional, and local workshops run by treatment literacy practitioners. In so doing, TAC assists people on antiretroviral treatment in understanding the nature of various monitoring tests and empowers them to engage with their doctors over side effects and treatment regimens. As Nathan Geffen (longstanding central TAC activist) comments: "Many of our members are able to explain, for example, what a nucleoside reverse transcriptase inhibitor is (and some of us will draw pictures to prove it too). . . . It is a patronising, racist . . . attitude to presume black people can't learn science" (Nattrass, 2007, p. 166).

The TAC fact sheet, "Talk about Antiretrovirals," presents common questions and answers. The answers are attributed to real people with names and photographs. In this sense, the strategy parallels public disclosure by HIV activists as a form of consciousness-raising. Thus, for example, Nontsikelelo Zwedala answers the question "How do ARVs work?" with the following:

They reduce the amount of virus in my blood. This helps my immune system to work properly again and to fight off infections that make people with HIV sick. I weighed 42kg when I started ARVs. I was close to death. Now I weigh over 60kg and am working and healthy. To meet the challenges of HIV, we must take responsibility to learn about the disease and become treatment-literate. It is not only our doctors and nurses who must understand our medical needs. We must understand them too. (http://www.tac.org.za/documents/arv-pamphlet.pdf)

An anthropologist observed that such testimonies "with their references to CD4 counts, viral loads and the role of TAC in giving 'new life' seem to blur the lines between science and religion, medicine and spirituality, and technology and magic" (Robbins, 2006). But while TAC is certainly revered in many parts of South Africa, the testimonies are more appropriately taken at face value as affirmations of the power of science to combat AIDS. Of course, not everyone is as fully trained as a TAC treatment literacy advocate, and probably not even all these activists have a good enough knowledge of science to educate others fully about the science of HIV and antiretroviral therapy. Furthermore, as Ashforth (2005) has shown, a scientific understanding of HIV does not necessarily purge the worry that possibly the disease was "sent" by an enemy. For many people, the search for healing may thus include traditional and biomedical strategies (Nattrass, 2005). The ongoing challenge for AIDS activists is to incorporate traditional healing strategies within a framework that privileges science.

## FIGHTING AIDS DENIALISM

Peter Duesberg, the leading AIDS denialist and member of President Mbeki's presidential panel, has been arguing since the mid-1980s that HIV is a harmless "passenger virus" and that AIDS is caused by recreational drugs, malnutrition, and even antiretroviral treatment itself (e.g., Duesberg, 1996; Duesberg et al., 2009). Such "dissident" views, including those of Joseph Sonnabend, a New York doctor who was sceptical of the early antiretroviral drugs and argued that AIDS was caused by multiple co-factor infections, were not unreasonable in the early days of the U.S. AIDS epidemic. But once the clinical benefits of antiretroviral treatment became clear, Sonnabend changed his stance toward them (2000) and later explicitly disassociated himself from the AIDS denialists. Although he can be criticized for doing this rather late in the day and for spinning rather than repudiating his earlier views (Mass, 2011), Sonnabend took the step Duesberg never did. To this day, Duesberg refuses to accept the scientific evidence that HIV causes AIDS and that antiretroviral help treat it. He also ignores the many scientific rebuttals of his argument (see, e.g., Blattner et al., 1988; Gallo, 1991; Cohen, 1994; Galea & Chermann, 1998; Chigwedere & Essex, 2010). This has earned him the label "denialist" rather than "dissident" and has resulted in HIV scientists and activists taking action against him in ways that go beyond the mere rebuttals of his claims. As discussed below, they have fought to undermine his credibility by limiting the extent to which his views can be seen as "scientific." As such, it forms part of the general "boundary work" conducted by scientists to protect the integrity of what is legitimately understood to comprise science (Nattrass, 2011).

Duesberg's reputation in the scientific community has been so damaged by his approach to AIDS that when *Scientific American* published an article by him on cancer, the editors posted the following disclaimer alongside the article:

The author, Peter Duesberg, a pioneering virologist, may be well known to readers for his assertion that HIV is not the cause of AIDS. The biomedical community has roundly rebutted that claim many times. Duesberg's ideas about chromosomal abnormality as a root cause for cancer, in contrast, are controversial, but are being actively investigated by mainstream science. We have therefore asked Duesberg to explain that work here. This article is in no sense an endorsement by *Scientific American* of his AIDS theories. (Disclaimer published alongside Duesberg, 2007)

The disclaimer is noteworthy for the distinction it draws between controversial views in a legitimate debate (defined as one that is being "actively investigated by mainstream science") and intransigent views flying in the face of rebuttals. Duesberg and his supporters, of course, regard *any* closure on the debate about HIV as the cause of AIDS as oppressive and ultimately "unscientific." The disclaimer in *Scientific American,* however, reflects the broader view within the HIV scientific community that Duesberg is no longer engaging with AIDS as a scientist.

A similar stance was adopted by John Maddox, the editor of *Nature,* 13 years earlier when he concluded that Duesberg no longer had the "right of reply" in his journal. At that time, early studies of the HIV-status of stored samples of donor blood and the development of AIDS among those who had received blood transfusions showed clear correlations between HIV infection and AIDS. Duesberg, however, refused to accept this evidence for the connection between HIV-infected blood transfusions and subsequent AIDS deaths among hemophiliacs—and posited a set of alternative unfounded speculations (about potentially contaminated clotting factors) as the cause of such deaths (see Cohen, 1994). Maddox became infuriated with Duesberg and in an unprecedented editorial in *Nature,* he announced that he would no longer be publishing Duesberg's letters and papers on the topic because of his unacceptable debating techniques, misreading of the work of others, and refusal to accept evidence contrary to his hypotheses (Maddox, 1993).

Maddox also complained about the way Duesberg "advertises" his position to the public, "thus giving many infected people the belief that HIV infection is not in itself the calamity it is likely to prove" (1993, p. 109). In a boldfaced line right under the title of his editorial, Maddox wrote, "Dr Peter Duesberg, the virologist-turned-campaigner, is wrongly using tendentious arguments to confuse understanding of AIDS and those in danger of contracting the disease. He should stop." As such, Maddox's editorial was a prequel of the public health concerns that motivated a subsequent action by HIV scientists 16 years later against the journal *Medical Hypotheses* (a fringe journal known for publishing controversial ideas without prior peer review) for publishing an article by Duesberg without subjecting it to peer review (Nattrass, 2011).

The paper in question, Duesberg et al. (2009), was a response to Chigwedere et al.'s argument (2008) that Mbeki's AIDS policies had caused hundreds of thousands of unnecessary deaths in South Africa. In their reply Duesberg et al. repeated their longstanding claims that antiretrovirals were causing harm and, ignoring the demographic literature on AIDS, argued that there was no evidence of an African AIDS epidemic. Initially submitted to JAIDS, the paper had been rejected after peer review for selective "cherry picking" and misrepresentation of scientific facts (Cartwright et al., 2010a). *Medical Hypotheses* subsequently published it without peer review.

John Moore, a virologist with a long track record of fighting AIDS denialism, mobilized a group of HIV scientists and AIDS treatment activists to write to the National Library of Medicine (NLM) requesting that *Medical Hypotheses* be reviewed for deselection from Medline on the grounds that articles were not adequately reviewed and that *Medical Hypotheses* had become a "tool for the legitimization of at least one pseudoscientific movement with aims antithetical to the public health goals of the NIH and the NLM, notably AIDS denialism." Moore and others also complained to the publisher, Elsevier, about Duesberg's paper and wrote to their university libraries requesting that subscriptions to *Medical Hypotheses* be canceled. Elsevier responded by setting up an expert panel (managed by *The Lancet*) to review Duesberg's paper. It unanimously recommended rejection, and Elsevier permanently withdrew the paper (http://www.ncbi.nlm.nih.gov/pubmed/19619953). This direct action against Duesberg and *Medical Hypotheses* can be understood as boundary work on the part of HIV scientists and AIDS activists to protect the integrity of what is seen to count as a "scientific" publication. In this instance, it forms part of their broader credibility battle against AIDS denialism.

Duesberg eventually managed to publish a reworked version of the article in an Italian journal, sparking further controversy and protest

resignations from a member of the editorial board (http://www.nature
.com/news/paper-denying-hiv-aids-link-sparks-resignation-1.9926), but
the main outlet for his work has been the media (facilitated especially by
sympathetic journalists, the "praise-singers" of AIDS denialism), and
increasingly also the Internet. This, in turn, has forced HIV scientists,
activists, and physicians to engage with AIDS denialism in new ways.
They have, for example, teamed up with AIDS activists to create a website, www.AIDStruth.org, dedicated specifically to countering AIDS
denialism. In fact, the first posting on AIDStruth.org (Gallo et al., 2006)
was a detailed refutation of an article published in *Harper's Magazine*
promoting Duesberg's views (Farber, 2006a). Scientists linked to AIDS
truth.org have also responded to HIV misinformation in videos, for
example complaining successfully to the British Broadcasting Corpora-
tion about a film falsely depicting antiretrovirals as having caused harm
to children in New York, and more recently posting a critique of the
documentary film *House of Numbers* for what they deemed its misrepresentation of AIDS science (Nattrass, 2012). Other pro-science websites
and bloggers also participate in the ongoing fight against AIDS denialism; for example, Ben Goldacre (a physician) on "Bad Science" (http://
www.badscience.net/), Seth Kalichman (a psychologist) on "Denying
AIDS" (http://denyingaids.blogspot.com/), and Nick Bennett (a physician) on "Correcting the AIDS lies" (http://aidsmyth.blogspot.com/).
Also important are blog postings by individuals in response to denialist
views expressed in blogs and chat rooms.

This popular defense of science and action against AIDS denialism
takes on a wider cast of characters than Duesberg. This is because in
addition to the role of the "hero scientist," AIDS denialism gains social
traction through the work of the "cultropreneurs," who peddle alternative therapies in the place of antiretrovirals, and the "living icons"–HIV-
positive people who seemingly provide proof of concept by appearing
to live healthily without them. I have discussed the importance of these
roles for AIDS denialism elsewhere (Nattrass, 2012). The key point is that
together they offer potential converts to AIDS denialism a seductive new
identity: as bold truth-seeker standing up to a corrupted AIDS establishment while doing well on natural-sounding remedies. But it also provides
targets for pro-science advocates and anti-AIDS denialists who expose the
pseudo-scientific claims of the cultropreneurs and publicize the deaths of
the living icons. Precisely because the living icons appear to offer proof of
concept, their deaths from AIDS-related illnesses undermine the credibility
of AIDS denialism.

Alternative and complementary medicine is important for AIDS denialists as it hooks into a broader social current of suspicion against medical science and speaks to the anxieties people living with AIDS have about their medical condition and fears about the side effects of antiretrovirals (Nattrass & Kalichman, 2009). But in supporting alternative remedies, the AIDS denialists are pretty indiscriminate—basically anything other than antiretroviral drugs is recommended. For example, Duesberg and the other AIDS denialists on Mbeki's panel recommended that "massage therapy, music therapy, yoga, spiritual care, homeopathy, Indian Ayurvedic medicine, light therapy and many other methods" (PAAPR, 2001, pp. 79, 86) be used to treat immune deficiency.

The connection between AIDS denialism and alternative therapists is reflected also in their overlapping organizational networks. For example, Duesberg sits on the boards of Rethinking AIDS, an organization that promotes his views about HIV, and Alive and Well, an organization founded by Christine Maggiore that "questions" HIV science and promotes alternative treatments. This organizational dimension of AIDS denialism is of particular concern for AIDS activists. As the founder of *AIDS Treatment News,* John James, observes:

> The denialists regularly deny that precautions against infection are necessary, deny that HIV testing is appropriate, deny that any approved treatments should be used (or CD4 or viral load tests to monitor disease progression), deny that treatment saves lives, and often deny that AIDS is a real epidemic, or even a real medical condition. The problem is not ideas, but the organized efforts to practice bizarre medicine, telling people with a major illness to reject care entirely. (James, 2000)

Precisely because AIDS denialism can kill people by encouraging them not to use antiretrovirals, HIV scientists get very upset with Duesberg, seeing his activism against HIV science as responsible for many unnecessary deaths. But Duesberg's supporters dismiss their concerns, seeing their complaints as part of a drug company–funded conspiracy against him. According to Celia Farber, Duesberg's leading praise-singer, "As AIDS grew in the 1980s into a global, multibillion-dollar juggernaut of diagnostics, drugs, and activist organizations, whose sole target in the fight against AIDS was HIV, condemning Duesberg became part of the moral crusade" (2006a).

Ironically, AIDS denialism can clearly be linked to a different set of commercial interests—notably the "cultropreneurs" peddling alternative therapies for which the conspiratorial move against HIV science functions as a convenient marketing device. Duesberg himself is funded by a venture capitalist with an interest in alternative therapies (Nattrass, 2007, p. 115).

Cultropreneurs, and indeed all alternative therapists, rely on anecdotal evidence and testimonies of people who were pleased with the treatment. The role of the "living icon," the person who through his or her very existence "proves" that HIV disease can be fought with alternative remedies, is thus crucial for their success (and the reason why AIDS activists contest their claims). The most important of these icons for the AIDS denialist movement was Christine Maggiore, who not only actively promoted the cause of AIDS denialism, but tragically also put her own health and that of her family on the line.

In the preface to her widely distributed book, *What If Everything You Thought You Knew about AIDS Was Wrong,* she says she lost faith in HIV science after a series of what she perceived to be a series of inconsistent HIV tests, but which were consistent with her being tested first during the early stages of HIV infection when tests are inconclusive (see http:// www.houseofnumbers.org/Maggiore_s_Labs.html). Dissatisfied with the state of HIV science, Maggiore conducted her own investigation "outside the confines of the AIDS establishment" and started Alive and Well to "share vital facts about HIV and AIDS that are unavailable from mainstream venues." Writing in 2000, she observed that her HIV status had been "decidedly positive" for five years, but that she was enjoying good health and was living "without pharmaceutical treatments or fear of AIDS" (Maggiore, 2000, p. 2).

When she was pregnant in 2002 with her second child, Maggiore was featured on the cover of *Mothering* (a pro–alternative healing and antivaccination magazine) with a red circle slash symbol over the letters "AZT" (an antiretroviral drug used to reduce the chances of transmitting HIV from mother to child) emblazoned across her abdomen. After the baby was born—a daughter called Eliza Jane—Maggiore increased the risk of transmitting HIV yet further by breastfeeding her. Tragically, Eliza Jane died at age three of what the Los Angeles coroner ruled to be AIDS-related pneumonia (http://www.aidstruth.org/documents/ejs-coroner -report.pdf).

Maggiore, however, denied that HIV had anything to do with the death—dismissing the presence of p24 capsid protein in Eliza Jane's brain (a clear indication of HIV infection) as being the result of a medical "scavenger hunt" designed to make an HIV diagnosis. Farber agreed, writing that the coroner had gone out of his way to make the death look as if it was AIDS-related simply because Eliza Jane was Maggiore's child (2006b). She attributed Eliza Jane's death to public anger against Maggiore— manifested in angry emails, Web postings, and even printed flyers—to "the impossibly censorious and even brutal treatment one can expect if one is branded an 'AIDS denialist.' Farber observed:

> I started to see the story as one that was less and less medical, more and more psycho-social—a story of an almost crushing kind of mob rule, where the victims have no rights. Few could resist the delicious temptation to condemn a "denialist" mother, or to appropriate EJ as their own tragic little girl. It was all done in the pitch-perfect tones of the AIDS morality play some of us know so well. (2006b)

Farber's argument is remarkable for its failure to consider that Eliza Jane was the victim in this instance, and that the "AIDS morality play" she sneers at is rooted in genuine social concern about the well-being of children. As Mark Wainberg, a microbiologist and past president of the International AIDS Society, put it: "Maggiore was so misguided in believing this concoction of bullshit, that it cost not only her life, which is her business, but also the life of her three-year old kid, and that is everybody's business" (Law, 2009).

According to psychologist Seth Kalichman (2009), AIDS denialists live in a state of encapsulated delusion—in a world that is impenetrable by facts. When Eliza Jane died, Maggiore told reporters: "I have been brought to my emotional knees, but not in regard to the science of this topic. . . . I am not second-guessing or questioning my understanding of the issue" (Ornstein & Costello, 2005). Maggiore remained in denial to the end, dying in 2009, aged 52, of bilateral bronchial pneumonia and disseminated herpes viral infection—both common AIDS-related opportunistic infections (http://www.aidstruth.org/new/sites/default/files/maggiore-death-certificate.pdf). That she was prepared to endanger her own life and that of her family speaks volumes about the passion and sincerity with which AIDS denialist beliefs can be embraced and to the powerful psychological forces at work.

The death of this important living icon was obviously a hard blow for organized AIDS denialism. Maggiore's organization, Alive and Well, posted a memorial notice when she died, but visitors to the website today are still greeted with a "message" from Christine Maggiore on the "about us" page, which gives no indication that she is dead (http://www.aliveandwell.org/html/top_bar_pages/aboutus.html). Activists running anti-AIDS denialist sites respond to such attempts to obscure and downplay the deaths of living icons by publicizing them—see, for example, http://www.aidstruth.org/denialism/dead_denialists. Other attempts have been made to create new "living icons"—for example, the people profiled on a website called We Are Living Proof (http://wearelivingproof.org/)—but none of them comes close to being able to replace Maggiore's symbolic and organizational power.

The symbolic importance of Maggiore—and now her death—is illustrated in this posting by a one-time AIDS denialist. He talks about how his "dissident" beliefs encouraged him to ignore his positive HIV test result, but that when he heard that Maggiore had died, alarm bells started ringing for him for the first time:

> In 2008 I had bumped into the website aidstruth.org and, while reading it in a "yeah blah blah whatever" kind of attitude, I saw the "denialists who have died" and "who the denialists are" sections. Something clicked. And very soon after I paid one of my usual visits to the Alive and Well site and found the memorial text about Maggiore's death. It didn't mention the cause (of course) so I Googled away thinking "please, let it be a traffic accident or something" and bam! Pneumonia.

> You know how denialists usually say it's just a coincidence, like "why not? Anybody can have pneumonia," but having recently read the list of dead denialists and wondering if those weren't too many untimely coincidences, for me Maggiore's death is where I drew the line. For me it was the "one too many" coincidence. That's where I secretly started to wonder if I had been wrong. (http://denyingaids.blogspot.com/2010/07/how-aids-denialism-can-kill-you-part.html)

Medical science is more trustworthy than "alternative" medicine precisely because the former is built on randomized controlled trials, whereas the latter rests on anecdotes and individual testimonies. It is thus somewhat ironic that a single death—Maggiore's—has possibly done more than scientific rebuttals to fight AIDS denialism. Precisely because this death was that of a living icon who rejected HIV science in favor of alternative therapies, it carried disproportionate weight for those tempted by AIDS denialism. It illustrates how the battle for science and reason is not always just about "the facts," as some facts, like the death of Christine Maggiore, are symbolically more important than others.

## CONCLUSION: THE BROADER STRUGGLE FOR EVIDENCE-BASED MEDICINE

The struggle against AIDS denialism has involved scientific rebuttals, action against publishers, and criticism on the Internet. Whereas in the past, boundary work in defense of science was conducted primarily by scholars seeking to develop and maintain public respect for science and to relegate pseudo-science beyond the pale of academia, today the battle is more diffuse, public, and decentralized—often fought at an individual level via cut and thrust debate on blog postings. This socially embedded struggle fought by what Damien Thompson calls "freelance defenders of the truth" (2008, p. 135) is becoming very important in defending HIV science and evidence-based medicine.

But how easy is it to persuade people through factual corrections of their misperceptions? The answer seems to depend a great deal on the individual. For example, AIDS denialists like Maggiore are impervious to corrective evidence about HIV science. They are impossible to argue with, and indeed, it may even be counterproductive to do so. According to recent research in political psychology, providing people who are ideologically committed to a particular view with "preference-incongruent information" can "backfire" by causing them to support their original argument even more strongly (Nyhan & Reifler, 2010). However, not all or even most AIDS denialists are as psychologically committed and through their own process of truth-seeking may well be open to changing their minds, as was the case with the person quoted above who started changing his mind after Maggiore died.

This, in turn, creates the space for pro-science activists to compete for the attention of those seeking information about health and healing. And, by doing this in the electronic world, through dedicated websites, blogs, and by posting comments in response to claims by cultropreneurs and the like, the Internet becomes a tougher place for people to sequestrate themselves in a comfortable cocoon of the like-minded. These days, a "Google search," the modern-day equivalent of practical seekership, catapults one from AIDS denialist to pro-science activist websites and exposes one to news (like Maggiore's death) that sites like Alive and Well prefer to downplay, if not hide.

The challenge for the pro-science advocacy movement is thus to keep an active presence on the Internet, both with regard to exposing the cultropreneurs and promoting evidence-based medicine. And, in order to be credible, they need to acknowledge that scientific practice can be biased and shoddy and that everyday scientific practice is shaped by social relationships, tacit forms of knowledge, and contestations over findings, and that it thus often, if not typically, falls short of the ideal "scientific method." Acknowledging the limitations of scientific practice and challenging all practitioners to produce better evidence are necessary to build public support for evidence-based medicine.

## BIBLIOGRAPHY

Ashforth, A. (2005). *Witchcraft, violence and democracy in South Africa.* Chicago: University of Chicago.

Barkun, M. (2003). *A culture of conspiracy: Apocalyptic visions in contemporary America.* Berkeley: University of California Press.

Barrell, H. (2000). "Mbeki fingers CIA in AIDS conspiracy." *Mail and Guardian.* October 6.

Blattner, W., Gallo, R., & Temin, H. (1988). "HIV causes AIDS." *Science* 241: 515–516.

Bogart, L., Galvan, F., Wagner, G., & Klein, D. (2010). "Longitudinal association of HIV conspiracy beliefs with sexual risk among black males living with HIV." *AIDS and Behavior.* Retrieved at http://www.springerlink.com/content/1q7622555j53k4j2/

Bogart, L. M., & Thorburn, S. (2003). "Exploring the relationship of conspiracy beliefs about HIV/AIDS to sexual behaviors and attitudes among African-American adults." *Journal of the National Medical Association* 95 (11): 1057–65.

Bogart, L. M., & Thorburn, S. (2005). "Are HIV/AIDS conspiracy beliefs a barrier to HIV prevention among African Americans?" *Journal of Acquired Immune Deficiency Syndromes* 38 (2): 213–8.

Bogart, L., Wagner, G., Galvan, F., & Banks, D. (2010). "Conspiracy beliefs about HIV are related to antiretroviral treatment nonadherence among African American men with HIV." *Journal of Acquired Immune Deficiency Syndrome* 53 (5): 648–55.

Bohnert, A. S., & Latkin, C. A. (2009). "HIV testing and conspiracy beliefs regarding the origins of HIV among African Americans." *AIDS Patient Care and STDs* 23 (9): 759–63.

Cartwright, J. (2010a). "AIDS contrarian ignored warnings of scientific misconduct." *Nature,* May 4. doi:10.1038/news.2010.210

Chigwedere, P., Seage, G., Gruskin, S., Lee, T., & Essex, M. (2008). "Estimating the lost benefits of antiretroviral drug use in South Africa." *Journal of Acquired Immune Deficiency Syndrome* 49: 410–415.

Chigwedere, P., & Essex, M. (2010). "AIDS denialism and public health practice." *AIDS and Behavior* 14 (2): 237–247.

Cohen, C. (1999). *The boundaries of blackness: AIDS and the breakdown of black politics.* Chicago: University of Chicago Press.

Cohen, J. (1994)."The Duesbergphenomenon." *Science* 266: 1642–1649.

Cooper, W. (1991). *Behold a pale horse.* Flagstaff, AZ: Light Technology.

Cullinan, K., & Anso, T. (eds.) (2009). *The virus, vitamins and vegetables.* Auckland Park: Jacana.

Duesberg, P., Nicholson, J., Rasnick, D., Fiala, C., & Bauer, H. (2009). "Withdrawn: HIV-AIDS hypothesis out of touch with South African AIDS—A new perspective." *Medical Hypotheses.*

Duesberg, P. (2007). "Chromosomal chaos and cancer." *Scientific American* 296 (5): 52–9.

Duesberg, Peter (1996). *Inventing the AIDS virus.* Washington: Regnery Publishing.

Epstein, S. (1996). *Impure science: AIDS, activism and the politics of knowledge.* Berkeley: University of California Press.

Farber, C. (1999). "Ignoring the flames." *Impression,* August. Retrieved from: http://www.virusmyth.com/aids/hiv/cfflames.htm

Farber, C. (2006a). "Out of control: AIDS and the corruption of medical science." *Harper's Magazine.* March: 37–52.

Farber, C. (2006b). "A daughter's death, a mother's survival." *LA City Beat,* June 8. Retrieved from http://www.lacitybeat.com/article/php?id=3887&IssueNum=157

Feinstein, A. (2007). *After the party: A personal and political journey inside the ANC.* Cape Town: Jonathan Ball.

Fourie, P. (2006). *The political management of HIV and AIDS in South Africa: One burden too many?* New York: Palgrave Macmillan.

Galea, P., & Chermann, J. (1998). "HIV as the cause of AIDS and associated diseases." *Genetica.* 104:133–142.

Gallo, R. (1991). *Virus hunting: AIDS, cancer and the human retrovirus. A story of scientific discovery.* New York: Basic Books.

Gallo, R., Geffen, N., Gonsalves, G., Jeffries, R., Kuritzkes, D., Mirken, B., Moore, J., & Safrit, J. (2006). *Errors in Celia Farber's March 2006 article in Harper's Magazine.* http://www.tac.org.za/Documents/ErrorsInFarberArticle.pdf

Garrett, L. (2002). "Anti-HIV drug poison, summit told." *The Age,* July 9. Retrieved from: http://www.theage.com.au/articles/2002/07/08/1025667115671.html

Geffen, N. (2010). *Debunking delusions: The inside story of the Treatment Action Campaign.* Cape Town: Jacana Press.

Geffen, N., & Cameron, E. (2009). "The deadly hand of denial: Governance and politically-instigated AIDS denialism in South Africa." Centre for Social Science Research, Working Paper number 257, University of Cape Town.

Gilbert, D. (2004). "AIDS conspiracy theories: Tracking the real genocide." In David Gilbert, *No surrender: Writings from an anti-imperialist political prisoner,* pp.129–50. Montreal: Abraham Guillen Press. Originally published in 1996 in *Covert Action Quarterly.* Retrieved from http://www.kersplebedeb .com/mystuff/profiles/gilbert/aidsconsp.html

Goldacre, B. (2008). *Bad science.* London: Fourth Estate.

Grebe, E. (2011). "The Treatment Action Campaign's struggle for AIDS treatment in South Africa: Coalition-building through networks." *Journal of Southern African Studies,* 37, 4: 849–868.

Grebe, E., & Nattrass, N. (2011). "AIDS conspiracy beliefs and unsafe sex in Cape Town." *AIDS and Behavior,* 16, 3: 761–773.

Hodes, R., & Holm-Naimak, T. (2011). "Piloting antiretroviral treatment in South Africa: The role of partnerships in the Western Cape provincial roll-out." *African Journal of AIDS Research,* 10, 4: 415–425.

James, J. (2000). "AIDS denialists: How to respond." *AIDS Treatment News,* 342. Retrieved from http://www.aegis.org/pubs/atn/2000/atn34210.html

Kalichman, S. (2009). *Denying AIDS: Conspiracy theories, pseudoscience and human tragedy.* New York: Springer Press.

Law, S. (2009). "In denial." *McGill Daily,* November 16. http://mcgilldaily.com/ articles/22781

Maddox, J. (1993). "Has Duesberg a right of reply?" *Nature* 363: 109.

Maggiore, C. (2000). *What if everything you thought you knew about AIDS was wrong?* 4th ed., revised. Studio City, CA: American Foundation for AIDS Alternatives.

Mass, L. (2011). "HIV denialism and African genocide." *The Gay and Lesbian Review,* 18, 3. http://www.glreview.com/article.php?articleid=339

Nattrass, N. (2005). "Who consults Sangomas in Khayelitsha? An Exploratory Quantitative Analysis." *Social Dynamics,* 31, 2.

Nattrass, N. (2007). *Mortal combat: AIDS denialism and the struggle for antiretrovirals in South Africa.* Pietermaritzburg: University of KwaZulu-Natal Press.

Nattrass, N. (2008). "AIDS and the scientific governance of medicine in post-apartheid South Africa." *African Affairs* 107 (427): 157–176.

Nattrass, N. (2011). "Defending the boundaries of science: AIDS denialism, peer review and the medical hypotheses saga." *Sociology of Health and Illness,* 33, 4: 507–521. doi:10.1111/j.1467-9566.2010.01312.x

Nattrass, N. (2012). *The AIDS conspiracy: Science fights back.* New York: Columbia University Press.

Nattrass, N., & Kalichman, S. (2009). "The politics and psychology of AIDS denialism." In P., Rohleder, L., Swartz, S., Kalichman and L., Simbayi, (eds.), *HIV/AIDS in South Africa 25 years on,* 123–134. New York: Springer Press.

Nyhan, B., & Reifler, J. (2010). "When corrections fail: The persistence of political misperceptions." *Political Behavior,* 32: 303–330.

Ornstein, C., & Costello, D. (2005). "A mother's denial, a daughter's death." *Los Angeles Times,* September 24.

Presidential AIDS Advisory Panel Report (PAAPR), (2001). *Presidential AIDS Advisory Panel Report: A synthesis report of the deliberations by the panel of experts invited by the President of the Republic of South Africa, the Honourable Thabo Mbeki.* Retrieved from: http://www.info.gov.za/otherdocs/2001/aidspanelpdf.pdf

Robbins, S. (2006). "Rights, passages from 'near death' to 'new life': AIDS activism and treatment testimonies in South Africa." *American Anthropologist,* 108, 2, June.

Ross, M., Essien, J., & Torres, I. (2006). "Conspiracy beliefs about the origin of HIV/AIDS in four racial groups." *Journal of Acquired Immune Deficiency Syndrome* 41 (3): 342–344.

Smith, R. A. & Siplon, P. D. (2006). Drugs into bodies: Global aids treatment activism. Westport, CT: Praeger.

Sonnabend, J. (2000). *Honoring with pride: 2000 honoree: Joseph Sonnabend.* Retrieved from http://www.amfar.org/cgi-bin/iowa/amfar/record.html?record=22

Thompson, D. (2008). *Counterknowledge: How we surrendered to conspiracy theories, quack medicine, bogus science and fake history.* London: Atlantic Books.

Tun, W., Kellerman, S., & Maime, S. (2010). *Conspiracy beliefs about HIV, attitudes towards condoms and treatment and HIV-related preventive behaviors among men who have sex with men in Tshwane (Pretoria), South Africa.* XVIII International AIDS Conference, Vienna, 2010 [abstract TUPE0656].

Volberding, P., & Deeks, S. (2010). "Antiretroviral therapy and management of HIV infection." *The Lancet* 376: 49–62.

Worobey, M., Gemmel, M., Teuwen, D., Haselkorn, T., Kunstman, K., Brunce, M., Muyembe, J, Kabongo, J., Kalengayi, R., van Marck, E., Gilbert, T., & Wolinksy, S. (2008). "Direct evidence of extensive diversity of HIV-1 in Kinshasa by 1960." *Nature* 455: 661–664.

# PART 2
# COUNTRY- AND REGIONAL-LEVEL HIV/AIDS ACTIVISM AND COMMUNITY MOBILIZATION

# 7

# The Challenges of Forming Associations of People Living with HIV in Low-Prevalence and High-Stigma Contexts: The Case of Sudan and Lebanon

*Jocelyn DeJong, Iman Mortagy, and Rana Haddad Ibrahim*

Internationally, groups formed by people living with HIV/AIDS have been critical in challenging and shaping the response to HIV. However, most of the research on such movements is based on the experience of high-income countries or of low- and middle-income countries with high HIV prevalence. In low-prevalence contexts, where strong stigma is often associated with HIV and the behaviors that increase exposure to it, the epidemic is typically hidden from public view and therefore absent from public debate. This is the case in the Middle East and North Africa (MENA) region where the mobilization of people living with HIV/AIDS in the response to the epidemic is at a relatively nascent stage and faces many barriers.

This chapter compares findings from interviews with members of an Association of People Living with HIV in Sudan (previously northern Sudan) with those from interviews with a support group for people living with HIV in Lebanon. Both are countries included in UNAIDS' definition of the Middle East and North Africa region. The chapter draws on two separate studies on each setting, the first carried out in 2005 in Sudan and the second, based on findings from the Sudan study, conducted in 2007 in Lebanon. Both studies aimed to analyze the experience of the establishment and growth of these associations for people living with HIV and the challenges they face from the point of view of those involved in them. In each setting the role and nature of each association have continued to evolve over time and therefore our findings do not reflect their present situation. Moreover, the epidemiological context, access to treatment, and the general response to HIV in each country have also changed. Nevertheless, the perspectives of HIV-positive members of these associations about the challenges faced in their respective contexts have lessons for other associations that are increasingly being formed in the Middle East and North Africa region as elsewhere. The chapter also analyzes the perspectives of people living with HIV that point to deficiencies in policy in these settings that have wider relevance to the rest of the region and to other contexts where HIV is both at low prevalence and associated with high levels of stigma. It demonstrates the importance of community-level mobilization to counteract HIV-related stigma and the role of such associations in advocacy for improved health and social policies and the realization of greater rights for people living with HIV. As countries aim to scale up access to treatment, such associations have a key role to play and can act as intermediaries between people with HIV and the health care system.

## ASSOCIATIONS OF PEOPLE LIVING WITH HIV/AIDS IN THE MIDDLE EAST/NORTH AFRICA REGION

As of 2009, there were an estimated 460,000 people living with HIV in the Middle East and North Africa region (Joint United Nations Program on HIV/AIDS [UNAIDS], 2010). Intense stigma around HIV and the behaviors that increase the risk of exposure to it and pervasive discrimination have been a major challenge to AIDS prevention efforts in the Middle East and North Africa region (Abu-Raddad et al., 2010; Akala & Jenkins, 2005). The United Nations Special Program on HIV/AIDS (UNAIDS) has held a series of meetings, beginning in Algeria in 2005 (Algiers Declaration, 2005), to increase the involvement of people living with HIV/AIDS. A review of the situation of people living with HIV summarizes: "Until very recently, people living with HIV in the MENA region were not organized and engaged in support groups, networks and NGOs, but remain fairly isolated" (Kay & Datta, 2010: p. 8). In general, however, groups from the region have only begun to be represented in global networks of people living with HIV. A number of Arab countries including Algeria, Egypt, Jordan, Lebanon, Morocco, and Sudan have seen the formation of associations of people living with HIV/AIDS but no published literature is available to our knowledge on their process of formation or on their role and impact. These associations vary in size, legal registration, and visibility. Many are initiating a transition from offering mutual support to a more collective and public role as advocates on behalf of those with HIV to improve health services and policy, but also to reduce AIDS-related stigma in society overall.

## The Sudanese Context

An Islamist regime has been in power in Khartoum since 1989. In 2005, the war between the Government of Sudan and the Sudan People's Liberation Movement based in the south of the country ended with the signing of a Comprehensive Peace Agreement. Under this agreement, a Government of National Unity was established with more autonomy delegated to the Government of Southern Sudan. A January 2011 referendum resulted in overwhelming support for separation of the north and south of the country, and South Sudan was declared an independent country in July 2011. During 2012, however, renewed tensions surfaced between the two now separate countries.

At the time the study was conducted, Sudan had a population of some 45 million (including over 8 million in the south). The population was ethnically and religiously diverse with a Muslim majority combined with Christians and animists originating from the south of the country. In total, about 70 percent of the population was estimated to be Sunni Muslim (in the north); Christians comprised about 5 percent of the population (mostly living in the south and in Khartoum); while those espousing indigenous or animist beliefs comprised 25 percent of the population (Index Mundi, 2011). The United Nations Development Program's (UNDP) 2006 *Human Development* report ranked Sudan 141st among 177 countries in terms of human development. Moreover, according to statistics from the UNDP/World Bank, 60–75 percent of the population in the north and 90 percent in the south are estimated to be living below the poverty line of less than U.S. $1 a day (UNDP, n.d.). It is estimated that only 61 percent of the population is literate (Index Mundi, 2011).

Sudan has the second highest HIV/AIDS adult prevalence in the Middle East and North Africa region, but the available limited information (constrained by years of civil conflict) indicates that only South Sudan may have a generalized epidemic (Abu-Raddad et al., 2010). In northern Sudan (now Sudan), there is evidence of a possible concentrated epidemic among injecting drug users and among men who have sex with men, but there is no evidence of a concentrated epidemic among female sex workers

(Abu-Raddad et al., 2010). According to a recent epidemiological and behavioral review of the HIV situation in Sudan (August, 2009) by the Sudan National AIDS Programme (SNAP), the overall HIV prevalence is estimated at 1.1 percent overall and 0.67 percent in the north (SNAP, 2010). In 2009, the total number of adults and children living with HIV was about 122,216 in North Sudan (SNAP, 2010). SNAP reported in its 2006–2007 report on North Sudan to the United Nations General Assembly Special Session on HIV/AIDS (UNGASS) that only HIV-positive 1,759 individuals were on antiretroviral treatment (SNAP, 2008).

Prolonged civil war, including ongoing warfare in Darfur, poverty, and displacement have severely limited both surveillance and the response to the epidemic. At the same time, action has been boosted by high-level political commitment that is unusual in the region, as well as significant foreign funding, particularly from the Global Fund to Fight AIDS, Tuberculosis and Malaria since 2005.

There is no published literature on HIV-related stigma in northern Sudan although existing unpublished literature attests to pervasive stigma: A survey of over 400 health care providers found that over 50 percent harbored negative feelings toward people with HIV (Health Alliance International, 2008). A needs assessment by the SNAP and UNAIDS in 2006 found that the main difficulties expressed by people living with HIV were in the areas of low socioeconomic status, stigma, education, rights, medical care, and psychological well-being (SNAP, 2008). A qualitative unpublished study on the experience of stigma among 38 HIV-infected individuals in Khartoum found that stigma resulted in a reluctance to seek the increasingly available voluntary and counseling testing services, thus "creating and increasing an invisible population with HIV who are unable or unwilling to access treatment and care" (Christian Aid, 2008, p. 5). Moreover, individuals with HIV reported extensive discrimination by medical providers toward them, which led to many concealing their HIV status from providers.

## The Lebanese Context

Lebanon, which has a population of approximately 4 million, is a small, middle-income country. During the last 35 years, Lebanon's history has been characterized by one of political instability and civil conflict relating to both internal inequities as well as geopolitical forces affecting the region. The Lebanese civil war, 1975 to 1990, was concluded through the Taif Accords of 1989, which retained the confessional system of governance initially established by the colonial powers, but stipulated a careful balance of power between religious sects. A Syrian military presence in Lebanon was maintained. Within this system, the president is a Maronite Christian, the prime minister a Sunni Muslim, and the Speaker of Parliament a Shi'ite Muslim. In 2005 the Lebanese former prime minister, Rafik Hariri, was assassinated, resulting in the resignation of the government, a series of assassinations of political figures, and the withdrawal of Syrian forces. In July 2006, Israel invaded Lebanon for 33 days, leading to over 1,000 Lebanese civilian deaths. In May 2008, further civil unrest erupted, albeit briefly.

As a result of this history, the state plays a minor role in the provision of social welfare in the country, with the main provider of social services being the private, for-profit sector. Civil society, however, often aligned along sectarian lines, is a major provider of social welfare in the country. Lebanon's human development indicators in 2009 placed it at the low end of "high human development," and the country is ranked 83 out of 183 countries (UNDP, 2009). Life expectancy is 71.7 years, infant mortality rate is 16.1, and the combined educational enrollment is 73.4 percent (UNDP, 2009).

In terms of the epidemiology of HIV in the country, over the 20-year period from 1989 until November 2009 there have been a cumulative number of 1,253 HIV cases reported to the Ministry of Public Health (National AIDS Program). The number of people estimated to be living with HIV in Lebanon in 2009 was 3,760 (1,700: 7,200) (UNGASS, 2012). The number of reported cases has risen in recent years, with a growing rate of infection among men who have sex with men in particular. A first HIV bio-behavioral survey among at-risk groups in HIV in 2008 found reported risky behaviors to be relatively high but prevalence to be low, except for among men who have sex with men (MSM), among whom the population prevalence was found to be 3.6 percent (Mahfoud et al., 2010).

Unlike Sudan, Lebanon has never had financial support from the Global Fund to Fight AIDS, Tuberculosis and Malaria for its national country program on HIV. Over 20 voluntary counseling and testing (VCT) centers have been operational in Lebanon since 2008, largely run by NGOs (such as SIDC) but under the supervision of the National AIDS Program. As in other areas of social welfare, NGOs play a major role in the response to HIV in Lebanon. Indeed, 55 percent of the HIV budget was spent by civil society organizations in 2011 (UNGASS, 2012). Lebanon is also exceptional in the region for having an NGO, HELM, founded in 2004 and actively promoting the rights and well-being of MSM. As of 2012, there are two support groups for people living with HIV, including Vivre Positif, the subject of this chapter, and another entitled Think Positive.

## METHODS

The first and second author conducted a qualitative case study on the Sudanese association. We recruited a convenience sample of members of the association by being present at the premises of the association after an initial introduction by the president of the association and staff at the SNAP. The second author conducted open-ended interviews with 15 HIV-positive members of the association mainly in Arabic (with three interviews in English with Southern Sudanese who did not speak Arabic) for a duration ranging from one to two hours and at a venue chosen by the interviewee. The second author recorded interviews with a digital recorder (with the consent of the interviewees), transcribed them verbatim, and simultaneously translated Arabic interviews into English. The first and second authors analyzed the transcribed interviews first separately and arrived at themes for analysis independently. A consolidated list of themes was then formed. We then analyzed the retrieved segments using content analysis.

The Lebanese study was designed by the first and third authors based on findings from the Sudan study. The third author conducted the interviews with 10 HIV-positive members of the Lebanese association in late 2007 in Beirut. The leadership of the support group based at the NGO, SIDC, agreed to provide information about the study to members of the support group at their regular meetings. Interviews were conducted in Arabic, recorded and transcribed verbatim, and then translated into English.

In both studies, we explained the purposes of the research carefully to the interviewees, and confidentiality was assured in that no names or identifiers were requested. Verbal informed consent was obtained and a private space was ensured. The study in Sudan was approved by UNAIDS in Khartoum and that in Lebanon was approved by the Institutional Review Board of the American University of Beirut, Lebanon.

## AIDS-Related Stigma, Recognition, and Redistribution

Studies on stigma in public health broadly owe their roots to the work of Erving Goffman (1963), who described stigma as an "attribute that is deeply discrediting" (as cited in Shamos, Hartwig, & Zindela, 2009, p. 1679) but who, unlike some who subsequently used his work, drew attention to the social processes and relationships creating stigma (Castro & Farmer, 2005).

HIV, however, has attributes that make it and the behaviors increasing expo-sure to it highly susceptible to stigma (Parker & Aggleton, 2003). Writers on HIV-related stigma have, over the last decade, endeavoured to shift attention away from attributing stigma to a static, individual level and more toward the social processes and power relations that generate stigma (see, for example, Mahajan et al., 2008; Parker & Aggleton, 2003). Thus Shamos and colleagues define stigma as a "social process conducted in a relative power structure that allows labelling and separation and that leads to status loss or discrimination" (Shamos et al., 2009, p. 1679). In calling for greater attention to the structural roots of AIDS-related stigma, Parker and Aggleton (2003) underscore the importance of community mobilization and activism by those stigmatized. Yet as they note, there has been relatively little documentation of collective processes for reducing stigma, at least in developing country contexts.

There is a substantial literature on the role of support groups and people living with HIV/AIDS associations in developed countries (see, for example, Crook, Browne, Roberts, & Gafni, 2005; Jankowski, Videka-Sherman, & Laquidara-Dickinson, 1996; Sandstrom, 1996; Spirig, 1998). The literature on movements in developing countries has understandably tended to focus on relatively high AIDS prevalence settings and on individual NGOs (such as, for example, The AIDS Support Organization, TASO, in Uganda—see Kaleeba et al., 1997—or the Treatment Action Campaign, TAC, in South Africa—see Robins, 2006). These have moved from supporting individual members to political activism on a national and even global level to widen access to treatment and promote the rights of those with HIV. Research on the Thai network for People Living with HIV/AIDS (TNP+) has shown how it has helped in the "social normalization of being HIV-positive" (Lyttleton, 2004, p. 3) but also to expand access to antiretroviral therapies (Lyttleton, 2004; Lyttleton, Beesey, & Sitthikriengkrai, 2007; see also Liamputtong, Haritavorn, & Kiatying-Angsulee, 2009, on the importance of support groups for women in Thailand).

Beyond health and within the realm of political philosophy, research-ers on the "politics of recognition," beginning with Charles Taylor (1994), have drawn attention to the cultural processes that prevent some groups in society from being recognized or from participating in normal social life and decision making. The social movements underlying the currently preeminent "identity politics" are said to engage in such a process of rec-ognition that aims at attributing value to cultural difference. Insofar as forming associations for people living with HIV is a process of forging a collective identity based on a shared health status—being HIV positive—such movements are engaged in a struggle for "recognition" in this sense. Nancy Fraser has argued persuasively, however, that the obstacles to such participation are usually not only a question of addressing social exclusion in terms of changing social attitudes. Rather, she argues that redressing the injustice of their exclusion typically requires not only social processes of recognition but also economic processes of redistribution (see, for example, Fraser, 1996). As we argue here, Fraser's work on "redistribution with recognition" is particularly relevant in the case of the challenge faced by members of these HIV support groups in both Sudan and Lebanon where individuals' sense of social exclusion and economic insecurity are interrelated. In what follows, we document the challenges faced by the two associations in Sudan and Lebanon to achieve "recognition." We also show, following Fraser, that AIDS-related discrimination in both settings had economic consequences and thus redressing stigma necessarily requires confronting both the social and economic basis of exclusion.

## FINDINGS

### Description of Sudan Sample

The sample of HIV-positive members of the Sudanese association was purposely selected to include both Muslims and Christians and men and women. The sample included eight HIV-positive women and seven HIV-positive men. The then-president, who was HIV-negative, was also interviewed. Interviewees come from different places of origin including South, east, central, and north Sudan but were living in Khartoum and the age range was 25–65 years old. The individuals' knowledge about their infection ranged from 3 months to 10 years.

### Description of Lebanon Sample

Given the smaller size of the support group in Lebanon, there was no attempt to select purposively. Of the 10 interviewed members of the support group in Lebanon interviewed in 2007, the majority (8) were men and 2 were female, reflecting the mainly male membership of the support group at that time. Seven were Christian and three Muslim, and they ranged in age from 23 to 67. Four were from Beirut but others came from other regions of Lebanon and had to travel for the regular meetings, which occur in Beirut. The educational levels ranged from no education and only able to read to a PhD. Out of the 10 people interviewed, 3 were working regularly, 3 were working irregularly, and 4 were not working. The period from which they had known their HIV status ranged from 9 months to 30 years.

## History of the Associations

According to interviewees, the Sudanese association grew out of a program sponsored by the Sudanese National AIDS Program (SNAP) and encouraged by UNAIDS, some faith-based organizations, and NGOs active in HIV/AIDS. Formally registered in 2003, it only succeeded in renting its own premises as of 2005. The initial impetus for the formation of the association was an individual who had died before we conducted this research from HIV/AIDS and whom interviewees described as a highly charismatic figure. Quite exceptional for the time in Sudan, this former president of the association was able to speak in public about his HIV status. He mobilized a small support group of infected and affected individuals and counselors calling themselves the Association of Patients' Friends, which met monthly. Having a strong vision for the association, he was able to lobby the government to register it legally despite having faced strong stigma from his own family.

The deputy of the association, himself an HIV/AIDS counselor but not HIV positive, subsequently took over as president. This reflected the fact that the facilitating role of HIV/AIDS counselors was critical in the history and formation of the association. Counselors were typically from nongovernmental organizations including faith-based organizations such as the Sudan Council of Churches. At the time that the interviews were conducted, the association had—at least on paper—roughly 250 members in the Khartoum base and 13 branches (in Khartoum, Bahr el Jabal, Juba, North Kordofan, Gadaref, Red Sea, White Nile, Unity, Kassala, Upper Nile, Elgezira, Sinar, River Nile, West Bahr Alzar).

The group of people living with HIV in Lebanon began in the late 1990s and was initially hosted by the NGO Soins Infirmiers et Developpement Communautaire (SIDC), but later grew into an independent institution entitled Vivre Positif. The support group applied for legal registration in 2007 and having received no objection is considered legal. As one member of the support group, himself a lawyer, explained Lebanese law:

> The law says that any three persons or more can create an organization; they have 15 days to notify the Ministry of Interior about the status of the organization and the Ministry of Interior has a two-month period to respond—to object or not to reply; if it doesn't object this means that the organization is operational.

At the time the interviews were conducted there were approximately 30 members of the Lebanese support group and it included both Muslims and Christians. Although members came from all over the country, all meetings and most activities took place in Beirut and there had been no formal effort to establish branches in other parts of the country. Four HIV-positive founding members of the support group were among the interviewees for the study reported here. Several members of the support group are also involved in HIV-related activities of the SIDC NGO. Unlike the support group in Sudan at the time, the Lebanon support group also has a website, which according to one interviewee was being referred to by at least 150 people.

## CHALLENGES OF RECOGNITION AND DEFUSING HIV-RELATED STIGMA

The following sections point to the commonalities expressed by interviewees of the associations in the two countries in terms of the challenges faced by the association in asserting what Nancy Fraser and other writers refer to as "recognition."

### Moving from Mutual Support to Advocacy

The literature on support groups across public health concerns refers to their crucial contribution to supporting individuals. Interviewees in both settings appreciated this function. However, the role of the associations under study here was also transcending the mutual support role to one of public advocacy. That is, there was an articulated goal of changing the way in which the issue of HIV in these settings is considered and to argue for an acknowledgment at a societal level of the challenges faced by those with HIV.

At the time the interviews were conducted, the Sudanese association had many functions including supporting its members, conducting home visits, and providing names of sympathetic medical providers to the newly infected. But it had also made the transition to engaging more in public education and advocacy. Its members traveled to meetings around the country talking about their experience of the illness and advising the public about HIV. As one interviewee described their impact at public gatherings:

We always ask doctors to give a summary about HIV and then we ask what if we had a person living with HIV with us here, what would you do to them? Some people respond: put them in prison, segregate them, burn them, why bring them here. After that when a PLHIV tells his experience the audience changes, and they apologize. They find out that the PLHIV is a father responsible for a family or a mother taking care of her children.

The same was true in Lebanon—the support group had evolved from one of mutual support and collective discussion to a more active and public role. As one interviewee there described it: "We are organizing activities, awareness sessions, and conferences. We travel abroad, we appear on TV. It grew a lot—before HIV was taboo."

Both in Sudan and Lebanon, however, the challenge of participating in such public education activities, which by its nature requires some disclosure of one's HIV status, posed dilemmas to the individuals concerned. Members of both organizations varied in the extent to which they had disclosed their status to their social networks and, even further, more publically. Some were quite open and able to give public testimonies whereas others preferred to remain anonymous. In Sudan, the large size of the country both geographically and demographically meant that anonymity was easier to maintain, whereas in Lebanon the small size of the country and its limited population made it harder to remain unidentified.

One interviewee in Lebanon described the way in which the association had divided roles to allow for this variation in disclosure levels. As he described it, those comfortable with disclosing their status would be willing to participate in awareness-raising sessions openly, whereas others preferred to work on brochures or staff the hotline run by SIDC. As he described their reluctance to participate, fearing that their identity might be revealed and its consequences: "Some people are employees and are afraid they might lose their jobs; some others have families." At the same time he was critical of this lack of disclosure, considering it a form of suicide: "Don't tell Mum, don't tell Dad, this thing staying within him. . . . How are you planning to live? How many personalities do you want to have?"

The same dilemma applied to the debate within each association as to whether the organization should be exclusively for people with HIV or also include affected and supportive individuals who are HIV-negative. This was also tied to the names given to the associations. In Sudan, the fact that the association includes both has been important for the many members who prefer to keep their positive HIV-status from their family and social networks. As one HIV-positive female member described it, this is particularly important to her as a woman:

I travel to awareness sessions for other branches. But in Khartoum, I don't like to present myself as HIV-positive because they will recognize me immediately. Once I had to give a lecture, but when I finished someone said we were all HIV-positive at the association. So immediately a high-ranking woman stood up and said that the association is made of positive but also nonpositive people and everyone is encouraged to join. She saved me because in the audience were former colleagues of mine at the university, who live in the same neighborhood as I do. It would have been a disaster for me.

Some considered the issue strategically and felt that the involvement of individuals such as counselors and others sympathetic to the plight of those with HIV helped to defuse stigma. As one female HIV-positive member argued, the larger the number of infected and noninfected people who join the association, the more understanding there would be about HIV/AIDS in society at large.

Interviewees in the Lebanon support group were also unanimous in their view that in principle HIV-negative individuals could be included, but several underlined the importance of a clear vetting process to ensure they have the best interests of the support group in mind. As one interviewee in Lebanon stated: "The more non-HIV-positive people join the better it is, but it should be done in an organized manner, in a way not to hurt the others and in a way that there would be a general agreement."

Overall, then, while in both settings most individuals saw the associations as a means of supporting individuals who are HIV-positive, they also recognized its larger role in public education and defusing stigma in society. As one Lebanese interviewee put it: "On a national level, I think that this is the first point for HIV positive people: to have a strong psychological immunity in order to speak their mind and prove that they are just like all other people, so that they manage to break this stigma and shame." At the same time, the interviews were replete with examples of the difficulty of disclosure that being involved in the association might entail. Some explicitly voiced this as a personal sacrifice that needed to be made for the sake of progress in the advancement in the rights of people with HIV. This same sentiment was expressed in Sudan, as one male interviewee stated:

The effort has to come from the people living with HIV/AIDS themselves. Nobody gives others their rights, whether social or material rights. They themselves have to ask for their rights so that they can obtain them, this is the only way. Changing the society needs a big effort from the infected people. Many of them will need to sacrifice their reputation. They need to meet with officials, talk in the media. It needs an effort from us first to ask for our rights.

To interviewees, not only did the very existence of such an organization help defuse stigma, but being a member of such organizations helped them to challenge discrimination experienced in their everyday lives. Both in Sudan and Lebanon, interviewees provided examples of how being a member of the support group gave them the courage to confront stigma and discrimination in different venues. One member in Lebanon, for example, described how, when he was attending a conference on HIV, a doctor moved his place when he discovered that the interviewee was HIV-positive. However, the latter confronted him, as he explains:

After the session ended, I went to him and talked to him, and told that I respect your decision to change your seat, but what I cannot respect is that you [are] here in order to discuss a decision that will affect the lives of certain people, that I am one of them; but changing your seat is not an honorable act for one simple reason: If you are here to discuss this issue and you are scared of me, you shouldn't have come in the first place.

To summarize, in both Sudan and Lebanon members of the associations saw the need for these organizations not only as a venue for providing mutual support but also recognized their potential, and indeed obligation, to redress HIV-related stigma in their societies. Nevertheless, this same imperative raised challenges for their members in that playing such a public role necessitated disclosure at an individual level of one's HIV status, which many feared doing.

## The Role of Family

Just like religion, the role of the family in the lives of the interviewees was a recurring theme, and participants in both settings expressed dilemmas about what role the associations could play vis-à-vis their members' families. Concerns among members focused on hesitation about disclosure and how to disclose their status to their family members, fear concerning infecting family members, and concern over the potential stigma family members would face. There was wide variation in both contexts in the degree to which they had disclosed their status to family members and the reaction of their families. These ranged from cases where the family had completely rejected them to others where a parent was actively encouraging the support group and encouraged his son to invite his colleagues from the support group home. For those who did not disclose their HIV status to their family, some justified this out of concern for them, as one Lebanese interviewee expressed it: "I love my dad to an extent that I know that if he finds out he's going to be very sad, meaning I am not afraid of him as much as I am afraid for him." In cases where their families had rejected them, other members of the association had sometimes intervened to try to mend relations.

In both countries, the lack of social safety nets means that the family becomes a major source of security. Therefore, for those rejected by their family the economic hardship was evident, while those who were still close to their families faced the burden of how they would fulfill the expected role of supporting parents in their old age. As one interviewee in Lebanon explained it: "So this is a kind of burden, I am his only son. I am the one who is supposed to help him in the future." At the same time, many of the younger interviewees expressed frustration at what they perceived as their lack of prospects for starting a family due to their HIV status. In both settings, some interviewees saw the association as a potential venue for meeting potential partners.

## HIV and Religious Discourse

In the Middle East and North Africa region generally, religion plays a major role in public debate. Members of the associations spoke of the need to challenge and engage religious discourse in order to overcome HIV-related stigma. Despite the difference in the religious composition of the interviewees of the support groups in Lebanon, religion was a recurring theme in both sets of interviews. One interviewee in Lebanon underlined the importance of religion in HIV-related stigma in Lebanon and asked, "I am an HIV-positive person; does that make me against religion?" Another explained how the issue was seen with moral reprobation across all religions in Lebanon: "I tell you once more that the first thing they think of is the moral side; because this issue is related to sex, and sex outside the wedlock is banned in our society and in all religions." Another answered, in response to the question of what makes people discriminate against people with HIV in Lebanon:

Because it has a certain background according to our Arabic, oriental, and religious culture; this topic is connected to sex, and premarital sex is forbidden, meaning it is forbidden religiously, socially, and morally; so there is more than one interrelated factor that would lead somebody to despise the person who contracted the virus; he deserves it, it was him who brought this upon himself, and he deserves no mercy.

At the same time, Lebanese interviewees stated that one thing that they liked most about the support group was its diversity, including its religious diversity, in a society deeply divided along sectarian lines. In Sudan also, the support group at the time of the interviews included both Northerners (who are predominantly Muslim) and Southerners (who are predominantly Christian).

Both in Sudan and Lebanon and among Muslims and Christians interviewed, faith was expressed by most interviewees as critical to their coping with their HIV status. We have already noted the critical role of religious organizations such as the Sudan Council of Churches in the formation of the association there. In Sudan, however, there was some articulated frustration with interactions with religious entities. There, interviewees expressed difficulties in the dealings of the association with the governmental Muslim charity department, Diwan al Zikat, which they implied treated them with discrimination. But they also reported a remarkable improvement as, they felt, stigma associated with HIV/AIDS was reduced. UNAIDS reported that the Diwan al Zakat later played a critical role in receiving private-sector donations for people living with HIV/AIDS, which it was able to pass on to the association (H. Hassan, UNAIDS, email message to authors, June 29, 2006). And in 2008, a UNDP-organized meeting brought together 100 Muslim and Christian religious leaders to discuss their role in responding to HIV/AIDS in Sudan. They produced a declaration of commitment on HIV/AIDS that emphasizes the urgency of responding to the AIDS epidemic, calling for awareness campaigns, outreach to vulnerable groups, and treatment and care for those infected and affected by HIV (SNAP, 2010). At that meeting, a representative of the Ministry of Guidance and Endowment stated that "an individual living with HIV/AIDS is someone passing through an ordeal and who God wished to test. He is our brother and we should not discriminate against him" (*Sudan Tribune*, 2008).

### Challenge of Expanding Membership

The enormity of the challenge of identifying and recruiting potential HIV-positive members of the organization was daunting to interviewees, as one interview described, since prevailing stigma effectively makes the epidemic hidden:

> One thing affects me a lot and that is that we cannot put our hands on what exactly is happening in Sudan. . . . Since last year we are talking about the 3 × 5 initiative, we are saying that Sudan has many thousands of PLHIV and many have died, but you can't know exactly how many die or not and you can't find out where the PLHIV live. In the association we only have 250 members, so where are the other thousands, where?

In Lebanon, interviewees expressed this same frustration about the need, but at the same time the difficulty, of reaching more people and the seeming invisibility of people with HIV. "Where are they?" asked one interviewee about other people living with HIV who might be potential members. Another described knowing others who could join but who remained reluctant: "I know a lot of people outside the group, but they are still afraid to join, and this fear is their own problem; how much more can we do?"

In Sudan, the association had already established several other branches in other geographic areas of Sudan, although it was not clear how active these were. In Lebanon, activities were restricted to Beirut, and interviewees were unanimous in the view that it was not sufficient to have a support group that was based in the capital, given transportation costs to Beirut and the difficulty of reaching those living in more peripheral areas. At the same time they recognized the resource needs of expansion. As one interviewee described it: "The thing is that the group is only present in Beirut and it is barely standing on its feet."

Several interviewees in Lebanon blamed the fact that doctors were not doing enough to share information about the support group. Indeed, of the 10 interviewees most had either heard about the support group by chance or through personal connections rather than information deliberately shared by the health care system.

### Economic Implications of HIV-Related Stigma and Their Impact on the Association

Despite their contrasting economic settings, a recurring theme emerging from interviews in both Sudan and Lebanon was the economic uncertainty and insecurity that interviewees felt was exacerbated by their HIV status. They also voiced fear about growing old in contexts of limited public pension provision. In Lebanon, where health care is highly privatized, this was intermingled with concerns over who would pay the costs of health care if they got sick, and the strain on their resources of paying for HIV viral load tests. For while the Lebanese government pays for antiretroviral treatment for all those who need it, this does not include the costs of HIV-related blood tests. One expressed the fear that if his health insurance company learned about his HIV status, his health insurance would stop.

In both settings, interviewees provided examples of either being dismissed from their work due to their HIV status, or their fear of being dismissed if they disclosed their status. As two Lebanese interviewees put it: "They will fire me as soon as I tell them" and "Most of the people who know that you are HIV-positive won't hire you." Interviewees in Lebanon also described a constriction in their chances of employment in the Gulf region, a common strategy in the region of outward migration to secure a better income, due to mandatory HIV testing for all migrants to those countries. As one interviewee in Lebanon described, his options in life had become limited due to his HIV status: "Decisions in my life that I have excluded. I canceled them. For example, if I was considering looking for a job in the Gulf countries, I excluded that." Another described how deportation from the Gulf region due to the discovery of his HIV status had completely disrupted his life and economic chances. That said, one interviewee in Lebanon described a more positive example in which he disclosed his HIV status to his supervisor, who was very supportive and even raised his salary.

Nevertheless, the fact that most of the interviewees in Lebanon were unemployed (only 4 out of 10 had regular work) was recognized by participants themselves as a constraint on the activities of the association. Several pointed to the limits of voluntarism in such a situation. As one said: "The concept of voluntarism is still very primitive in Lebanon. Meaning you are not providing anything for this volunteer when he becomes unemployed, you are not securing enough funds in order to motivate him and keep him persistent in the work and in the awareness activities." Those who were unemployed could not afford to do unpaid work on a voluntary basis, particularly if it entailed transportation expenses, and they were preoccupied with securing employment.

## CONCLUSION

The above discussion has underscored the common challenges, despite their different contexts, faced by the associations in Sudan and Lebanon.

These have centered on the challenge of moving from a mutual support role to one including public education and advocacy to defuse the stigma associated with HIV. As shown in both the Lebanese and Sudanese contexts, individuals' reluctance to disclose their status publically, precisely because of this stigma, in turn constrained these more public functions of the associations. That said, at the same time interviewees recognized the importance of so doing and the need for people with HIV to mobilize collectively to articulate their rights. Moreover, in both contexts, the roles of religion and the family were central both to interviewees' discourse about HIV-related stigma in their settings and to the challenges faced by these associations in reducing stigma.

Members of both organizations were also frustrated with the limited reach of their respective associations and complained about the seeming invisibility of people with HIV. That is, in both cases, the association had not yet achieved a national coverage and become known widely among institutions in the country. This suggests the need to strengthen the two-way relationship between such associations and the health care system. Reinforcing those links more formally would allow individuals newly diagnosed with HIV to be referred to support groups but would also provide scope for such support groups to take a more active role in helping individuals negotiate the health care system and thereby increase their access to treatment.

Finally, interviews with both Sudanese and Lebanese HIV-positive members of the associations studied revealed the perceived interrelationship between HIV-related stigma and economic insecurity. Individuals' economic security, which was exacerbated by their HIV status, in turn constrained the public action of the organizations in defusing societal-level stigma. This is despite the difference in per capita income between Sudan and Lebanon.

Despite these commonalities, however, certain differences also emerged between the two settings. For example, the history of these associations was quite different. Whereas in Sudan it emerged spontaneously, led by individuals living with HIV themselves, in Lebanon the support group was encouraged by an NGO already active in HIV prevention and support. In Sudan, support from the Global Fund to Fight AIDS, Tuberculosis and Malaria has helped to strengthen the response and to encourage the involvement of people living with HIV. In Lebanon, however, no funding has been available at a country level from the Global Fund, and indeed funding for HIV is fairly limited to the country. Civil society has taken the lead in both settings in supporting and representing people living with

HIV, but in both countries securing funding for this work has been a continual challenge.

A final difference of relevance to the formation of the associations is that in Sudan, being a much more populous country with a higher (although still low) HIV prevalence than Lebanon, there are many more individuals infected with HIV. The large size of the country both geographically and demographically allows scope for more anonymity, as interviewees illustrated with examples.

Irrespective of these commonalities and differences between these two settings, however, the findings of interviews with both these two associations have many lessons of relevance to other settings. First, a focus on the formation of such organizations draws attention to the intersection between the situation and efforts of individuals and those of the societies in which they live. Horton (2006) has pointed out that the discourse on HIV/AIDS has become polarized between the focus on the individual and the biomedical on the one hand and public health approaches focused on populations on the other, with little focus on the intermediate, community level of action. The literature on stigma has called for such community-level mobilization of those who are stigmatized if the roots of HIV-related stigma are to be addressed. The challenges faced by such associations illustrates this process, which has not been sufficiently documented.

In Sudan and Lebanon, as is the case in most developing countries, AIDS-related interventions currently focus on those with HIV as individuals. Yet in the cultural context of both countries and indeed the larger region, addressing the wider family would arguably be beneficial. Rotheram-Borus, Flannery, Rice, and Lester (2005) have argued that because of the history of the epidemic in the West, there has been resistance to seeing the importance of family interventions. Yet there are strong arguments—particularly in developing countries where the family is often the only reliable social safety net—that one should be helping families, not only individuals, to cope with the disease.

Such data also points to the need for improvement in HIV-related policies beyond the health sector. Interviewees pointed to the unnecessary and unfair hardships experienced in securing and maintaining employment because of employment-related discrimination. In both settings, then, interviewees described their economic marginalization and uncertainty that was exacerbated by their HIV status and raised expectations of its members. This in turn impeded the activities of the associations in pointing to the plight of those with HIV and in the challenge of "recognition." In this sense, our findings are consistent with Fraser's arguments that cultural recognition to redress the loss of status is not sufficient to redress the social exclusion brought by stigma, but that addressing the concomitant economic exclusion is also necessary. Indeed, as she argues, "Economic harms that originate from the status order have an undeniable weight of their own. Left unattended, moreover, they may impede the capacity to mobilize against misrecognition" (Fraser, 1996: p. 21). In other words, with HIV exacerbating economic insecurity, the challenge of counteracting stigma and discrimination becomes all the more difficult. Given that their HIV status exacerbated poverty, the HIV-positive members of the association were not in a position to engage fully in unfunded activities of the association to mobilize against stigma and discrimination, thus affecting its operations in a vicious circle.

Our findings reinforce the need in all settings for a major involvement of people living with HIV/AIDS in the response to HIV. Interviews have provided insights about barriers to testing and delays in diagnosis and treatment that are instructive for improvement in the health care system. This is particularly important as Lebanon and Sudan, as elsewhere, endeavor to roll out treatment more broadly. Indeed, the Middle East and North Africa currently has the lowest proportion of those on treatment out of those who need it of any region, at only 11 percent (UNAIDS, 2012). As one interviewee in Lebanon expressed it: "As long as any governmental, civil, or international organization deals with the AIDS issue without taking the opinion of those living with AIDS, I know that it will not reach the desired solution."

## BIBLIOGRAPHY

Abu-Raddad, L., Akala, F. A., Semini, I., Riedner, G., Wilson, D., & Tawil, O. (2010). *Characterizing the HIV/AIDS epidemic in the Middle East and North Africa: Evidence on levels, distribution and trends. Time for strategic action. Middle East and North Africa HIV/AIDS epidemiology synthesis project.* Washington, DC: The World Bank. doi:10.1596/978-0-8213-8137-3

Akala, F. A., & Jenkins, C. (2005). *Preventing HIV/AIDS in the Middle East and North Africa: A window of opportunity to act.* Washington, DC: The World Bank. doi10.1596/978-0-8213-6264-8

Algiers Declaration (2005). *UNAIDS regional workshop on empowerment of people living with HIV/AIDS in the Middle East and North Africa (draft declaration).* Algiers: Author.

Castro, A., & Farmer, P. (2005). Understanding and addressing AIDS-related stigma: From anthropological theory to clinical practice in Haiti. *American Journal of Public Health, 95,* 53–59. doi:10.2105/AJPH.2003.028563

Christian Aid (2008). *Condemned, invisible and isolated: Stigma and support for people living with HIV in Khartoum* (Unpublished report). Retrieved from http://www.christianaid.org.uk/images/stigmatisation.pdf

Crook, J., Browne, G., Roberts, J., & Gafni, A. (2005). Impact of support services provided by a community-based AIDS service organization on persons living with HIV/AIDS. *The Journal of the Association of Nurses in AIDS Care: JANAC, 16*(4), 39–49. doi:10.1016/j.jana.2005.05.003

DeJong, J., & Mortagy, I. The struggle for "recognition" of an association for people living with HIV/AIDS in a low-prevalence country: The case of Sudan (accepted, *Qualitative Health Research*).

Fraser, N. (1996). *Social justice in the age of identity politics: Redistribution, recognition, and participation* [PDF document]. Retrieved from The Tanner Lectures on Human Values, Stanford University website: http://www.intelli genceispower.com

Hassan, W. (for Health Alliance International, SNAP, and UNFPA) (2008). *Knowledge, attitudes and practice of Sudanese health care providers toward HIV/AIDS and HIV/AIDS patients in state and federal general hospitals.* Presentation by Wisan Hassan (for HAI, SNAP, and UNFPA) at the International AIDS Conference, Mexico.

Horton, R. (2006). A prescription for AIDS 2006–10. *The Lancet, 368*(9537), 716–718. doi:10.1016/S0140-6736(06)69266-0

Index Mundi (2011). *Sudan demographics profile 2012.* Retrieved from http://www.indexmundi.com/sudan/demographics_profile.html

Jankowski, S., Videka-Sherman, L., & Laquidara-Dickinson, K. (1996). Social support networks of confidants to people with AIDS. *Social Work, 41*(2), 206–213. Retrieved from http://www.cinahl.com/cgi-bin/refsvc?jid=662&accno=1996034035

Kaleeba, N., Kalibala, S., Kaseje, M., Ssebbanja, P., Anderson, S., Van Praag, E., . . . Katabira, E. (1997). Participatory evaluation of counselling, medical and social services of the AIDS support organization (TASO) in Uganda. *AIDS Care, 9*(1), 13–26. doi:10.1080/09540129750125307

Kay, A., & Datta, S. (2010). *Paths to leadership for people living with HIV in the Middle East and North Africa.* Washington, DC: Futures Group, Health Policy Initiative, Task Order 1.

Liamputtong, P., Haritavorn, N., & Kiatying-Angsulee, N. (2009). HIV and AIDS, stigma and AIDS support groups: Perspectives from women living with HIV and AIDS in central Thailand. *Social Science & Medicine, 69*(6), 862–868. doi:10.1016/j.socscimed.2009.05.040

Lyttleton, C. (2004). Fleeing the fire: Transformation and gendered belonging in Thai HIV/AIDS support groups. *Medical Anthropology, 23*(1), 1–40. doi:10.1080/01459740490275995

Lyttleton, C., Beesey, A., & Sitthikriengkrai, M. (2007). Expanding community through ARV provision in Thailand. *AIDS Care, 19*(1), S44–53. doi:10.1080/09540120601114659

Mahajan, A. P., Sayles, J. N., Patel, V. A., Remien, R. H., Sawires, S. R., Ortiz, D. J., . . . Coates, T. J. (2008). Stigma and the HIV/AIDS epidemic: A review of the literature and recommendations for the way forward. *AIDS, 22*(2), 567–579. doi:10.1097/01.aids.0000327438.13291.62

Mahfoud, Z., Afifi, R., Ramia S., El Khoury, D., Kassak, K., El Barbir, F., Ghanem, M., El Nakib, M., & DeJong, J. (2010). HIV/AIDS among female sex workers, injecting drug users and men who have sex with men in Lebanon: Results of the first bio-behavioral surveys. *AIDS. Special Issue on HIV/AIDS in the Middle East and North Africa, 24* (Supp 2): S45–S54. doi:10.1097/01.aids.0000386733.02425.98

Parker, R., & Aggleton, P. (2003). HIV and AIDS-related stigma and discrimination: A conceptual framework and implications for action. *Social Science & Medicine, 57*(13), 24. doi: 10.1016/S0277-9536(02)00304-0

Robins, S. (2006). From "rights" to "ritual": AIDS activism in South Africa. *American Anthropologist, 108*(2), 312–323. doi:10.1525/aa.2006.108.2.312

Rotheram-Borus, M. J., Flannery, D., Rice, E., & Lester, P. (2005). Families living with HIV. *AIDS Care, 17*(8), 978–987. doi:10.1080/09540120500101690

Sandstrom, K. L. (1996). Searching for information, understanding, and self-value: The utilization of peer support groups by gay men with HIV/AIDS. *Social Work in Health Care, 23*(4), 51–74. doi:10.1300/J010v23n04_05

Shamos, S., Hartwig, K. A., & Zindela, N. (2009). Men's and women's experiences with HIV and stigma in Swaziland. *Qualitative Health Research, 19*(12), 1678–1689. doi:10.1177/1049732309353910

Spirig, R. (1998). Support groups for people living with HIV/AIDS: A review of literature. *The Journal of the Association of Nurses in AIDS Care: JANAC, 9*(4), 43–55. doi:10.1016/S1055-3290(98)80044-7

Sudan National AIDS Control Program (SNAP) (2008). *HIV/AIDS in North Sudan. United Nations General Assembly Special Session on HIV/AIDS (UNGASS) Report 2006–2007.* Retrieved from http://www.unaids.org/en/regionscountries/countries/sudan/

Sudan National AIDS Control Program (SNAP) (2010). *HIV/AIDS in North Sudan. United Nations General Assembly Special Session on HIV/AIDS (UNGASS) Report 2008–2009.* Retrieved from http://www.unaids.org/en/regionscountries/countries/sudan/

*Sudan Tribune* (2008, February 26). Sudan religious leaders campaign in favour of people living with HIV/AIDS. *Sudan Tribune.* Retrieved from http://www.sudantribune.com/spip.php?article26135

Taylor, C. (1994). The politics of recognition. In A. Gutmann (ed.), *Multicultur-alism: Examining the politics of recognition*. Princeton: Princeton University Press.

UNAIDS (2010). *Fact sheet. Middle East and North Africa. Increasing HIV prevalence, new HIV infections and AIDS-related deaths*. Retrieved from http://www.unaids.org/documents/20101123_FS_mena_em_en.pdf

UNAIDS (2012). *Together we will end AIDS*. Retrieved from http://www.unaids.org/en/media/unaids/contentassets/documents/epidemiology/2012/20120718_togetherwewillendaids_en.pdf

UNDP (n.d.). *Sudan: Achieving the MDGs and reducing human poverty*. Retrieved from http://www.sd.undp.org/focus_poverty_reduction.htm

UNDP. 2009. National Human Development Report, Lebanon 2008–2009: Towards a Citizens' State.

UNGASS (2012). *Country progress report: Lebanon, narrative report*. Retrieved from http://www.unaids.org/en/dataanalysis/knowyourresponse/countryprogressreports/2012countries/ce_LB_Narrative_Report[1].pdf

# 8

# How to Exit an Epidemic: Philanthrocapitalism, Community Mobilization, and the Domestication of Sexual Dissidence in South India

*Robert Lorway*

> Unless philanthrocapitalism digs more deeply into social change, it is in danger of replicating, not transforming, existing patterns of power and inequality, even if people have access to loans, medicine . . . they so desperately need.
>
> —Michael Edward, *Small Change*

"Don't boil the ocean" is a comment directed to me by a Harvard-trained MBA business manager of the Gates Foundation–sponsored AIDS in India initiative, Avahan, while I was conducting AIDS research among sex workers in South India. "Boiling the ocean" is a North American business term meaning that too much nuance distracts us from the bottom line. The manager then proceeded to inform me, rather emphatically, "There is that one moment, Robert, when someone is about to come into contact with HIV and there has to be someone there to intervene." For the Avahan manager, HIV prevention appeared to be quite a straightforward matter. When I suggested the possibility that people may move in and out of various contexts of risk over the course of their life, our meeting came to an abrupt end.

In this chapter, I specifically examine how particular business logics that were employed in Avahan programs combine with epidemiology to constitute "regimes of intervention" (Marcus, 2005) that govern the access of sex workers to specialized health services. Specifically, I suggest that the form of managerialism enacted through Avahan programs, although "effectively" mobilizing sex workers for STI reduction, simultaneously diminishes the potential political force of sexual dissidence. Furthermore, the way Avahan conceptualizes social life in simplistic terms, vis-à-vis new philanthropic managerial discourses and practices referred to as "philanthrocapitalism" (Bishop & Green, 2008), may actually jeopardize sex worker–run community-based organizations (CBOs) from taking the lead. At the moment when Avahan programs transition to a publically funded system (Rao, 2010), the ability of the community to sustain key areas of the intervention's operation is a central concern of Avahan allies and opponents alike.

While the role of philanthropic organizations and private-sector thinking in economic and health development is by no means new, philanthrocapitalism can be defined by the *intensified* emphasis placed upon measuring and tracking of the donor's investment in development through ongoing mandatory reporting and the employment of business metrics, which define progress and performance of projects in quantitatively measurable terms; there is, furthermore, "an augmented pattern of interaction between the donor (or 'investor') and the recipient (or 'investee') . . . in which investors facilitate skill and technical resource transfer, sustained relationship building and organizational support" (Moran, 2009, p. 7). What this has meant in the case of Avahan is that the Gates Foundation not only provides ongoing financial support to India's HIV prevention programs, but MBA-type personnel (mostly from the global management consulting firm McKinsey & Company, who are without any kind of health studies background) also *directly manage* the intervention so as to track the progress of the foundation's investment. In particular, this chapter will show how the deployment of business metrics melds remarkably well with the epidemiologically oriented monitoring and surveillance techniques, such that both perspectives cannot always be readily distinguished.

Replication and coverage (or scaling up) of Avahan's service delivery model is a central aim that guides the managerial approaches of the intervention. In a published interview, Avahan program officer Aparajita Ramakrishnan, a graduate of Harvard Business School, explicitly draws an analogy between optimal health service coverage and the running of a successful large business.

Large businesses do not just implement in one little place, otherwise they don't make enough money. . . . Similarly, with impact [of HIV prevention programs], I think you want to have a greater span. One of the ways to achieve this is . . . to be able to build an implementation pyramid. In other words, to be able to deliver services simultaneously across large geographies and across many populations. Then, some of the questions you can ask are: How do you manage the supply side to ensure that the product's sales force, in this case peer educators, are in the right place at the right time? Are they doing the right things? Is their job performance being measured? Do they have accountability? (Asthana, 2008, para. 4–5)

This illustrates a core ideology at work in Avahan's business model for health development, one that is based on management expert C. K. Prahalad's (2006) "Bottom of the Pyramid (BOP)" theory. This theory is a key guiding text of philanthrocapitalism that purports that there are unmapped markets ("a fortune") that lie at the base of the social economic pyramid—among the world's poor. By supplying them with goods that they can buy and sell, they will not only be lifted out of poverty but will be socially and politically transformed. In the case of Avahan's goals, impoverished sex workers are viewed as an untapped marketing resource (referred to above as the "sales force"). By "sales force" Ramakrishnan means that the participation of sex workers in the intervention is expected to generate demand for health services—liberating a market force that will sustain the delivery of HIV prevention to highly stigmatized populations. Thus, Avahan managers such as Ramakrishnan insist that "the reframing of development as enterprise, or targeting the poor as consumers, can contribute 'lasting solutions' that cannot be provided by traditional charitable relief" (Moran, 2009, p. 7). For this reason, Avahan's vision of "success," in terms of sustainability, has come to hinge upon the participation of sex workers, as Ramakrishnan explains:

It's similar to any business model that you can find in the private sector, where there's a focus on the customer as the beneficiary of the services being sold—or delivered in the case of health. In the private sector that's buying toothpaste; in the public sector it might be the impact in terms of lives saved. In the context of HIV prevention in India, the recipients of prevention services (sex workers, men who have sex with men, injecting drug users) need to be part of the delivery, as peer workers (a "sales force") and leaders of community-based organizations delivering the interventions. So the question is "Are you measuring everything you do?" which is a very critical piece of any good business (Asthana, 2008, para. 3)

The community mobilization techniques devised by Avahan, which follow the business logics described by Ramakrishnan, have certainly proven effective for increasing health services access to highly stigmatized communities on a grand scale. Moreover, it is important to note that the employment of this model has also yielded some striking results with respect to the reduction of curable STIs and HIV prevalence (see *AIDS Special Supplement 5*, 2008, which is devoted to a review of Avahan's outcomes). However, such thinking fails to take critical stock of how capitalist forces actually rely upon and intensify the production of social and political inequalities (related to gender, sexuality, race, ethnicity, etc.). The fact that Avahan's approach to community mobilization lacks any informed or complex analysis around social movements raises serious questions about the sustained agency of "the community" beyond this intervention.

As the managerial infrastructure transitions to a publicly funded system, criticism of Avahan as a lavishly overfunded intervention is now coming to a head. Controversies erupt over how the public system will be able to sustain the successes demonstrated by the Avahan-supported infrastructure of specialized clinical and outreach services delivered to vulnerable populations. In 2003, the original target set for community mobilization by Avahan was that 50 percent of CBOs (run by sex workers) would take over TIs in India. However, only a much smaller fraction of CBOs are regarded by the state as being prepared to assume leadership. More recently, consultants working for the publically funded National AIDS Control Organization (NACO) and who have been evaluating Avahan programs have assessed a number of local NGOs and community-based organizations as unfit to assume leadership over targeted interventions in their district. The downgrading of frontline organizations working directly with sex workers is also greatly abetted by larger global health trends toward the medicalization of HIV prevention (Nguyen, Bajos, Dubois-Arber, O'Malley, & Pirkle, 2011), which have led NACO to execute increasingly intrusive and coercive modes of surveillance. The following excerpt from a publically released draft letter, composed by the Lawyers Collective HIV/AIDS Unit, National Network of Sex Workers, Indian Harm Reduction Network, and the Integrated Network for Sexual Minorities, helps to illustrate the turbulence that swirls around the state's deployment of monitoring and evaluation techniques to govern India's most-at-risk populations (MARPs):

> Organizations implementing TIs have confirmed that the inability to meet testing targets leads to a negative evaluation by the Technical

Surveillance Unit (TSU) and/or State AIDS Control Society (SACS), triggering a series of adverse consequences. These include downgrading of performance rating, reduction in the size of population to be served under subsequent grants, decline in funding and even disqualification from running TIs. This despite the fact that the TI may be performing well on other indicators such as coverage through outreach, referral to STI screening and delivery of condoms or sterile needles.

As a result, organizations operating TIs are reportedly resorting to coercive or compulsive methods to test MARPs in order to meet the prescribed testing targets. In some places, access to services provided by the TI has been made conditional upon undergoing HIV testing. . . . Still others are reportedly organizing "health camps" to test persons with no reported high risk behavior in order to fill in numbers of people tested for HIV. The priority of the intervention has evidently shifted from explaining HIV risks and encouraging safer behaviors to instructing people to get tested (Tandon, 2010, pp. 1–2).

The letter then continues by criticizing NACO's mandatory "line-listing" procedures:

Project staff in TIs are mandated to record the name, address and other contact information of MARPs and share this data with TSU/ SACS. The practice is ostensibly to improve follow up as well as monitoring of the TI, at the cost of client confidentiality. . . . We would like to reiterate that respecting client confidentiality is not only a legal requirement but also a good public health strategy, as it improves attendance at clinics, enables clients to reveal medical or related risks and facilitates correct diagnosis and treatment. Safeguarding privacy and confidentiality assumes greater importance for MARPs on account of the stigma and criminality associated with sex work and drug use (Tandon, 2010, p. 3).

The culture of measurement initiated by Avahan and intensified under NACO policies not only overshadows the social inequalities that these communities must transform for more lasting improvement to health services access, but it also may inadvertently constitute a new system of domination as the political energies of sex workers become bound to the enumerative procedures of accountability.

Although there are certainly important local success stories of social transformation, such as the Ashodaya Samithi collective in Mysore

(Argento, Reza-Paul, Lorway, & O' Neil, 2011; Dixon, Reza-Paul, O'Neil, & Lorway, 2012) the fact that far fewer than expected CBOs have received the grade to take the lead of local TIs has certainly raised questions about the sustainability of community participation schemes more generally. Some state officials I spoke with informally toward the beginning of the transition expressed concern that the community lacked the kind of capacity that Avahan had originally envisioned. Furthermore, for some program managers I have interacted with in Karnataka more recently, the problem has begun to shift from a concern for how the community will be able to take the lead of TIs to how the community can be more effectively governed to ensure the success of TIs beyond the transition. Those who have the most at stake in this controversy are, of course, the communities whose lives have been dramatically altered by mobilization schemes that govern access to vital HIV-related services.

I suggest that the problem of sustainable community mobilization does not lie in the inherent capacity—or incapacity—of CBOs or the community to take control over the course of their own destiny with respect to HIV prevention. Rather, the problem resides in the form and enactment of various managerial and market-oriented logics, which are grafted onto epidemiological techniques of surveillance; *they neither fully account for nor prepare these communities to confront more deeply socially embedded forms of sexual stigma.* Sexual stigma, which reiterates across kinship relations and through hegemonic notions of ideal citizenship, poses a major occlusion to achieving social justice for male and female sex workers. However, non-normative sexualities cannot be readily harnessed in the promotion of the Avahan brand to a wider mainstream public. This became particularly evident in June 2012 when a more senior representative from Avahan visited the sex worker collective known as Ashodaya Smithi before a press meeting to officially announce that he would be stepping down from his directorship. While videographers were shooting him as he sat on the floor among a group of male and female sex workers, two transgender (male-to-female) *hijras* came to sit next to him, one on either side. An accompanying Avahan manager monitoring the shoot quickly scolded the group to alter their arrangement, declaring, "That doesn't look good! We need to have the women sit next to him." The *hijras* eventually withdrew to the background.

Although the HIV epidemic is widely understood among Avahan partners and epidemiologists alike as a "localized epidemic" that primarily infects marginalized "core groups" (sex workers, MSM, and *hijras*), stigma reduction campaigns sponsored by Avahan have tended to construct public awareness around the imagery of a generalized epidemic affecting "normal" people. This is exemplified in the Hero's Project, which launched a series of awareness campaigns featuring film and sports stars. In collaboration with wealthy Indian philanthropist Parmeshwar Godrej and the U.S.-based Henry J. Kaiser Family Foundation, the Avahan-sponsored project forms the largest nongovernmental media campaign and claims to have "garnered nearly fifty-percent of the media exposure on HIV & AIDS in India . . . [and] engaged nearly one hundred celebrities and trained nearly five hundred writers and producers in creating HIV & AIDS messaging" (Kaiser Foundation 2006). One series of ads that were run for the Heroes Project visually depicts AIDS-related stigma by employing the metaphor of a cage to represent the social bondage of many persons living with HIV and AIDS. In one ad, a young HIV-positive child, whose movement is encumbered by living inside a cage, attends school where he is rejected by his fellow students and their parents who refuse to socialize or have physical contact with him. A second ad shows a pregnant mother, also encaged, who is attending a hospital. This character is refused services when the attending health worker learns about her HIV-positive status. A third ad in the series portrays a young encaged man preparing to remove his office belongings after being dismissed from work for being HIV-positive. This line of ads is quite compelling in the manner in which it portrays institutional stigmatization. Yet, the message they convey appeals to a general public, as the background of the characters remains unclear. While the ads do not occlude the possibility that the pregnant woman is a sex worker, that the office worker is in a same-sex relationship, and that the student is the child of a sex worker, there is a preferred reading conveyed in the ads— that these are just ordinary HIV-positive people who are most deserving of the audience's sympathy: a young boy without friends, a pregnant mother with an absent spouse, and a once economically mobile young man now unemployed. Like many other national antistigma HIV-related campaigns in India, these ads veer away from confronting the multiple layers of sexual stigma that surround HIV and AIDS and that lie at the root of the forms of discrimination encountered by people living with AIDS—including those who are not sexual minorities. The point here is not to suggest that by simply representing sexual minorities in the media sexual stigma will necessarily be mitigated or overcome; instead, what is important to note is how such normative portrayals of people living with HIV actually mobilize and reinforce wider notions of social acceptability, rather than unsettling them.

The mainstreaming of stigma reduction works in tandem with the market-oriented managerial approaches of Avahan, which strive to create "active and pulsing demand for prevention services among the core groups" (Ashana, 2006, para. 12) and the enumerative practices of accountability imposed by NACO. Together, they stand in tension with the political potential of sexual transgression—a more radically transformative resource that will likely be needed to challenge sexual stigma as well as confront emerging forms of governance in the public health system. The mobilization of sexual subversion is certainly not something that readily lends itself to measurement, the regulatory procedures of management science, or social marketing schemes. Although the Avahan umbrella includes numerous sexual minority rights organizations, which mobilize sexual subversion in their human right demonstrations and public protests, the ways that Avahan's managerial system enlists the political energies of social movements into the project of health governance and measurement, I argue, serves to stifle sexual dissidence. Before demonstrating this point, I first briefly describe the architecture of Avahan.

Avahan's $338 million program has provided funding and administrative infrastructure to six of India's high-HIV-prevalence states, most of which are in the southern region. It exemplifies the *intersectoral blending* that Michael Moran (2009) describes with respect to new forms of social entrepreneurship taking place in international development, led by Google, the Acumen Fund, and the Skull Foundation; they invest in, connect with, and celebrate networks of social entrepreneurs. The important transnational players within Avahan's managerial structure are as follows: the National AIDS Control Program (NACO), which is the HIV prevention and care policy center in Delhi that is directly accountable to India's health minister; the various international NGOs (INGOs) or state-level partners that hold multiple ties with Western academic institutions and that flow Avahan funds to the local organizations running the TIs on the ground. Then, there are the local NGOs that, much like the INGOS, continually respond to—and become transformed by—the changing rhythms of the Global Fund, USAID, and PEPFAR in their capacity-building work with community-based organizations run by sex workers, men who have sex with men (MSM) and *hijras*. Currently, the intervention program that Avahan implemented is being transitioned to the state AIDS control societies (the publically funded health system).

In what follows, I offer a brief glimpse into the contemporary history of community mobilization by referring to two particular techniques utilized in Avahan programs to manage large populations of sexual minorities. These techniques not only enable epidemiologists to identify the most-at-risk populations and locations of sex workers, but also enable Avahan managers to render sexual minority subpopulations *measurable,* allowing managers to track the returns on their investment. Although I focus particularly upon MSM, *hijras* and male sex workers, much of the same logic is at play in interventions that target female sex workers in this region and elsewhere in India.

## MANAGING THE NEW GEOGRAPHY OF SEXUAL MINORITIES

The first technique pertains to how the geography of sexual difference is charted. Intervention managers mobilize particular notions of space in their management of risk among those deemed to be the most vulnerable to infection. Based upon the mapping of key locations where people pursue sexual partners (defined as epidemiological "hotspots"), public health practitioners have set up networks of specialized spaces and clinics to attract sexual minorities (Pandey et al., 2009). As part of the Avahan initiative, these most-at-risk populations are recruited to mobilize their peers at hotspots, with the expectation that these communities will become better connected to prevention and treatment services for sexually transmitted infections (STIs) and HIV infection (Verma et al., 2010). It is expected that these peer outreach workers (who receive a part-time salary) will be able, through promotion, to generate demand for clinical services in their community through their daily outreach work with fellow sex workers. These community mobilizers are at times guided by managers to employ mapping procedures to plan their outreach work. During my ethnographic work at three urban sites in Karnataka State, I regularly witnessed peer educators spending considerable time counting their contacts in hopes of reaching their daily target, filling out spreadsheets with program staff and participating in weekly community guide meetings that evaluate their performance.

This spatialized approach to HIV epidemic prevention has indeed transformed cruising spots where MSM share erotic intimacies into places that also track and connect MSM to STI treatment and HIV prevention services. The following excerpt, based on the participant observations of a local community outreach worker during a community research project I led, helps to reveal how everyday sexual life has become intertwined with the intervention and how the community has become drawn into the project of governing everyday sexual risk (Du Plessis, Reza-Paul, Pasha, & Lorway, 2011, p. 55).

"Hi, did you get your presumptive therapy?" I asked. We exchanged pleasantries [at the park] and then he said, "Where is the satellite clinic where we [two] can get [STI treatments]?" So, we went to the clinic. [The STI physician] was there and she said "Hi, long time no see. This person needs presumptive therapy, it is due. OK, bring the register from that room, get the ID number for the both of them." So I went with the card to the doctor. After we took the [treatment] and came to the market, the two left by bus. It was calm, people traded and waited for the buses. I had field work at the park and passed through the bus-stand. There itself I met a few *kothis* [feminine males]. One told me "Sister, give me chocolate [condom], a *panthi* [client] is calling me." "I told her to be careful and to go only with decent guys as there are more instances of bullying these days." [Mysore]

The next community researcher account illustrates how cruising spots have come to serve as avenues to identify and recruit new CBO members.

A train had just arrived at the station. It was 4 p.m. Travelers were busy getting their luggage off the train and calling the auto rickshaw drivers. Many of them were also waiting with their bags and baggage for their respective trains to board. *Kothis* make a very common sight at the railway station. Our CFs [community facilitators] had gone there to distribute condoms to *kothis*. We saw a *kothi* with a very unusual gait and strange mannerism passing by. We clapped to draw her attention. She looked at us and smiled, this time we called her. She came and introduced herself. Our CFs also did the same. We told her about our DIC [drop-in center] office and the activities we have there. She asked, "Everybody who visits your office is a *kothi*?" She further asked in a tone filled with apprehension and fear, "What will I do if your staff wants to have sex with me?" We tried to convince her by saying that a lot of *kothis* visit our office frequently. We also told her that a doctor comes to our office regularly and we also organize events. We suggested meeting the doctor in case she wants to get a check-up done and she can obtain flavored condoms from our office. I also advised her to use condoms while having sex. This perked her up and she asked if she could take her friends along with her when she visits our office. [Belgaum]

The second technique widely utilized across the Avahan program to efficiently govern access to prevention services for male and transgender

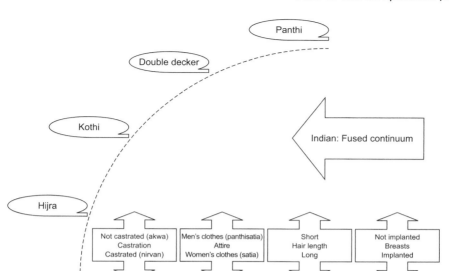

**Figure 8.1**  Sexual typology utilized by intervention specialists

sex workers has been through the deployment of local cultural categories for Indian homosexuality. Figure 8.1 appears in a set of unpublished meeting notes, which were given to me in 2006 by a former program officer working for Karnataka Health Promotion Trust in Bangalore, with the intention of assisting my orientation to the local context. The diagram was adapted from the Naz Foundation International literature on sexual typologies, which has been used to mobilize sexual minority rights development programs throughout India. As anthropologist Lawrence Cohen (2005) reminds us, widespread indigenous categories (such as *kothi* and *panthi*) are, with the exception of *hijras,* a relatively recent invention, having proliferated through sexual minority rights development work in the 1990s (also see Boyce, 2007). Whether authentic or not, these categories, along with mapping procedures, enable intervention managers and epidemiologists to *conceptualize* MSM and transgender people as definable, calculable—*and therefore governable*—subpopulations. They also enable them to *visualize* the discrete locations where the HIV epidemic can be imagined to reside (Legg, 2007).

These two techniques—the mapping of hotspots and the typologization of sexual difference—articulate together, making possible what I refer to as *inspection tours,* which are demonstrations of the intervention's effectiveness. To illustrate what I am talking about here, I provide a short excerpt taken from my field notes composed shortly after my first arrival in Bangalore:

On the first day of my orientation to Avahan programs, as a prospective postdoc, a health promotion manager guided me to a small office room in the NGO in Bangalore and rhymed off the labels and definitions for MSM and transgender people: *kothi, panthis, double-deckers, hijra,* etc. He explained in an irritated tone that many of the MSM didn't, in fact, know their "real" identity and proceeded to tell me that their NGO was trying to get vocal coaches for *hijras* so that they would be able to speak in a higher voice. I was then introduced to a group of frontline staff and community outreach workers who were waiting in an adjoined meeting room to further my orientation to their intervention. The public health staff introduced themselves using their names and educational credentials while each community member rhymed off their name and sexual identity label. For instance, one sex worker rose and introduced himself by saying, "I am Raju and I am a *double-decker* because I am sexually versatile"; another man announced, "I am Rakesh, and I am a *kothi* because I feel like a woman." This all seemed quite rehearsed. When I was later taken by the community leaders to one of their small drop-in centers to meet with more than 50 members, each person rose proudly, introducing themselves with their names and sexual identity label. But more interestingly was the fact that *hijras,* who were very feminine in their appearance, bellowed instructions to the groups of men in deep masculine voices. They were clearly leaders who commanded great respect from the rest of the group. Moreover, the dissonance between their feminine appearance and masculine voice seemed to be part of what made them empowered commanders during the meetings. I then wondered why it was so urgent for the public health professional to have them receive voice lessons to speak more like "normal" women.

On the second day of my orientation, the KHPT manager insisted that I should join a team of other prevention specialists for a field visit to Cubban Park to view how they had mobilized the community. I moved about the popular MSM cruising spot, as they called it, on a late Saturday afternoon with four other health promotion managers who began pointing at individuals and firing out identity labels: "That one there is an MSW [a male sex worker], and that one is a *hijra,* she is transgender. The one waiting by the banyan tree is a CSW, a commercial sex worker. The one walking like a woman is called a *kothi.* And over there, he is a *puka panthi* [client], a real macho man!" I felt like I was on safari. Then they said, "Here are two of our community guides. Let's stop and talk with them and they can tell us about their work today." We stopped the car to meet with a small group of outreach workers who told us about how many condoms they had given out and how many "contacts" they had reached for that day. They were most pleased because they had exceeded their daily target.

These regimes of intervention create the imaginary idea that sexual minorities are readily identifiable and manageable, and therefore make them *available* for the promotion of Avahan's intervention. These inspection tours enable people working on the Avahan program, then, to demonstrate their skill in spatially managing sexual minorities and, by association, to manage sexual risk. The manner in which the sexual life of community members is put on display not only creates the illusion of order and control, but for Avahan these regular inspection tours also allow for the workings of the intervention to be viewed by local and foreign monitoring and evaluation specialists as well as prospective funders. I have frequently witnessed how field visits impressed visiting donors to such a degree that they became the selling point for them to invest in the intervention. Inspection tours, therefore, function to foster confidence in the Avahan brand.

As some of the targeted interventions I became familiar with matured over the coming years, community members too began to demonstrate their mastery over the emergent geography of intervention. During one occasion I recall a young male sex worker, who was well accustomed to providing tours of community hot spots, leading a field visit for an international consortium of health scientists and international donors in Bangalore:

[This] is an MSM park where they practice sex work, although sometimes we take our clients to the nearby lodge for anal sex; that bus stop, over there, is where you'll find male sex workers looking for clients, this is primarily the commercial circuit; down there you will find the "double-deckers" [men who are sexually versatile] and MSM who are "officials" [well educated]. They are part of the pleasure circuit. And over there, in the public toilets, that is where older MSM can be found; they mostly have hand sex and sometime oral sex. [Field notes, June 2007]

Placing the community at the forefront of inspection tours is designed to show sexual minorities in a "positive light"—taking responsibility for community health. But these regimes of intervention reproduce highly sanitized and one-dimensional portraits of sexual life; in effect, they domesticate sexual dissidence by rendering sexual subversion docile. This is not unlike the violence of self-discipline that Michel Foucault (1975) describes in *Discipline and Punish* in relation to the supposedly "more humane" ways of treating prisoners through the implementation of daily routines and itineraries.

## The Phantom Phallus and the "High-Tech *Hijra*"

*Hijras,* referred to by some academics and rights activists as a "third sex," have occupied a socially accepted religious role since ancient times (Nanda, 1990). Today they continue to perform and give blessings during weddings and births and earn a living through *basti* work (blessing shops for a small fee). Nevertheless, *hijras* have also become extremely socially marginalized, impoverished, and, coupled with their regular practice of sex work, extremely vulnerable to HIV infection (Reddy, 2005). It is worthwhile noting that in neighboring Pakistan, *hijra* sex workers now feature centrally within national prevention programs, yielding positive outcomes with respect to HIV testing practices and reported behavioral outcomes such as condom use (MOH, 2010). HIV prevention work with *hijras* in Pakistan has been abetted by the Supreme Court of Pakistan's ruling in 2009 that grants *hijras* full citizenship rights and that enables them to access state social welfare services and financial support programs.

With the descent of public health interventions upon the state of Karnataka, the notion of *hijras* as a culturally distinctive sex has begun to shift toward more Western biomedical definitions of transgender bodies. Historically, *hijras* have undergone castration by removing the external genitalia through a ritualized process that posed significant health risks, and which leaves only an opening for urination. Increasingly, *hijras* are now electing to take hormonal replacement, have breast implants, and undergo partial or full vaginal reconstruction, depending on how much money they are able to save.

The fostering of new norms of health service–seeking among gender-nonconforming males has certainly increased their access to safer castration procedures. Medical professionals in more cosmopolitan cities like Bangalore provide castration surgeries and vaginal reconstruction on medical grounds to get around laws prohibiting castration. In much smaller and less cosmopolitan cities, such as Bellary, some local doctors have also begun to perform these surgeries, as doctors can earn more than

300,000 rupees (roughly U.S. $7,500) per operation. Thus a new and unexpected enterprise has arisen around the Avahan intervention. The increased access to biomedical technologies also holds serious implications for local community support networks.

Historically young aspiring *hijras,* or *chelas,* became part of *hijra* clans (a hierarchical social structure between *gurus* and *chelas*). Over an extended period of time and through ritualistic social practices that establish their membership within a particular clan, *chelas* eventually may elect to undergo traditional castration ceremonies. More recently, however, among some of the young males who actively participate in the intervention, I have witnessed the acceleration in the process of undergoing castration made possible by medical operations. A few young men I have come to know have expressed considerable regret after too hastily having made the choice to become castrated. For example, one young man I will call Raju, who is a leading community mobilizer for his CBO, went in one day, spoke to the doctor, booked his operation, and then a few days later received the castration surgery. His friends were deeply upset that he had had the surgery without consulting with them to make sure that he was certain of his decision. And Raju himself was at a loss to explain how quickly it had all happened. On one occasion, Raju spoke with me about his amputated body and how he would wake up in the middle of the night, feel that his genitalia were still present, and then realize, regretfully, what he had done.

The rather extreme example of Raju's "phantom phallus" is not intended to suggest that doctors are coercing young males to undergo these operations or that the larger intervention is somehow responsible for the tragedy experienced by individuals like Raju, per se. It does, however, vividly call attention to the increasing speed through which sexual minorities are being "made," as biomedical technologies smooth the social pathways to assuming sexual identifications. These are, in other words, inadvertent negative side effects of Avahan's regimes of intervention that can be linked to the ethics of expediency, the concomitant compression of time, and emerging desires to be counted among those who can take responsibility for epidemic prevention and saving lives. Through the enumeration of daily life, sociality and modes of being are rapidly transforming in ways that neither afford individuals the time to adequately negotiate their place in the community nor to reflect upon the new meanings and values that are attaching themselves to ideas of selfhood.

The ironic individualizing effect of community mobilization is also exemplified in the emergence of a new identity, known locally as "the high-tech *hijra.*" These *hijras* are called "high tech" because they connect with their clients through cell phones and do not distribute their earnings through the traditional clan system. Local community members frequently criticize them as acting as though they are above "ordinary *hijras.*" One *hijra* explained to me that high-tech *hijras* operate more like individuals while her friend continued by saying: "They have wealthy clients and some can even afford to have full vaginal and facial reconstruction." The high-tech *hijras* I was introduced to all dressed in clothes that were noticeably more expensive than those of the many *hijras* I witnessed roaming the streets of various urban centers in Karnataka.

The emergence of high-tech *hijras,* particularly in Bangalore, can be tied to the unprecedented urbanization and economic transformation that has occurred in the region due to the boom in the information technology industry (Srinivas, 2001); there are more intense circulations of financial capital that can be captured through sex and *basti* work. However, these new identities are also ushered in through the networks of health promotion organizations working in association with Avahan. Various district-level program managers I have met have celebrated the success of their work with *hijras* and female sex workers by suggesting how they have come to start to resemble and even become indistinguishable from the more middle-class female staff working with them. On one hand, the regular contact between middle-class intervention managers and *hijras* and other sex workers has positively changed how many *hijras* come to see their relation to society—as being less marginal. However, within the context of the intervention the emergence of the "high-tech *hijra*" as one who distances herself from the previous *guruchelas* clan system, both economically and socially, points to locations where community networks of solidarity—the very resources that intervention specialists seek to cultivate—are breaking apart.

## Spoiled Selves

During my ethnographic work, I also grew most concerned by how community members who regularly participated in local programs described their own sexualities. Qualitative interview respondents in three different districts reported overtly self-stigmatizing perceptions. Even some community leaders I was working with, who actively participated in the day-to-day operations of the intervention (and who were extremely capable peer educators), referred to their own sexuality as an addiction, as a vice, and as something that spoiled their identity. Here are a few examples of such narratives (Du Plessis, Reza-Paul, Pasha, & Lorway, 2011, p. 43):

It is like an addiction. Some smoke, some drink. I don't do those. But this is my addiction. I can't get over that.

We feel very guilty about being what we are. We feel that our lives are wasted.

This is a dirty thing to do. Not good. . . . I am scared about my family coming to know about it. All my gay activities are outside home. I am scared, whether my family will come to know. So, I come outside to do sex.

Within the context of a large-scale and mature intervention that has invested tremendous resources into improving the health and well-being of sexual minorities, it is indeed troubling that these community leaders would conceptualize their own sexualities in such negative, pathological, and negative-moralistic terms.

In a broader sense, I consider these self-stigmatizing narratives as an important starting point for thinking through why some organizations led by sex workers and MSM may be unable to assume leadership of TIs. Indeed, these narratives point to a major shortcoming in Avahan's business model. Avahan's programs cast "the social" in uncomplicated, unreflexive, and decontextualized terms to suit the aim of generating quantitative "indicators of success"; this approach profoundly ignores how sexual stigma is deeply rooted in patrilineal notions of caste and reproduced through what anthropologist Guyatri Reddy (2005) refers to as local moral economies of respect and shame. This everyday reality was expressed by many young men who participated in qualitative interviews.

Interviewer: What would your family say of you having sex with men?

Respondent: They may throw us out from the house or they may beat us and all such things will happen. When I was standing and talking with someone, my brother scolded me that I was standing and speaking with him [another MSM]. He had beaten me, and asked why I was talking and putting my hands on him. So it is difficult to show [my identity] in the house and we have to keep such things far from the house. If we keep it in the house the name of the family will get spoilt and I will lose honor and all will scold me.

A highly experienced and well-respected community mobilizer confided in me that he could never imagine disclosing his identity to his family because as a young man he was expected to get married in order to receive his employment and inheritance. Although he was HIV-positive, he felt he still needed to get married to protect the family name. To otherwise abandon this social trajectory would not only disgrace the family but also leave him completely without financial and family support. For him this would lead to a form of social death. Although the repeal of the sodomy laws in Delhi's Supreme Court in 2009 was met with great celebration among MSM community networks throughout India, for many of the working class MSM I came to know in Karnataka, little had changed in how stigma continued to shape their everyday experience of having to manage a spoiled identity (Goffman, 1963).

## CONCLUSION

The Avahan program has shown many impressive gains in terms of enabling communities of sexual minorities to mobilize around HIV epidemic prevention. The long-term pouring of human, technical, and financial resources into the region is certainly impressive and for this, Avahan should be commended. What I have sought to illuminate in this chapter is an important dimension that has tended to be overlooked and which must be addressed to further mitigate the vulnerability of marginalized groups of sexual minorities and to enhance and sustain community participation in HIV prevention work.

Avahan's vision of community mobilization, which has been adopted and reinforced within NACO's policies, is lacking in any complex analysis around sexuality as informed by feminist, queer, and postcolonial thinkers. There is an inattention to how sexual dissidence can potentially nourish transformative modes of political resistance. According to the Avahan model, sexual minorities are viewed in a depoliticized way as a sales force that is responsible for generating lasting returns on the Gates Foundation's considerable investment. Sexual minorities are viewed as a subpopulation needing to be governed and tracked through enumerative techniques. These communities are not explicitly cast as a politically disenfranchised group in need of emancipation from the bondage of intense social stigmatization (although it is assumed by Avahan that generating demand for services on the ground will inevitably solve wider social problems). In large part, the problem lies in Avahan's deployment of universalistic ideas of capitalist market forces—as dislocated from local social, cultural, and political economic realities.

At this critical juncture of transition and uncertainty, understanding the problems and tensions mounting around the sustainability of Avahan's brand of community mobilization in India requires a more thorough and nuanced examination of how business-oriented managerial practices interact with and unintentionally submerge the local moral and political worlds of sex workers. I do, therefore, call for a kind of "boiling of the ocean" that we social scientists tend to do and which Avahan mangers have so firmly avoided, in the name of expedience, from the inception of the program.

## BIBLIOGRAPHY

Argento, E., Reza-Paul, S., Lorway, R., & O'Neil J. (2011). Confronting structural violence in sex work: Lessons from a community-led HIV prevention project in Mysore, India. *AIDS Care, 23*(1), 69–74.

Asthana, A. (2008). *Avahan India AIDS initiative: Interview with Aparjita Ramakrishnan.* Retrieved from http://globalhealthdelivery.org/2008/08/avahan-india-aids-initiative-interview-with-aparajita-ramakrishnan/

Bishop, M., & Green, M. (2008). *Philanthrocapitalism: How the rich can save the world.* New York: Bloomsbury Press.

Boyce, P. (2007). "Conceiving kothis": Men who have sex with men in India and the cultural subject of HIV prevention. *Medical Anthropology, 26,* 175–203.

Cohen, L. (2005). The Kothi wars: AIDS, cosmopolitanism, and the morality of classification. In V. Adams & S. L. Pigg (eds.), *Sex in development: Science, sexuality, and morality in global perspective* (pp. 269–303). Durham, NC: Duke University Press.

Dixon, V., Reza-Paul, S., O'Neil, J., & Lorway, R. (2012). Increasing access and uptake of clinical services at an HIV prevention project for sex workers in India. *Global Public Health,* doi:10.1080/17441692.2012.668918

Du Plessis, E., Reza-Paul, S., Pasha, A., & Lorway, R. (2011). *Final report: Individual, social and environmental barriers to HIV risk reduction among men who have sex with men (MSM) and transgender populations in India (CIHR).* Centre for Global Public Health, University of Manitoba.

Foucault, M. (1975). *Discipline and punish: The birth of the prison.* New York, NY: Random House.

Goffman, E. (1963). *Stigma: Notes on the management of spoiled identity.* Upper Saddle River, NJ: Prentice Hall.

Kaiser Family Foundation (2006). *News release: STAR INDIA and the Heroes Project announce extension of media partnership at the 2006 International AIDS Conference.* Retrieved from http://www.kff.org/hivaids/phip081406bnr.cfm

Legg, S. (2007). *Spaces of colonialism: Delhi's urban governmentalities.* Oxford: Blackwell.

Marcus, G. E. (2005). The anthropologist as witness in contemporary regimes of intervention. *Cultural Politics, 1* (1), 31–49.

Ministry of Health (2010). *UNGASS Pakistan Report, Progress report on the Declaration of Commitment on HIV/AIDS for UNGASS.* National AIDS Control Program, Government of Pakistan.

Moran, M. (2009). *New foundations, the new philanthropy and sectoral "blending" in international development cooperation.* Paper presented to the Australasian Political Studies Association Conference, Macquarie University, Sydney, Australia, 7. Retrieved from http://www.pol.mq.edu.au/apsa/papers/Refereed%20papers/Moran%20New%20foundations,%20the%20new%20philanthropy%20and%20sectoral%20%91blending%92%20in%20international%20development%20cooperation.pdf

Nanda, S. (1990). *Neither man nor woman,* 2nd ed. London: Wadsworth.

Nguyen, V. K., Bajos, N., Dubois-Arber, F., O'Malley, J., & Pirkle, C. M. (2011). Remedicalizing an epidemic: From HIV treatment as prevention to HIV treatment is prevention. *AIDS, 25,* 291–293.

Pandey, A., Dandu, C. S., Reddy, D. C. S., Ghys, P. D., Thomas, M., Sahu, D., Bhattacharya, M., Kanchan, D., Maiti, K. D., Arnold, F., Kant, S., Khera, A., & Garg, R. (2009). Improved estimates of India's HIV burden in 2006. *Indian J Med Res, 129,* 50–58.

Prahalad, C. K. (2006). *The fortune at the bottom of the pyramid: Eradicating poverty through profits.* Upper Saddle River, NJ: Wharton School.

Rao, P. J. (2010). Avahan: The transition to a publicly funded programme as a next stage. *Sex Transm Infect, 86,* 7–8.

Reddy, G. (2005). Geographies of contagion: *Hijras,* kothis, and the politics of sexual marginality in Hyderabad. *Anthropology & Medicine, 12* (3), 255–270.

Srinivas, S. (2001). *Landscapes of urban memory: The sacred and the civic in India's high-tech city.* Minneapolis: University of Minnesota Press.

Tandon, T. (on behalf of the Lawyers Collective HIV/AIDS Unit, the National Network of Sex Workers, the Indian Harm Reduction Network, and the Integrated Network for Sexual Minorities) (2010). Draft letter to NACO on testing and line listing in TIs. Retrieved from http://groups.yahoo.com/group/infosem/message/2163

Verma, R., Shekhar, A., Khobragade, S., et al. (2010). Scale-up and coverage of Avahan: A large-scale HIV-prevention programme among female sex workers and men who have sex with men in four Indian states. *Sex Transm Infect, 86,* 76–82.

# 9

# Mobilizing Men and Boys in HIV Prevention and Treatment: The Sonke Gender Justice Experience in South Africa

*Wessel van den Berg, Dean Peacock, and Tim Shand*

Efforts to understand men's health-seeking behaviour are poorly understood in the AIDS epidemic, and encouraging men to get tested and into treatment is a major challenge, but one that is poorly recognized. Addressing these issues effectively means moving beyond laying blame, and starting to develop interventions to encourage uptake of prevention, testing, and treatment for men—for everyone's sake. While there has been an expectation of gender inequality that favors men, the evidence indicates that we are doing a disproportionately poor job of providing them with the medical assistance they need. (Mills, Ford, & Mugyenyi, 2009)

There is mounting evidence that men are at a distinct disadvantage in the roll-out of ART in sub-Saharan Africa. Disproportionately fewer men than women are accessing ART across Africa. Men are starting ART with more advanced HIV disease, men are more likely than women to die on ART, to interrupt treatment and to be lost to follow-up on ART. Despite this evidence of gender inequity in access to ART, most international and national ART-related policies and programmes in Africa are still blind to men. (Cornell, McIntyre, & Myer, 2011)

The fact that men represent a "blind spot" in the global AIDS response is self-evidently bad for men's health. Put bluntly, men get sick and die unnecessarily. It is also bad for other men, for women, their families and communities, and for public health systems. When men do not know their HIV status they are less likely to change their sexual practices, less likely to use condoms, and thus much more likely to infect their partners. They are also less likely to access treatment and more likely to need ongoing care and support—initially at home where the burden of care is usually borne by women, and then later by public health officials who attend to men with alarmingly compromised immune systems who are hard to treat and who often require expensive treatment to restore to health.

The "blind spot" that men represent needs urgent attention. Bringing men into focus in the global response to HIV and AIDS should be an international public health priority. *The Lancet* puts it succinctly: "Addressing these issues effectively means moving beyond laying blame, and starting to develop interventions to encourage uptake of prevention, testing, and treatment for men—for everyone's sake."

Sonke Gender Justice Network is working to accomplish this. Based in South Africa but working across Africa, Sonke has developed an innovative model to build government, civil society, and citizen capacity to effectively engage men for HIV prevention, treatment, and care—and to mobilize men as AIDS activists. The authors present this model and suggest that it is imperative to engage with men and engage systemically if advances are to be made in gender equality, HIV prevention, and the delivery of antiretroviral treatment. The chapter closes with the suggestion of a set of organizational capacities that have proven useful in this endeavor.

## THE TWIN EPIDEMICS OF HIV AND GENDER-BASED VIOLENCE

In spite of tremendous advancements toward preventing HIV and the inclusion of gender equality in global goals—now stated in numerous UN conventions and the Millennium Development Goals—much progress remains to be made. The UN estimates that globally, 30 percent of women suffer physical violence at least once from a male partner, and in multi-country studies nearly 20 percent of women say that their first sexual experience was forced. Approximately 100 to 140 million girls and women in the world have experienced female genital cutting, with more than 3 million girls in Africa annually at risk of the practice. Rape continues to be used as a weapon of war, affecting hundreds of thousands of women (UN Women, 2011). Sub-Saharan Africa is still the epicenter of the HIV epidemic, with the highest global new infection rate, affecting mostly women (UNAIDS, 2010). This disparity is especially pronounced in sub-Saharan Africa, as shown in Figure 9.1.

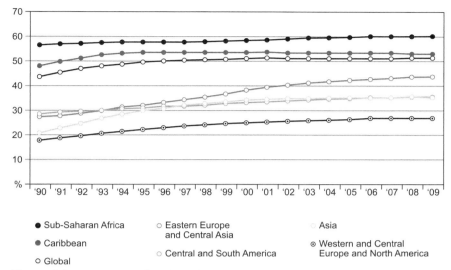

● Sub-Saharan Africa    ○ Eastern Europe      ◌ Asia
                 and Central Asia
● Caribbean                           ⊚ Western and Central
               ○ Central and South America    Europe and North America
○ Global

**Figure 9.1**    Percentage of adults (15 years and over) living with HIV who are female, 1990–2007 (UNAIDS 2008 Global Update)

Sub-Saharan Africa faces a number of well-documented public health challenges, most notably high levels of HIV and gender-based violence. It is fair to say that they have in fact become twin epidemics. All too often rigid gender norms and expectations condone male violence against women and girls, grant young and adult men the power to initiate and dictate the terms of sex, and make it extremely difficult for women and girls to protect themselves from either HIV or violence. These same gender norms also discourage men and boys from seeking health care services including vital HIV testing and treatment, and then leave women and girls with the burden of providing care and support to people sick with AIDS-related opportunistic infections.

## HIV and AIDS in South Africa

Almost one-third of sexually active women (31 percent) in South Africa reported that they had not wanted their first sexual encounter and that they were coerced into sex (Pettifor, Rees, & Stevens, 2004). A 2004 national survey of over 250,000 school-aged youth found that 8.6 percent of respondents said they had been forced to have sex in the past year, with younger boys and older girls reporting greater pressure than younger girls and older boys (Andersson et al., 2004). South Africa has among the highest rates of domestic and gender-based violence in the world. Research conducted by the South African Medical Research Council (MRC) in 2004 shows that every six hours, a woman was killed by her intimate partner. This is the highest rate recorded anywhere in the world (Mathews et al., 2004).

UNAIDS estimates that, at the end of 2009, the national HIV prevalence was 17.8 percent among 15–49-year-olds, with around 5.6 million South Africans living with HIV (UNAIDS, 2010). Violence against women and the unequal power it reflects between men and women is one of the root causes of the rapid spread of HIV in South Africa. As a result of the high rates of coercion to have sex, young women in South Africa are much more likely to be infected than men and in 2004, women made up 77 percent of the 10 percent of South African youth between the ages of 15 and 24 who were infected with HIV (Pettifor, Rees, & Stevens, 2004). Women and girls are vulnerable to a dual burden: They are more likely to be infected, and they disproportionately bear the burden of care.

It should be emphasized that this imbalance in health impacts and power disparities is related to gender norms that rigidly define masculinity and manhood to be equated with dominance, power, and appearing strong. These norms inform both gender-based violence and risky sexual behavior (Dunkle et al., 2004).

## THINKING ABOUT MEN

Men commit the majority of all acts of domestic and sexual violence against women and children. Men's violence against women does not occur because such men lose their temper or because they have no impulse control. Men who use violence do so because they equate manhood with aggression, dominance over women, and sexual conquest. Often they are afraid that they will be viewed as less than a "real" man if they apologize or share power. Instead of finding ways to resolve conflict, they resort to violence. This mindset also leads to the high levels of violence used by men against men (Ratele, Smith, van Niekerk, & Seedat, 2011).

With regard to intimate partner violence, a representative survey conducted in South Africa by the South African Medical Research Council found that 27 percent of men reported having raped a woman and 42.4 percent of men reported having used domestic violence against an intimate partner in their lifetime (current or ex-girlfriend or wife). Fully 14 percent or nearly one in six (95 percent, CI 12.4, 15.7) disclosed that they had perpetrated physical violence against a woman in the past year. Those men who disclosed violence were much more likely to have engaged in a range of risky sexual behavior, as well as to have raped and been

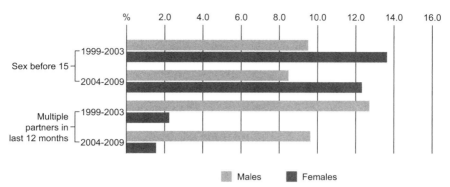

**Figure 9.2**    People aged 15–25 years who had sex before age 15 years and who had multiple partners in the past 12 months. (UNAIDS 2010 Global Report)

raped. The study also found associations between physical intimate partner violence and HIV. Using logistic regression, it was found that men who had been physically violent to a partner on more than one occasion were almost two times more likely to have HIV (odds ratio 1.48, 95 percent confidence intervals 1.01, 2.17, p = 0.04) (Jewkes, Skweyiya, Morrell, & Dunkle, 2009). These outcomes mirror results from other studies within South Africa, finding that women with violent male partners are at increased risk of HIV infection (Dunkle et al., 2004).

However, alongside these alarming statistics, other research also shows that many men are deeply concerned about South Africa's sky-high rates of violence and that they often do not know what to do about it. Research also shows that many men are in fact beginning to live more gender-equitable lives with their partners and with their children, but that rather than being celebrated or serving as examples to others, these activities often remain unacknowledged and hidden, often because of an attempt to succumb to the dominant traditional norms of manhood (Montgomery, Hosegood, Busza, & Timæus, 2005).

While women bear the brunt of men's violence, a deeper analysis reveals that along with the privileges bestowed on men by patriarchy, men are also negatively affected by harmful gender norms of masculinity. High male mortality due to violence (Ratele et al., 2011:45), risky sexual behavior, and low participation in and utilization of health services are some of the negative effects on men's lives. Men tend to have far more sexual partners than women, often concurrent, placing both themselves and their partners at high risk of HIV infection. This is evident in Figure 9.2, which shows that while young women have had sex more often before age 15 than young men, young men have many more sex partners than young women. This has, however, decreased significantly in the two periods monitored.

Traditional gender roles also lead to more negative condom attitudes and less consistent condom use and promote beliefs that sexual relationships are adversarial (Noar & Morokoff, 2001). As we have seen, traditional gender roles also decrease the likelihood that men will seek health services, including critical HIV-related health services. As a result of patriarchal beliefs, then, men are underrepresented in HIV testing and access treatment late and often very ill—at huge costs to themselves and also to the women who usually take care of them. In 2001, men accounted for only 21 percent of all clients receiving VCT (Magongo, Magwaza, Mathambo, & Makhanya, 2002). This improved slightly over the following decade. In the intensive HIV Counselling and Testing (HCT) campaign of 2010 to 2011, a total of 12,961,000 people were tested and only 30 percent of testers were adult males (DoH RSA, 2011:38).

In terms of men's access to, participation in, and utilization of health services much evidence exists showing that men's attitudes about manhood limit uptake of health services. There is also a wealth of evidence from many studies that shows that obstacles can be created by service providers and health facilities (Beck, 2006). It can be seen as both a demand side problem, with men avoiding health services, and a supply side problem, with the health system not being oriented to offer vital services to men. The consequences of this have been devastating.

## Men and ART

On the demand side, in terms of antiretroviral treatment, disproportionately fewer men than women are accessing ART across Africa (Muula et al., 2007). In some regions the differences are much starker (Cornell, McIntyre, & Myer, 2011). When men do access treatment, they often start ART at a late stage with advanced HIV-related disease (Cornell et al., 2009; Stringer et al., 2006). Consequently, men are more likely than women to die while on ART (Cornell et al., 2011; Taylor-Smith et al., 2010; Mills, Ford, & Mugyeni, 2009). Men are also more likely to interrupt treatment (Kranzer et al., 2010) and more likely to be lost to follow-up on ART (Ochieng-Ooko et al., 2010). These gender discrepancies in ART uptake may reflect men's beliefs that seeking health services is a sign of weakness or vulnerability, and that such services may not be perceived as male-friendly (Nachega et al., 2006).

In South Africa, 55 percent of those living with HIV are female but more than 66 percent of patients receiving public-sector ART are female (UNGASS, 2008; Cornell et al., 2011). In Zambia, 54 percent of those living with HIV are women yet 63 percent of adults starting ART in Lusaka were female (Stringer et al., 2006). Both countries have detailed national strategic plans yet neither identifies male access as a gap or includes plans to address it.

## Men and PMTCT

The 2010 South African health systems approach to the prevention of mother-to-child transmission (PMTCT) is another example of obstacles, or rather gaps, on the supply side.

Mother-to-child transmission of HIV can occur during pregnancy, labor, delivery, or through breastfeeding. In 2010, around 390,000 children under 15 became infected with HIV, mainly through mother-to-child transmission (UNAIDS, 2011). About 90 percent of children living with HIV reside in sub-Saharan Africa where, in the context of a high child mortality rate, AIDS accounts for 8 percent of all under-five deaths in the region (UNAIDS, 2010; UNICEF, 2004).

Multiple studies show that health outcomes are better for women, children, and men when men are involved in PMTCT. An evaluation of the Men As Partners and PMTCT program in South Africa showed a 46 percent increase in men testing with their partners and an 87.6 percent increase in the number of men joining their partners for PMTCT visits.

The gap in men's knowledge of PMTCT is immense. The 2009 South African National Communication Survey found that only 10 percent of men know that exclusive formula feeding prevents transmission and only 1 percent knew the same about exclusive breastfeeding. Despite the evidence of benefits and the gap in knowledge, the number of times the words "men, man, male, father, parent, fatherhood, dad" appeared in the 2010 South African National PMTCT Guidelines was *zero* (DoH RSA, 2011a).

The consequences of not addressing harmful male gender norms within the context of both beneficiaries and providers of health services have been disastrous. Men have much higher HIV-related mortality rates than women, where crude mortality rates (of deaths per 1,000 person years) were 26.9 for women compared to 43.9 for men. This is supported by an emerging body of literature that shows consistent shortcomings in the involvement of men in treatment programs (Mills, Ford, & Mugyeni, 2009).

While men often have more economic, political, and cultural privileges than women, in terms of HIV-related health services, men are not being provided with or accessing the medical assistance they need. Both women and men stand to benefit from an increase in men's uptake of health services (Mills, Ford, & Mugyeni, 2009).

## Advances toward Healthier Gender Norms

Men are negatively implicated in health and human rights crises and men are also essential for their successful resolution. The global response to the HIV epidemic has, however, too often neglected how gender stereotyping plays out in the lives of men and boys—to the detriment of women, and to the detriment of men and boys. One way to engage effectively with these challenges is to involve men as active role players towards the improvement of human rights, gender equality, and health.

South African men are by no means unique when it comes to defining manhood in ways that contribute to violence and poor health-seeking behaviors. Data from a 2011 survey confirms that these ideas about manhood are found across the world, and that there is some indication of progress toward healthier gender norms.

Between 2009 and 2010, a household-based survey on men's attitudes and practices, called the International Men and Gender Equality Survey (IMAGES), was conducted across Brazil, Chile, Croatia, India, Mexico, and Rwanda (Barker et al., 2011). HIV and health-related findings from the survey provide some insight into men's gendered engagement with the epidemic.

It was clear from the data that irrespective of a man's age, male respondents who displayed more conservative understandings of masculinity and gender were often also the male respondents who were more likely to report use of violence against a partner, suffering from sexually transmitted infections, and previous arrest or drug or alcohol abuse (Barker et al., 2011:18).

Between 17 and 39 percent of male respondents in reporting countries reported perpetrating violence against women. Women were also asked questions about surviving men's violence and except for India, women's reports of surviving IPV were consistently higher than men's reports of perpetrating IPV (Barker et al., 2011:45).

Again male respondents had relatively low rates of HIV testing, consistently lower than women's rates of testing. The exception was Rwanda, where men's seeking of HIV testing was high (87 percent). In the study, higher education and support for more equitable gender norms were associated with men's greater likelihood to have been tested for HIV. Particularly in Croatia, India, and Mexico male respondents with more gender-equitable attitudes were also more likely to have been tested for HIV (Barker et al., 2011:36).

Importantly, the survey found that among participants, gendered change is in process (Barker et al., 2011:60) and there are clear indicators that rigid masculinities (and femininities) are adapting to a more gender-equitable social order. There is, for example, the indication that policy and service provision has enabled individual men to rethink their behaviors as men (Barker et al., 2011:28–36),

In terms of global policy, other advances have also been made. Governments and UN agencies, through regional and international commitments, have affirmed the need to involve men and boys in reducing HIV and AIDS, achieving gender equality, reducing violence against women and girls, preventing sexual exploitation, and promoting the rights and well-being of girls, women, and boys and men themselves. Many countries have affirmed their support for work with men in a number of international commitments. Examples of such platforms and commitments are the International Conference on Population and Development (1994), the Programme of Action of the World Summit on Social Development (1995) and its review held in 2000, the Beijing Platform for Action (1995), the twenty-sixth special session of the General Assembly on HIV and AIDS (2001), the United Nations Commission on the Status of Women in 2004 and 2009, UN Security Council Resolution 1325, and the Rio Declaration from the Global Symposium on Engaging Men and Boys on Achieving Gender Equality in 2009. These commitments require policymakers in signatory countries to develop and implement policies and programs working with men, and also provide civil society activists with leverage to demand rapid implementation.

In terms of program interventions, the recognition of the valuable role that men have to play in health and human rights has emerged across the world and multiple examples of success have developed. Program interventions at the local level have shown tremendous success in engaging men and boys in promoting their own health and well-being and the health and well-being of women and girls.

A recent World Health Organization review of 57 evaluated programs engaging men and boys in health-based interventions found that the majority were either effective or promising in demonstrating changes in men's attitudes and behaviors (WHO, 2007).

The review examined the effectiveness of program interventions engaging men and boys in sexual and reproductive health; HIV prevention, treatment, care, and support; fatherhood; gender-based violence; maternal, newborn, and child health; and gender socialization.

While some programmatic efforts within each of the intervention categories examined (group education, health services, and community mobilization and engagement) showed significant results, those programs that combined different types of intervention, particularly with community outreach, mobilization, and mass-media campaigns, were most effective in producing behavioral or health outcomes (including increased condom usage, delayed sexual debut, decreased violence, and lower rates of STIs) (WHO, 2007).

However, despite international commitments and the growing base of program experiences and evaluation, most initiatives to engage men and boys in achieving gender equality have been small-scale and short-term. In order to transform the pervasive gender inequalities, a scaling-up and widening in scope of the programs and models already known to be effective is imperative. The two values of engaging men and working systemically to scale up existing interventions therefore need to be combined as one holistic intervention. The remaining part of this chapter describes the work of an organization based in South Africa that exemplifies the successful combination of these two values.

## SONKE GENDER JUSTICE: AN EXAMPLE OF SYSTEMIC ACTIVISM FROM SOUTH AFRICA

Sonke Gender Justice Network (Sonke) is a South African–based nongovernmental organization (NGO) that works across Africa to strengthen government, civil society, and citizen capacity to support men and boys in taking action to promote gender equality, prevent domestic and sexual violence, and reduce the spread and impact of HIV and AIDS. Using a human rights framework to achieve gender equality, Sonke endeavors to create the change necessary for women and men to access equitable, healthy, and happy relationships that contribute to the development of just and democratic societies.

Activism refers to campaigning to bring about political or social change. To achieve change, Sonke engages in various forms of activism across levels of a socio-ecological framework that Sonke calls the Spectrum of Change. This approach toward achieving gender equality, health, and human rights is inspired first by a particular conceptual framework called the Spectrum of Prevention, and second by several examples of other activist organizations from across the world.

### The Spectrum of Change

The Oakland, California–based Prevention Institute developed the Spectrum of Prevention in the late 1990s to assist practitioners to develop multifaceted approaches to injury prevention (Cohen & Swift, 1999).

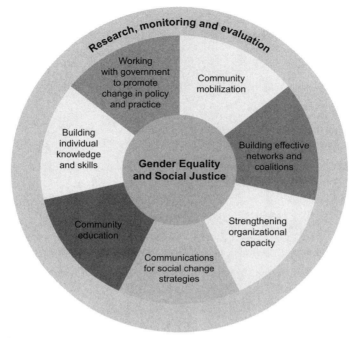

**Figure 9.3**   The Sonke Spectrum of Change

This approach is informed by the social ecological perspective, which regards social elements as constantly interacting and affecting each other on various levels (Oetzel, Ting-Toomey, & Rinderle, 2006). The approach emphasizes the integration of different change strategies to address the many forces in social systems that shape individual behaviour (Hawley, 1950; Rousseau & House, 1994; Stokols, 1996).

As noted earlier, work with men and boys often focuses on only one level, mostly direct educational work with individuals, and a broader, systemic approach is necessary to effect change. The socio-ecological perspective is often used for research and analysis; the Spectrum of Prevention moves from analysis to implementation and guides action. The Sonke-adapted version of the Spectrum of Prevention, called the Spectrum of Change, identifies seven mutually reinforcing social change strategies that move beyond an exclusive reliance on individual or small-group change to additionally promote changes at the social, political, and economic levels of people's lives. The seven levels are (as shown in Figure 9.3):

- Building individual knowledge and skills
- Providing community education

- Strengthening organizational capacity including work with service providers
- Community mobilization
- Communicating for social change through media
- Working with government to promote change in policy and practice
- Building effective networks and coalitions

An eighth dimension completes the spectrum and supports all of the other levels. This is the level of research, monitoring, and evaluation. Each of the levels depends on current research and keeps an active discipline of monitoring and evaluation going in order to ensure that the levels are evidence-related.

Working with an emerging network of organizations and beginning with work done through educational workshops, Sonke increasingly implemented interventions on all of the levels of the spectrum. Through the global network of organizations that were doing similar work, a few examples emerged of practices that supported the approach to have integration at a systemic level, with an explicit focus on engaging men and boys. These examples confirmed the various methods that were emerging from Sonke's implementation of the spectrum approach.

## OTHER CASES OF STRATEGIC ACTIVISM

### Community Mobilization: The Treatment Action Campaign

The Treatment Action Campaign (TAC) has perhaps become the best-known HIV and AIDS–related activist organization in South Africa. Through groundbreaking activism the campaign achieved a remarkable improvement in access to ART by enabling the production and distribution of generic medicine to people living with HIV (Robins & von Lieres, 2004).

In addition to campaigning for access to treatment, TAC advocates for gender equality and access to a wider range of human rights. The Lorna Mlofana case exemplifies the strategies that TAC employs to achieve change. Lorna Mlofana, a 22-year-old TAC member, was raped and killed on December 13, 2003, by a group of five men outside a tavern in an informal settlement just outside of Cape Town. Consequently members and community structures of TAC (including Positive Men United) mobilized to advance this case and work toward achieving justice. They pressured the police to take action, ensured that evidence was secured, and opposed bail applications. They organized large demonstrations at related court hearings and insisted that the criminal justice system take the case seriously. The criminal justice system did take the case seriously and the perpetrators were convicted, one receiving a life sentence.

In addition to the justice that was achieved through the conviction of the perpetrators, on the anniversary of Lorna's death, TAC held a rally that insisted that the local health services be improved for rape survivors. As a response, a rape crisis center was established, and now it provides counseling and postexposure prophylaxis to rape survivors (Peacock, Khumalo, & McNab, 2006; Peacock & Budaza, 2006).

The successful community mobilization that TAC achieved inspired in part the inclusion of the community mobilization process within the Sonke model. Along with training and capacity building, community mobilization makes up the part of the organization that engages most immediately and proximally with activists, community members, and beneficiaries. The Sonke model regards mobilization, however, in a wider sense, where protests outside court only form one part. The ideal envisioned is that whole communities are ready to act in a variety of ways to promote justice in their locality.

## Policy and Advocacy: Men's Action to Stop Violence Against Women (MASVAW)

Men's Action to Stop Violence Against Women (MASVAW), based in Lucknow, India, provides an example of advocacy to support implementation of hard-won policy gains. MASVAW provided a case that confirmed the way in which the Sonke model was developing in terms of policy advocacy work. The 2005 Protection of Women from Domestic Violence Act (DVA) came into force in late 2006 and provides "protection against physical, verbal and sexual abuse and the right to shelter and economic freedom" (Dhawan, 2006). The government's failure to budget for the necessary protection officers or to educate the general public about the provisions of the DVA left advocates concerned about how effectively it would be implemented and led a number of Uttar Pradesh–based NGOs to form the Domestic Violence Act U.P. Campaign. In collaboration with women's rights organizations, MASVAW coordinated the 2007 *Ab To Jaago!* (Wake Up Now!) campaign. This campaign was conducted in 41 districts across the state and provided rights-based education to urban and rural communities about the provisions of the DVA and holding tribunals in each community to gather information about implementation. This information was used to maintain pressure on the government for full implementation (Domestic Violence Campaign, 2007).

Two aspects here have been developed in the model employed by Sonke. First, a vital link between the training and capacity building on one hand and policy advocacy work is the education of communities about their rights. This ensures that when communities mobilize, it is in an informed manner with correct reference to their rights. Second, MASVAW presents a useful example of holding government to account for the policies that have been enacted.

South Africa boasts a constitution and legislative framework that have been recognized as progressive in terms of acknowledging human rights. Within this context, similar to MASVAW and TAC, Sonke plays a role of monitoring policy compliance, or advocating for policy change where necessary. The training, capacity building, and community mobilization work are thereby integrated with and connected to research, policy and advocacy work.

## Fostering Coalitions: Men's Association for Gender Equality—Sierra Leone (MAGE-SL)

The Men's Association for Gender Equality—Sierra Leone (MAGE-SL) is a third example of activism within the field of working with men and boys that informed the model Sonke employs. MAGE-SL is a network of organizations working with men and boys toward the promotion of gender equality. This is done through conducting advocacy, dialogue, and raising awareness on gender policies, women's rights, and empowerment in Sierra Leone.

MAGE-SL strives to circumvent the traditional academic approach to gender promotion and advocacy by adopting a bottom-up approach of grassroots strategies from within family settings of Sierra Leone. From 1991 to 2002 Sierra Leone was ravaged by civil war, political conflict, and violence that took the lives of tens of thousands and left millions displaced. This unrest damaged an already unstable infrastructure, consequently negating human rights.

The work of MAGE-SL can be described as a "two-attack approach." In the rural districts where they are based, they provide support to vulnerable women by providing safe places and shelter for women who are survivors of violence. On a larger scale, they use a network of grassroots initiatives to address the social causes that make women vulnerable. These include discriminatory cultural beliefs that favor men and power imbalances in gender relations.

MAGE-SL also united with a coalition of civil society organizations, known as the Task Force, to lobby for three new laws known as "the Gender Acts." These were the Domestic Violence Act, the Devolution of Estates Act, and the Registration of Marriage and Divorce Act. The acts were expected to provide protection for women and address men's behavior toward women. They used various creative communication and media tactics to popularize the Gender Acts across the country.

The multilevel approach that MAGE-SL used is similar to the Sonke Spectrum of Change model. The direct work with vulnerable women matches the community mobilization work done by Sonke, while the MAGE-SL network of grassroots initiatives for cultural and policy shifts is echoed in the coalition and network-building approach that Sonke uses. More importantly, it is the *combination* of these levels that has been proven to work well to effect change. In this example, being involved with female survivors of violence allows MAGE-SL to keep the policy work grounded in current challenges and prevents the advocacy from becoming abstract. In terms of Sonke's work, the policy work is likewise connected to engagement with and feedback from a network of grassroots organizations and individuals through the training, capacity building, community mobilization, and networking aspects of the model. Sonke's efforts to educate the broader public about provisions in key gender laws and the organization's efforts to monitor government implementation of laws such as the 2007 Sexual Offences Act draw on and reflect MAGE-SL's inspiring pioneering efforts.

As we've seen, these cases informed and confirm the way in which Sonke has developed the systemic model of social change it implements. The Spectrum of Change was laid as a foundation, and then cases like TAC, MASVAW, and MAGE-SL provided inspiring examples of approaches and methods in which to develop the appropriate levels of the Spectrum and the ways in which to integrate them.

## MOBILIZING MEN AND BOYS FOR HIV PREVENTION USING THE SONKE MODEL

Two important external influences played a role in the development of the Sonke model for social change. These were:

- The identified need: Emerging lessons from the field of HIV prevention that work with engaging men and boys are necessary.
- Examples of success that confirmed Sonke's strategies: TAC, MASVAW, and MAGE-SL.

In addition to these external influences, two major internal influences also contributed to the shaping of the model:

- The ability of a relatively new organization to adapt.
- An organizational philosophy based on the Spectrum of Prevention.

It is worth noting that in addition to the effect on program development, a more significant effect was the shaping of the *organizational structure* of Sonke.

The external and internal influences prompted the development of five different organizational capacities. These capacities have proven valuable for a systemic approach to mobilizing men and boys for HIV prevention. The lesson that the Sonke model offers is that it is possible to develop all five capacities within one organization. The capacities are to:

1. Engage directly with community members.
2. Shift social norms through media.
3. Build coalitions.
4. Affect the policy environment.
5. Maintain a resilient organization.

## First Capacity: Engaging Directly with Community Members

Within the Sonke model, a dedicated team focuses on implementing direct educational activities and grassroots community activism. Educational activities help men and women to broaden their attitudes about gender norms and health, and take action in their own lives to promote healthy relationships. The educational work is connected to community activities and mobilization.

The main community education campaign is the One Man Can campaign. It presents a set of practical, proactive educational and skills-building activities to communities that are motivated to act in the interests of involving men and boys in health and gender justice. An evaluation of the campaign conducted in 2009 found that there is significant scope for involving men in campaigns like the One Man Can campaign. The evaluation indicated significant changes in short-term behavior in the weeks following OMC activities. Twenty-five percent of respondents had accessed voluntary counseling and testing, 50 percent reported an act of gender-based violence, 61 percent increased their use of condoms, and over 80 percent talked to friends or family members about HIV, gender, and human rights issues (Colvin, 2009).

## Second Capacity: Shifting Social Norms through Media

In the Sonke model, the capacity to use media to shift social norms forms a vital part of systemic activism and mobilization. This capacity depends on two aspects. The first is the ability to use mass media platforms such as television and radio to create a wide spread of particular messages and to saturate these platforms with affirming and healthy norms. The second is the ability to use controversy to spark and drive national debate through news media.

An example of a mass media campaign supported by Sonke is the Brothers for Life campaign. The campaign focuses on communicating HIV and gender-based violence prevention messages to men. A typical annual estimated audience of the campaign is 15 million viewers or listeners. The campaign is a high-quality media campaign and utilizes billboards, regular radio shows, and television advertising spaces. The campaign also supports television series with advice and technical assistance in the developing of storylines that address HIV and gender-based violence themes.

An example of Sonke's deliberate courting of controversy to generate discussion and debate in the media is the Equality Court case Sonke brought against one of South Africa's best-known political leaders. In January 2009, Julius Malema, the outspoken youth leader of the African National Congress youth league, addressed a student audience and suggested that the woman who had accused President Zuma of rape had a "nice time" with him because "when a woman didn't enjoy it, she leaves early in the morning. Those who had a nice time will wait until the sun comes out, request breakfast, and ask for taxi money." Many people and organizations were outraged at the remark. In March 2009, Sonke filed a complaint at the South African Equality Court against Malema. Similar to the South African Human Rights Commission and the Commission for Gender Equality, the Equality Courts are institutions that serve as human rights watchdogs. The Equality Court found in favor of Sonke, and Malema was charged to deliver a public apology and pay a fine to an organization that supports survivors of gender-based violence. He fulfilled both obligations.

The case had substantial media and public attention with frequent coverage in almost all of South Africa's radio, television, and print outlets. Sonke also used community mobilization to amplify media attention. Sonke organized demonstrations outside the court during hearings, sometimes mobilizing people outside the Cape Town High Court even though the case itself took place in Johannesburg because of the conversation and coverage this generated.

## Third Capacity: Building Coalitions

Building coalitions enables organizations to learn from one another, craft shared agendas, and make convincing and powerful arguments for policy change. Within the Sonke model, such coalition building provides an important bridge between the direct engagement with communities and the capacity to affect policy.

In South Africa, Sonke serves as secretariat to the men's sector within the South African National AIDS Council (SANAC). The men's sector is a coalition within SANAC that seeks to address the involvement of men and boys in HIV prevention and treatment. The men's sector works to ensure that the South African National Strategic Plan on HIV and AIDS includes an explicit focus on engaging men to improve their and their partners' HIV-related outcomes.

## Fourth Capacity: Affecting the Policy Environment

The fourth organizational capacity that is important in the Sonke model is the ability to affect the HIV and AIDS–related policy environment. This is a dual task, where it first depends on the ability to assist with refinement of policies that compromise health, gender equality, and human rights, and second to monitor the implementation and compliance of good existing policies.

On World AIDS Day, December 1, 2011, SANAC launched the South African 2012–2016 National Strategic Plan for HIV, STIs and TB, which had been in development for the preceding year. The plan is the most important document for the South African national response to the epidemic and acts as a central guide for all HIV-related policies and implementation. The plan has ambitious goals, including the reduction of new HIV infections by at least 50 percent using combination prevention approaches; and getting at least 80 percent of eligible patients on antiretroviral treatment (ART), with 70 percent alive and on treatment five years after initiation (DoH RSA, 2011).

Sonke worked with and through the SANAC Men's Sector to ensure that language that addresses men's involvement was included within the NSP. Due to this work as a coalition, the following language was incorporated within the 2012–2016 final NSP document:

- Efforts must be made to increase men's health-seeking behavior.
- Challenge the gender roles, norms and inequalities that increase women's vulnerability to HIV and compromise men's and women's health.

- . . . address the position of women in society, particularly their economic standing; and engage with men on changing socialisation practices.

## Fifth Capacity: Maintaining a Resilient Organization

Similar to the Spectrum of Change dimension of research, monitoring, and evaluation, a fifth, general capacity, completes the Sonke model. This is the capacity to maintain operational resilience. A sound ability to maintain good governance and operational practice provides an organization with a secure, long-term ability to develop the other four capacities. The organizational structure was thus framed around five capacities, in a manner that ensures that all the levels of the spectrum are addressed. This has proven to be useful in the work of engaging boys and men for health.

A significant outcome of working with the Sonke model is that it does not only allow the multiple levels to be addressed, but also enables the actions on different levels to contribute to one another across levels.

Using the first capacity of engaging directly with community members, for example, assisted significantly with the ability to generate debate in the media around the aforementioned case against Julius Malema. Hundreds of young men and women, through the OMC campaign, joined protests and public debates to voice outrage about the case. The second capacity to use the media to shift social norms reinforced this grassroots engagement, where radio listeners and television viewers witnessed the OMC participants. Ultimately this dual engagement strengthened the power behind the case to achieve its outcome.

A second example of how actions on multiple levels reinforce one another was the ability to adapt the language of the 2012–2016 NSP for South Africa. The fact that the men's sector had been established, using the capacity to foster coalitions, enabled the eventual shift in policy (using the fourth capacity to influence policy). Again, the effect was positively reinforcing the men's sector coalition, where the new language in the NSP gave the sector an increased and better-defined mandate.

The Sonke model presents a valuable case that demonstrates that such integration is possible within one organization. Table 9.1 shows the Sonke model and where levels of the Spectrum of Change have been matched to the different organizational capacities. Note how this is an integrated association, and that each capacity complements the others and in turn depends on the others.

**Table 9.1** The Sonke Model of Systemic Activism

| Spectrum Level | | Organizational Capacities | |
|---|---|---|---|
| Research, monitoring, and evaluation | Building individual knowledge and skills<br><br>Providing community education | Engaging directly with community members | Maintaining operational resilience |
| | Strengthening organizational capacity<br><br>Community mobilization<br><br>Communicating for social change | Shifting social norms through media | |
| | Working with government to promote change in policy and practice | Affecting the policy environment | |
| | Building effective networks and coalitions | Working with other organizations to build coalitions | |

## CONCLUSION

The Sonke model offers lessons for researchers and practitioners in terms of the seven levels of the Spectrum of Change and the five organizational capacities required to work on these levels. The field of engaging men and boys in promoting gender equality and preventing HIV and gender-based violence remains relatively new. In order to move forward, scaling up this work beyond small and short-term interventions is essential. Successful models for large-scale and sustainable programming examples exist, such as the work of Sonke, which not only highlight the potential and importance of engaging men but also the necessity of such interventions employing a systemic and gender-transformative approach. These models can and must be replicated to effectively engage men and boys in the struggle to curb and eventually overcome the HIV pandemic.

# BIBLIOGRAPHY

Achyut, P., Bhatla, N., Singh, A., & Verma, R. (2011). *Building support for gender equality among young adolescents in school: Findings from Mumbai, India.* Washington, DC: International Center for Research on Women.

Andersson, N., et al. (2004). National cross sectional study of views on AIDS among South African school pupils. *BMJ* 329, 952.

Barker, G., Contreras, J. M., Heilman, B., Singh, A. K., Verma, R. K., & Nascimento, M. (2011). Evolving men: Initial results from the International Men and Gender Equality Survey (IMAGES). Washington, DC: International Center for Research on Women (ICRW) and Rio de Janeiro: Instituto Promundo.

Barker, G., Nascimento, M., Segundo, M., & Pulerwitz, J. (2004). How do we know if men have changed? Promoting and measuring attitude change with young men: Lessons from Program H in Latin America. In S. Ruxton (ed.), *Gender equality and men: Learning from practice.* Oxford: Oxfam GB, 147–61.

Beck, D. (2006). *Men and ARVs: How does being a man affect access to antiretroviral therapy in South Africa? An investigation among Xhosa-speaking men in Khayelitsha.* Centre for Social Science Research, University of Cape Town.

Cohen, L., & Swift, S. (1999). The spectrum of prevention: Developing a comprehensive approach to injury prevention. *Injury Prevention* 5, 203–207.

Colvin, C. (2009). *Sonke Gender Justice Network report on formative research conducted in seven South African provinces on men's attitudes and practices related to gender and HIV.* Sonke Gender Justice.

Cornell, M., McIntyre, J., & Myer, L. (2011). Men and antiretroviral therapy in Africa: Our blind spot. *Tropical Medicine and International Health* 16.7, 828–829.

Cornell, M., Myer, L., Kaplan, R., Bekker, L., & Wood, R. (2009). The impact of gender and income on survival and retention in a South African antiretroviral therapy programme. *Tropical Medicine and International Health* 1–10.

Department of Health, Republic of South Africa (Doh RSA) (2010). *South African national PMTCT guidelines.* Retrieved October 2, 2011 from http://www.fidssa.co.za/images/PMTCT_Guidelines.pdf

Department of Health, Republic of South Africa (Doh RSA) (2011). *South African national strategic plan on HIV, STIs, and TB 2012–2016.* Retrieved from http://www.sanac.org.za/index.php/nsp-2012-2016/national-strategic-plan

Dhawan, H. (2006, October 27). Act is alright, but will it be implemented? *The Times of India.*

Domestic Violence Campaign (2007). Retrieved from http://dvactupcampaign2007.blogspot.com/2007/12/lucknow.html

Dunkle, K. L., Jewkes, R. K., Brown, H. C., Gray, G. E., McIntyre, J. A., & Harlow, S. D. (2004). Gender-based violence, relationship power and risk of HIV infection in women attending antenatal clinics in South Africa. *The Lancet* 363, 1415–1421.

Gupta, G. R., Whelan, D., & Allendorf, K. (2003). *Integrating gender into HIV and AIDS programs: Review paper for expert consultation.* Geneva: WHO. Retrieved from http://www.who.int/gender/hiv_aids/en/Integrating%5B258KB%5D.pdf

Hawley, A. H. (1950). *Human ecology: A theory of community structure.* New York: Ronald Press.

Klein, K. J., Tosi, H., & Cannella, A. A. (1999). Multilevel theory building: Benefits, barriers, and new developments. *Academy of Management Review* 24, 243–248.

Jewkes, R., Nduna, M., Levin, J., Jama, N., Dunkle, K., Koss, M., Puren, A., & Duvvury, N. Impact of Stepping Stones on HIV, HSV-2 and sexual behaviour in rural South Africa: Cluster randomised controlled trial. *British Medical Journal* (submitted).

Jewkes, R., Sikweyiya, Y., Morrell, R., & Dunkle, K. (2009). *Understanding men's health and use of violence: Interface of rape and HIV in South Africa.* Medical Research Council.

Jewkes, R., Wood, K., & Duvvury, N. "I woke up after I joined Stepping Stones": Meanings of an HIV behavioural intervention in rural South African young people's lives. *Social Science & Medicine* (submitted).

Kranzer, K., Lewis, J. J., Ford, N., Zeinecker, J., Orrel, C., Lawn, S. D., Bekker, L. G., & Wood, R. (2010). Treatment interruption in a primary care antiretroviral therapy program in South Africa: Cohort analysis of trends and risk factors. *Journal of AIDS* 55(3):e17–23.

Magongo, B., Magwaza, S., Mathambo, V., & Makhanya, N. (2002). *National report on the assessment of the public sector's voluntary counseling and testing program.* Durban: Health Systems Trust.

Mathews, S., Abrahams, N., Martin, L., Vetten, L., van der Merwe, L., & Jewkes, R. (2004). *"Every six hours a woman is killed by her intimate partner": A national study of female homicide in South Africa.* Gender and Health Research Group, Medical Research Council.

Mills, E., Ford, N., & Mugyenyi, P. (2009). Expanding HIV care in Africa: Making men matter. *The Lancet* 374, 275–276.

Montgomery, C., Hosegood, V., Busza J., & Timæus, I. M. (2005). Men's involvement in the South African family: Engendering change in the AIDS era. *Social Science and Medicine* 62.10, 2411–2419.

Muula, A. S., Ngulube, T. J., Siziya, S., et al. (2007). Gender distribution of adult? patients on highly active antiretroviral therapy (HAART) in Southern Africa: A systematic review. *BMC Public Health* 7, 63.

Nachega, J., Hislop, M., Dowdy, D., Lo, M., Omer, S., Regensberg, L., Chaisson, R., & Maartens, G. (2006). Adherence to highly active antiretroviral therapy assessed by pharmacy claims predicts survival in HIV-infected South African adults. *Journal of Acquired Immune Deficiency Syndromes* 43(1), 78–84.

Noar, S. M., & Morokoff, P. J. (2001). The relationship between masculinity ideology, condom attitudes, and condom use stage of change: A structural equation modeling approach. *International Journal of Men's Health* 1, 1.

Ochieng-Ooko, V., Ochieng, D., Sidle, J. E., et al. (2010). Influence of gender on loss to follow-up in a large HIV treatment programme in western Kenya. *Bulletin of the World Health Organization* 88, 681–688.

Oetzel, J. G., Ting-Toomey, S., & Rinderle, S. (2006). Conflict communication in contexts: A social ecological perspective. In J. G. Oetzel & S. Ting-Toomey (eds.), *The SAGE handbook of conflict communication.* Thousand Oaks, CA: Sage.

Peacock, D., & Budaza, T. (2006). "Justice for Lorna Mlofana": The Treatment Action Campaign's AIDS and gender activism. In A. Ndinga-Muvumba (ed.), *Moralizing to preventive action: HIV and AIDS and human security in South Africa.* Cape Town: Center for Conflict Resolution.

Peacock, D., Khumalo, B., & McNab, E. (2006). Men and gender activism in South Africa: Observations, critique and recommendations for the future. *Agenda 69,* 71–81.

Pettifor, A., Rees, H., & Stevens, A. (2004). HIV & sexual behaviour among young South Africans: A national survey of 15–24-year-olds. Johannesburg: University of the Witwatersrand.

Pulerwitz, J., & Barker, G. (2008). Measuring attitudes toward gender norms among young men in Brazil: Development and psychometric evaluation of the GEM Scale. *Men and Masculinities* 10, 322–338.

Ratele, K., Smith, M., van Niekerk, A., & Seedat, M. (2011). Is it race, age or sex? Masculinity in male homicide victimization in South African cities. *National and international perspectives on crime and policing—Conference Proceedings,* 34–47. Institute for Security Studies.

Robins, S., & von Lieres, B. (2004). Remaking citizenship, unmaking marginalization: The Treatment Action Campaign in post-apartheid South Africa. *Canadian Journal of African Studies/Revue Canadienne des Études Africaines* 38, 3, 575–586.

Rousseau, D. M., & House, R. J. (1994). Meso organizational behavior: Avoiding three fundamental biases. In C. L. Cooper & D. M. Rousseau (eds.), *Trends in organizational behavior* 1, 13–30. New York: John Wiley.

Stokols, D. (1996). Translating social ecological theory into guidelines for community health promotion. *American Journal of Health Promotion* 10, 282–298.

Stringer, J. S., Zulu, I., Levy, J., et al. (2006). Rapid scale-up of anti-retroviral therapy at primary care sites in Zambia: Feasibility and early outcomes. *JAMA* 296, 782–793.

Taylor-Smith, K., Tweya, H., Harries, A. D., Schoutene, E., & Jahn, A. (2010). Gender differences in retention and survival on antiretroviral therapy of HIV-infected adults in Malawi. *Malawi Medical Journal* 22, 49–56.

UNAIDS (2010). *2010 Report on the global AIDS epidemic.* Geneva: WHO.

UNAIDS (2011). *Joint United Nations programme on HIV/AIDS (UNAIDS) World AIDS Day report 2011.* Retrieved from http://www.unaids.org/en/resources/presscentre/pressreleaseandstatementarchive/2011/november/20111121wad2011report/

UNGASS (2008). *UNGASS Country Progress Report: Republic of South Africa 2007.*

UNICEF (2004). *Progress for children: A child survival report card.* Retrieved from http://www.unicef.org/publications/index_23557.html

UN Women (2011). *Say no, unite to end violence.* Retrieved from www .saynotoviolence.org/issue/facts-and-figures

World Health Organization (WHO) (2007). *Engaging men and boys in changing gender-based inequity in health: Evidence from programme interventions.* Geneva: WHO.

# 10

# Crisis and Chronicity: How Treatment Is Changing Activism in South Africa and Beyond

*Christopher J. Colvin*

## ACUITY AND CHRONICITY IN AIDS ACTIVISM

Since its early days in Europe and the United States in the 1980s, AIDS activism has embodied a tension between the normal and the exceptional. On one hand, the dominant narrative of the disease has been one of crisis. This was a story of the unexpected eruption of a "premodern" plague across a landscape that was still "high on the hype of Reaganomics, deregulation and the end of the Cold War" (Comaroff & Comaroff, 2011: p. 173). AIDS was an emergency, a rupture in time and history, inexplicable in its capacity to bring early, gruesome, inevitable death into a world that imagined it had begun to conquer such terrors (Engel, 2006; Shilts, 1988).

For much of the public, the exceptional, terrifying character of the epidemic was quickly sublimated by casting those afflicted as the exception. The cruel mnemonic "4H" that defined those affected by AIDS as heroin addicts, Haitians, homosexuals, and hemophiliacs tried to map the disease onto the bodies of those outside the community of the moral and the healthy (Centers for Disease Control and Prevention, 1983). AIDS was the exceptional catastrophe of those whose non-normative bodies and behaviors placed them beyond the control (and protection) of rational science and governance.

Activists, of course, strongly resisted this narrative of exclusion and alterity but nonetheless operated in the same mode of exception. HIV catalyzed a movement of people, gay and straight, and inspired new activist, social, and memorial forms (Treichler, 1999). The gay community asserted its presence and its right to make claims at the center of public health policy and practice in a radically new way. AIDS activists inserted themselves into the process of scientific knowledge production and health policymaking in ways that other health activists before them had never imagined possible (Epstein, 1996). They insisted on both rights-based approaches to HIV testing that strongly protected individual confidentiality and advocated for community-based approaches to education and prevention that challenged stigma and denial head on.

One of the outcomes of this dramatic and creative activism was the fast-tracking of drug development for treating HIV infection. AZT, the first antiretroviral (ARV) approved by the FDA, became available in 1987 after one of the shortest periods of clinical testing and regulatory approval for any drug on record (Broder, 2010). As soon as this early treatment became available, talk of the promise of chronicity emerged among AIDS activists, researchers, and clinicians. Samuel Broder of the National Cancer Institute famously said in 1989 that HIV should now be considered a chronic illness and treated like cancer. The book *AIDS: The Making of a Chronic Disease* (Fee & Fox, 1992) was published in 1992 and made the same argument that HIV had been converted, through intense activism and remarkable scientific achievement, from an acute and consistently fatal disease to one whose progress could be significantly delayed through long-term drug therapy.

The introduction of highly active antiretroviral therapy (HAART) in the mid-1990s was the next dramatic shift in treatment efficacy from the remarkable but ultimately limited power of ARV monotherapies to a treatment strategy that could potentially extend the lifespan of those with HIV by several decades. It was with the stunning success of HAART that HIV's status as a chronic, manageable disease was finally cemented in the public's and medical community's imagination.

Activists have thus long been engaged in investing HIV with an aura of manageability, of normality, and of invisibility. In this register, they argued that HIV should be seen as unexceptional, as "just another chronic disease" (Mandell, 2010). The rise of antiretroviral treatment and its promise to convert the acuity of HIV infection into chronicity did not mean that activists abandoned the notion of the exceptional nature of HIV. Rather, there was a shifting of the balance between these two narratives, narratives that remained, and still remain, in tension in much of AIDS activism.

In Southern Africa, a similar medical and activist history has played out more recently, with the same narrative tensions between AIDS as an acute crisis and a chronic condition (Colvin, 2011). The crisis in this case was the lack of access in southern Africa to "triple therapy" HAART, the cocktail of ARVs that had proven to be the real breakthrough in keeping HIV infection at bay over the long term.

The founding outrage of AIDS activists in this region, most of whom who were assembled in South Africa under the banner of the Treatment Action Campaign (TAC), was the unaffordability of these first-world ART regimens. Activists understood this unaffordability to stem from both the intransigence of global pharmaceutical companies who wanted to protect profits and patent rights as well as the neglect and corruption of local states that did not want to make the political and financial commitments necessary to save the lives of their citizens (Nattrass, 2004).

While lack of access to treatment was what instigated the local AIDS movement, it was the "denialist" position taken by the Mbeki government in South Africa that really ratcheted up the anger among activists, communities, health professionals, and others involved in the fight against HIV (Geffen, 2010). Caught between profiteering drug companies, negligent and conspiracy-minded politicians, and rapidly growing numbers of dying compatriots, activists operated in a perfect storm of crisis, one that was described by many in South Africa as the "new struggle" that had replaced the epic struggle against apartheid (Vliet, 2001).

But then, seemingly as quickly as it had started, the crisis appeared to some to be over. In late 2003, the Mbeki administration changed tack and announced it would make ART available in the public sector. The rollout of this program in its first few years was agonizingly and unnecessarily slow (Mauchlin, 2009). With Jacob Zuma's assumption of the presidency and the replacement of Mbeki's hated minister of health, however, South Africa soon found itself in possession of the world's largest ART program. The "treatment gap" is still there (Zachariah, Van Damme, Arendt, Schmit, & Harries, 2011) but it is slowly being closed, as it is elsewhere in southern Africa and around the world (UNAIDS, 2010). AIDS activists have moved, therefore, in the span of a few short years, from a situation of intense crisis and uncertainty to one where the central problem is not *if* but *how* better to deliver treatment and encourage prevention.

Again, this shift from crisis to chronicity has not meant a replacement of one mode of activism by the other. Rather, they coexist and there remains a question within AIDS activism as to the right balance and relationship between these frames for understanding the epidemic. But there is also concern that the rise of treatment and its seemingly mundane, long-term challenges will dissipate the critical energies that once animated AIDS activism in the region. Put another way, some activists are wondering if treatment will "kill activism" (Robins, 2005). If the challenges of addressing HIV and AIDS were largely over, this dissipation of activist energy would be appropriate, even welcome. HIV's chronicity, however, introduces a host of new challenges around long-term adherence and viral resistance as well as the cost and complexity of delivering life-long treatment in struggling health systems. Activists fear that these problems, familiar in the world of chronic disease, may be harder to mobilize around.

This chapter addresses this question of the impact of treatment on activism, of the role of chronicity in reshaping the politics of disease. It begins with a case study of TAC's response to the recent provision of ART in South Africa's public-sector health system. This case study outlines how TAC activists have reconfigured their political energies and strategies to address some of the broader, structural drivers of the HIV epidemic, including norms around gender, sexuality, and gender-based violence; housing and labor policies; the governance and functioning of the health system; and local provision of sanitation and other basic services. For TAC, treatment access didn't kill activism but allowed it to engage in a more multifaceted struggle against the epidemic.

The next two sections examine how treatment activism and prevention activism, respectively, will likely change in the context of chronicity and treatment availability. Initiation of antiretroviral treatment is only the first step in maintaining lifelong treatment success. Treatment activism will continue to be necessary to support the expansion, affordability, and effectiveness of treatment programs, strengthen health care delivery systems and other forms of care and support, and address continuing challenges of stigma, denialism, and treatment adherence.

Prevention activism, on the other hand, has to contend with the fact that few prevention efforts up to now have had anything like the success of antiretroviral treatment. Adequate funding for prevention research and programming is also hard to come by. Recent successes in medical and pharmaceutical interventions have raised hopes that prevention may soon be as effectively deployed as treatment, but these interventions also run the risk of reducing the conversation around prevention back to narrow, technical strategies to the problem.

The final section explores how recent changes in the field of global public health, many of which were the result of earlier AIDS activism, shape the contemporary political conditions of possibility for AIDS activists. Growing interest, for example, in "horizontal" health interventions and health systems strengthening, noncommunicable disease, and the social determinants of health are all potentially welcome developments for AIDS activists interested in sustainable solutions to the epidemic. These shifts, however, also threaten to upset the traditionally exceptional status long afforded to HIV in global public health circles. The global financial crisis has also reduced available funding and revealed how "institutionalized" and dependent on particular forms of financing global AIDS activism has become.

The research for this chapter is based on several different ethnographic research projects with AIDS and other health activists in South Africa, including the Treatment Action Campaign, the People's Health Movement, the Social Justice Coalition, and the Khululeka Men's Support Group. It is also informed by qualitative research and policy work I have undertaken in South Africa as part of health systems development projects. The chapter also draws on a review of the secondary literature on AIDS activism after treatment access.

## NAVIGATING THE POST-ART LANDSCAPE: THE TREATMENT ACTION CAMPAIGN

The experience of South Africa's Treatment Action Campaign (TAC) highlights many of these issues around how AIDS activists have responded to a post-treatment landscape of fewer resources and more competing global health priorities. TAC began in 1998 when a group of activists gathered to protest the death of gay rights activist and veteran of the apartheid struggle, Simon Nkoli, from AIDS. At the time, ART was available in the private sector in South Africa for those who could afford it but the vast majority of those infected remained without access to treatment. TAC soon emerged as not only the major AIDS activist organization in the country but can be counted among the few significant social movements to have emerged in South Africa since the end of apartheid (Colvin & Robins, 2009). It had a charismatic leader, the HIV-positive Zackie Achmat; a broad grassroots support base, especially among women in the poorer urban and rural communities across South Africa; and it creatively combined a wide range of legal, media, political, and community-level strategies in its activism (Geffen, 2010).

Thanks largely to TAC's efforts, the public-sector rollout of ART began in 2004. TAC initially described its new role vis-à-vis the government as maintaining pressure and ensuring as rapid a rollout as possible. This proved to be prescient since the government failed to expand access to treatment as quickly as many observers considered possible. Citing short-term financial constraints and safety and quality control concerns over too rapid an expansion, the Department of Health developed a rollout plan that guaranteed the steady but slow expansion of services (Department of Health, 2004). Health facilities that wanted to offer ART had to be formally "certified," specialist staff had to be appointed and in place, and financing through the provincial health budgets had to be secured before they could offer ART services. TAC maintained its pressure on government to expand more quickly, arguing that this could be done safely and sustainably at a more rapid pace. They engaged government around recruitment policies, pharmacy regulations, and clinic infrastructure constraints that they argued unnecessarily impeded the rollout.

TAC also began broadening its efforts to improve the health services and opportunities for people with HIV. During this period, for example, they started including TB care and treatment in their set of concerns in more substantial ways and began developing policy proposals around social grants, the health status of refugees, and even chronic diseases. And like previous generations of AIDS activists in the United States and United Kingdom (Berridge, 1996; Epstein, 1996), they became increasingly involved in policy work at the national and provincial levels. Most prominently, Mark Heywood, TAC's national secretary, was appointed deputy chairperson of the South African National AIDS Council (SANAC) in 2007.

Many of these new interests were driven by aspects of the implementation of the ART program. However, they also moved TAC in new directions, beyond its central focus on securing ART treatment access and increasingly into the more "technical" realms of health service provision, scientific knowledge production, health policymaking and planning, and the political governance of health science and practice. More recently, they have issued press releases on improving monitoring and evaluation methodologies in the health system, mathematical modeling of TB transmission in prisons, the dangers of the Protection of State Information Bill (the so-called "secrecy bill"), gaps in health department procurement policies and procedures, bottlenecks in drug distribution logistics, the crisis of funding in the national laboratory services, and political inter-ference in the regulatory review of certain heart medications (see TAC's website, www.tac.org.za, for examples).

While TAC has always had a multidimensional understanding of the challenges of addressing HIV, especially in the context of a struggling health system, these recent efforts do mark a significant extension in the ways it understands and engages with the current HIV-related health challenges.

There have also been lingering traces of the "AIDS war" TAC fought with Mbeki that have brought out the old TAC. Churches promoting spiritual healing for HIV, German doctors selling vitamin cures, and traditional healers claiming to have developed nontoxic, "African" alternatives to

ART have all brought swift condemnation and even legal action from TAC (Cullinan & Thom, 2009). But these kinds of fights are fewer and farther between as treatment access expands and more people experience or witness its transformational potential.

In 2008, an unexpected crisis in South Africa also pushed TAC in new directions. In May of that year, xenophobic violence broke out in many places across South Africa. Long-simmering conflicts and resentments about the presence of non–South African Africans in the country erupted into several weeks of looting, assaults, evictions, and even killing of Africans from other countries who were living in South Africa townships (Neocosmos, 2010).

While the police and social services did mount a response to these attacks, attempting to quell the violence and protect its victims, civil society organizations also responded in significant but fairly uncoordinated fashion. In Cape Town, in particular, the internal displacement of people represented an additional and serious humanitarian crisis. Unlike those in the northern parts of the country who could flee across the border to other countries, most of those displaced in Cape Town did not have the means to leave the province and instead flooded into churches, community centers, and other safe havens in the city itself.

In the first few days of the chaotic response to the crisis, TAC emerged as a key platform through which the civil society response could be organized. TAC began by offering its office space in Cape Town as a place for local NGOs to meet and coordinate their activities. Soon, however, they were centrally involved in coordinating this civil society response, communicating with key actors and the public, and advocating to the state and international community for a more effective and sustained intervention in the violence. TAC's broad presence in communities, its professional and organizational capacity at its headquarters, and its political legitimacy all meant that TAC was the natural choice for organizing the local community response (Robins, 2009).

Besides now playing a more expansive leadership role in the civil society landscape, TAC's involvement in the response to the xenophobic violence also provoked a reflection on and recognition of some of the broader structural forces that fueled both HIV/AIDS as well as the recent violence. Lack of access to basic services, poor safety and security, crumbling schools, insufficient housing, and exclusion from local forms of political participation were all identified as problems of social justice that influenced both the spread of HIV (and the experience of ART) as well as the social tensions behind the xenophobic violence.

One consequence of this reflection was the founding of the Social Justice Coalition and Equal Education, new activist organizations, inspired by TAC's strategies and staffed by many of its key personnel, that seek to address these structural determinants of health. Recently, Zackie Achmat and others have also started another new project called *Ndifuna Ukwazi* (I Want to Know), which trains young activists to be literate in the technical knowledge and processes that undergird budgeting, the drafting of legislation, and the litigation of socioeconomic rights. Similarly, the AIDS Law Project, historically a close partner of TAC's, recently rebranded itself as Section 27, after Section 27 of the South African Constitution that guarantees a range of socioeconomic rights.

Thus, in addition to moving more deeply into some of the technical and administrative dimensions of the ART rollout itself, TAC and the partners it has inspired have also broadened their scope and begun to address some of the intersecting structural drivers of the HIV epidemic. While these developments are certainly in part the product of individual personalities and particularly the sociopolitical context in South Africa, they were also made possible by the space opened up by treatment access. Rather than killing activism, public-sector ART has made it possible for TAC and other activists to continue to address more deeply and more broadly some of the enduring health challenges in the country. This shift was not inevitable. And in the end, it may not produce the kinds of dramatic successes of the denialist-era TAC. But it does point to the potential for AIDS activism to transform itself in the process of shifting from acuity to chronicity.

## MOVING FROM TREATMENT ANARCHY TO PATIENT ADVOCACY

As the TAC case reveals, the creation and normalization of large-scale treatment programs does not remove the need for treatment activism. Some barriers to effective treatment, such as stigma, denialism, and poor adherence, continue to require intervention. Long-term treatment, however, also introduces a whole range of new challenges as well, including supporting and expanding treatment; ensuring it is effective, affordable, and equitable; strengthening the systems for delivering treatment; and maintaining a sufficiently broad and deep social safety net for those who will continue to require care and support.

As the TAC case study above makes clear, the provision of ART in the public sector is not a matter of simply writing policy, distributing drugs, and providing treatment. There are significant logistical and health system challenges to scaling up such a significant new service in any health system. TAC was frustrated by the unnecessarily slow pace of the rollout but even a politically supported and enthusiastically driven rollout in South Africa would have confronted serious roadblocks in terms of human resources, drug supply chain management, information systems, laboratory logistics, and clinic infrastructure (H. Schneider & McIntyre, 2003).

Such a roll-out would also require careful planning and effective communication at all levels of government, resources that are in short supply in many contexts. Indeed, the confusion and lingering denialist sentiments surrounding the initial rollout have been described by one commentator as "treatment anarchy" (Nattrass, 2007), a situation that arose from a combination of contradictory political messages, weak planning and communication, and the many barriers embedded in a struggling health system.

Activists thus have a role in ensuring ART policy decisions have continuing political commitment behind them and are thoroughly and correctly implemented. They can also lobby for improvements in the health system itself that would enable a swifter and more effective scale-up of ART (as well as supporting improvements in other services). Over time, AIDS activists may also need to maintain pressure for political commitment as new issues arise and competing priorities, both within health and in other departments, come to the fore. TAC has been involved in all of these capacities as a way to make sure the rollout proceeded as quickly and effectively as possible.

Challenges around intellectual property also do not disappear with treatment access. TAC won some spectacular reductions in cost of ARVs from the drug companies but in many cases, these victories took the form of settlements with or concessions by these companies, ones that could be taken away if and when the political climate shifts (Friedman & Mottiar, 2005). Similarly, success in securing affordable first-line regimens does not necessarily translate into easy access to affordable second- and third-line medications. As the treatment program matures, treatment failure will grow in scale and confrontations with pharmaceutical companies over price are likely to continue absent other legal interventions.

Beyond challenges of political will, health systems weakness, and drug pricing, activists will also increasingly confront the individual-level problem of adherence and treatment failure. Early indications have been that ART can be provided in the public sector with very good rates of early adherence in the first five years. However, there are growing concerns as the rollout continues that these early successes will be hard to sustain and that adherence will increase in scale and complexity as a clinical problem (Boulle et al., 2010).

Rather than large-scale political or legal activism, promoting and sustaining adherence will require community mobilization and strengthening of individual- and community-level services for those on ART. One organization in Cape Town, for example, has developed a model of "patient advocates," community health workers (CHWs) who support adherence in patients on ART on an ongoing and holistic basis (Igumbor, Scheepers, Ebrahim, Jason, & Grimwood, 2011). This dimension of treatment will indeed require "patient advocacy" both in the sense of advocacy *for* patients and advocacy *with* patience.

TAC already has a useful model for promoting patient empowerment through its "treatment literacy" program and has encouraged the development of CHW programming for ART adherence support. But effectively sustaining up to 2–5 percent of the population on lifelong treatment will require a much broader and deeper social safety net than any one organization can provide. Activists will need to both develop models for this kind of support as well as lobby for the social, political, and economic conditions that would make such support more broadly available.

Whatever the new challenges of adherence, though, many of the old challenges to treatment still persist. Stigma, for example, has slowly retreated in many communities in the face of time, political activism, community mobilization, and treatment access but it is still a very real barrier to treatment. Activists will need to continue to mobilize against stigma both in communities and in health facilities.

Similarly, denialism and "quackery" in many of the forms TAC resisted also persist. The social, cultural, and political forces that produce these conflicts over the interpretation of illness and the accepted forms of response are not specific to any one disease (Kalichman, 2009). Rather, the forces behind denialism are generic, and access to ART will not significantly change this fact. While the main-stage battle with President Mbeki and his supporters over AIDS denialism may have been won by TAC, uncertainty, confusion, denial, and outright fraud in the response to HIV will continue to emerge and pose a challenge to activists.

Finally, though initial ART access in the public sector and continuing pressure from activists to deepen coverage have resulted in a dramatic shift in whose lives are considered politically worthy of saving, treatment will also inevitably generate new lines of exclusion (Comaroff & Comaroff, 2011). Treatment, like all health care resources, is generally perceived as a scarce resource, and most health systems understand it to be their task to monitor and police who qualifies for access to these life-saving resources (Berger, 2002; People's Health Movement, Medact, & Global Equity Gauge Alliance, 2011).

As treatment programs mature, these new lines may be drawn with refugees, with undocumented workers, with the elderly, with the childless, or with "defaulters." It will be up to activists to name and critique these new forms of exclusion. In the longer term, activists will also have the opportunity to challenge ways of thinking about health care that are rooted in naturalized notions of scarcity.

Some of these challenges, like lack of political will, competing therapies, and forms of exclusion from the body politic, are familiar to AIDS activists and will persist as treatment scales up and patient cohorts enter their second decade of ART. Others, like adherence support and health systems strengthening, will require new, more sustained and patient forms of advocacy with individuals and communities.

## PREVENTION POLITICS, OLD AND NEW

Now that treatment access and activism in many countries has become more a question of "how" rather than "if," the public health and activist conversation around HIV has also noticeably shifted in the direction of prevention. Prevention was, of course, the original challenge of HIV before treatment was available. But starting with the development of the first monotherapies in the late 1980s, many felt that prevention activism became the poor cousin of treatment activism. Even now, prevention activists face a host of challenges including a poor record of success so far for most prevention strategies along with difficulty securing funding for both prevention research and programming. Technical interventions such as male medical circumcision and a range of "treatment-as-prevention" strategies do offer some hope, but activists may struggle to situate these interventions within broader goals of social, political and economic change.

Attention to prevention has increased in South Africa, however, not only because of the breathing room afforded by the rollout of ART but also because of the realization that little progress was being made in bringing down rates of HIV incidence (Shisana et al., 2009). Prevention efforts have clearly not been as successful as many had hoped, and the epidemic appears set to continue steadily reproducing itself in the population. This, in a way, is another form of chronicity, where the epidemic becomes endemic, where the crisis becomes chronic, self-perpetuating, and seemingly inescapable.

Of course, fate does not determine the shape of epidemics and activists have rightly argued that the time is ripe for paying proper attention to prevention. They are limited in this pursuit, however, by a range of factors, not least of which is the lack of proven, effective prevention strategies at the population level. The ABC approach, rooted in condoms and behavior change, is not without power or potential. But it has proven relatively ineffective in the South African context (Harrison, Newell, Imrie, & Hoddinott, 2010). Similarly, large-scale public awareness and education campaigns have raised the profile of HIV and may have greatly improved population knowledge about the disease but have not made a clear impact on transmission (Rehle et al., 2006).

Funding for prevention also remains the challenge it has always been. The power of treatment is easier to recognize and reward politically and the existence of the largest ART program in the world means that money for HIV prevention in South Africa will always be set against the need to maintain and extend successes in the treatment program. It can also be difficult to secure research funding for prevention work. Even pharmaceutical solutions, such as microbicide gels, have failed to attract industry sponsorship and have instead relied on donor and state funding for their research and development (Philpott, Slevin, Shapiro, & Heise, 2010).

There have been a significant number of promising developments in South Africa in the field of prevention, however, almost all of them in the form of biomedical or pharmaceutical interventions, often involving ARVs. Male medical circumcision (MMC) has been recently recognized as an effective form of prevention for men (Siegfried, Muller, Deeks, & Volmink, 2009). Activists in South Africa have been quick to promote MMC services in the public sector though they have also had to contend with concerns around gender equity and potentially damaging commercial interests in these services (AVAC: Global Advocacy for Prevention, 2010).

Activists searching for a woman-controlled forms of prevention were similarly excited when the CAPRISA 004 trial showed for the first time that microbicide gels that included an ARV could work as a relatively effective form of prevention (Abdool Karim et al., 2010). ARVs as prophylaxis have also been used in a number of other forms. Preexposure prophylaxis (PrEP) and postexposure prophylaxis (PEP) both provide ARVs to HIV-negative people to prevent HIV inoculation from establishing itself as infection in the body. The latest innovation is treatment-as-prevention (TAP), an approach that delivers ART to HIV-positive people with high CD4 counts (i.e., sooner than they would usually start treatment) in the hopes that their reduced viral load will translate into reduced rates of infection of others (Seale, Lazarus, Grubb, Fakoya, & Atun, 2011).

These promising new prevention strategies, many of them rooted in treatment technologies, have been championed by activists who have long despaired of trying to find and promote effective ways of stopping HIV transmission. And fascinating debates have emerged among researchers, public health practitioners, and activists around the scientific process of testing and certifying these interventions as safe and effective. Many of the activists, for example, who heard the dramatic announcement of the results of the CAPRISA 004 vaginal microbicide trial at the 2010 International AIDS Conference in Vienna were quick to push for registration of the gel. Others cautioned that trial results needed to be confirmed and that regulatory processes would require a second trial. When the VOICE trial subsequently failed to demonstrate the effectiveness of the microbicide gel, activists were understandably disappointed though many maintained, just as the earliest AIDS activists did, that the current process of scientific review and regulatory approval of new interventions was still unnecessarily slow and cumbersome (McEnery, 2011).

Again, most of the progress and enthusiasm in new forms of prevention has centered on biomedical and pharmaceutical interventions. This is perhaps not surprising given the vivid power of treatment and the lack of clear success in efforts to change social norms and individual behavior. This situation represents both a threat and an opportunity for AIDS activism. While these new strategies hold real promise—and may also require significant activist energy to bring to full fruition—they also reinforce global business and health science interests in technological solutions to health problems. Bypassing the social, cultural, political, economic, and individual dimensions of prevention may be appealing in the short term but carries a real risk for activists who might otherwise advocate for a more holistic, long-term, and critical vision of the production and prevention of diseases.

## RECALIBRATIONS IN GLOBAL PUBLIC HEALTH

The two previous sections have recounted how South Africa's public-sector ART program and the global progress being made in closing the treatment gap have forced AIDS activists to adjust to a host of challenges, new and old, with respect to both treatment and prevention. These sections have surveyed some of the risks and prospects for activism in this new landscape of widespread ART access. The rise of large, public-sector ART programs, however, has coincided with a number of other important changes in global public health, changes that also represent potential threats and opportunities for AIDS activism. These changes include increasing interest in primary health care, health system strengthening, and aid harmonization as well as renewed emphasis on noncommunicable diseases and the social determinants of health. The global financial crisis has also reduced funding for HIV and forced activists to confront the institutionalization of AIDS activism and its dependence on particular forms of funding for their work.

Many of these changes in thinking about global public health were themselves initially catalyzed by the global response to the AIDS epidemic. In fact, in many ways, the response by northern countries, intergovernmental institutions, and private philanthropies to the epidemic in the late 1990s and 2000s was one of the main forces behind the emergence of the field of "global health" and the significant structural changes in the financing and governance of health seen in the last 10 years at a global level (Ravishankar et al., 2009).

Not surprisingly, however, many of the changes inspired by the response to HIV have begun to exceed their original intention and challenge conventional thinking and practice with respect to HIV and AIDS. The intense interest and generous funding around HIV, for example, initially produced responses that were highly "vertical" in nature, programs and policies that were devoted to funneling resources specifically to HIV-related services, bypassing in many cases dysfunctional health bureaucracies and systems that activists and policymakers feared would dilute the impact of donor funding (Levine & Oomman, 2009). This approach was rooted in a crisis-oriented narrative of AIDS that demanded an exceptional response.

While this strategy was an understandable response to the emergency of HIV, it quickly drew criticism for a range of unintended effects on local health systems including internal brain drain (as human resources were shifted to HIV services), service fragmentation, and unnecessary duplication of systems and bureaucratic procedures (Garrett, 2007). The impact of "stove-piping" of HIV programs into horizontally structured primary health care systems has been an important catalyst for much of the recent interest in and development of "systems thinking" in public health (Savigny & Adam, 2009). Increasingly, health policymakers, donors, and AIDS activists are being asked to rethink the exceptionality of HIV and AIDS programming and design ways to provide HIV services in a more integrated, horizontal, and systems-oriented approach.

The urgent global response to HIV also tended to far exceed the capacity of many public sectors, especially in Southern Africa, to spend money and implement new programs. Local health systems were often too weak or too slow to respond to the pressing concerns of global donors. One consequence was the flourishing of civil society organizations as an implementing partner for a wide variety of HIV-related interventions, ranging from community awareness and grassroots mobilization to the direct provision of large ART programs (Kelly & Birdsall, 2010). Donors effectively bypassed the state in many cases and delivered services directly via the nonprofit sector.

This strategy of short-circuiting local states proved effective in the short term for delivering emergency aid to individuals and communities. But it has also resulted in considerable duplication of services, fragmentation of care, competition and lack of coordination among implementing partners, and conflict with national policies and priorities. As a consequence, the last few years have seen growing priority placed on the harmonization of aid and the use of "country coordinating mechanisms" to better coordinate the flow of money, the activity of various roleplayers, and provision of services within a country (Hill, Dodd, Brown, & Haffeld, 2012).

For activists, these new interests in health system strengthening and the improved coordination of aid and development initiatives represent an opportunity to translate the exceptional responses to HIV into more sustainable, efficient, and systemic changes in health and health systems. The recently renewed interest in the "social determinants of health" is a similar development that promises to introduce some critical and holistic thinking, long absent in public health policy, about the structural conditions necessary for good health. These kinds of expanded notions of health, health systems, and health determinants should resonate with the political perspectives of many AIDS activists who understand HIV to be a symptom of deeper crises in the global political and economic order.

On the other hand, however, improving weak health systems and addressing the social determinants of health are formidable, long-term challenges, much more complicated than figuring out how to provide vertical ART services. And state-led coordination of overseas and private funding and interventions runs a real risk of cooptation and bureaucratization. Activists will need to consider what kind of balance to advocate for between long-term and short-term goals, between vertical and horizontal strategies, and between government facilitation and independent action in the field of HIV and health more broadly. Many of these strategic decisions in turn hinge on what activists decide is the best balance between crisis and chronicity as a way to understand the epidemic.

Another significant sea change in the world of global health is one that was entirely unexpected by most observers. The global financial crisis has had a number of profound effects on AIDS activism, not the least of which is the recent funding crisis in HIV. Besides the broader economic and health effects of the crisis, activists have been worried primarily that reductions in donor funding will undermine the recent successes in treatment and severely damage efforts to refocus on prevention (K. Schneider & Garrett, 2009). And indeed, the recent cancelling of the Global Fund's 2011 funding cycle and the general pullback in donor spending in the last couple years have put serious pressure on governments, civil society, and activists alike.

Besides the direct cuts to HIV funding, one indirect effect of the crisis has been to bring into sharper relief the institutionalization of activism, and indeed the entire "AIDS industry," and its reliance on a particular set of global financial relationships for support (Gillett, 2003). TAC, for example, has experienced several critical funding shortages recently that have threatened to close its doors. This is a dramatic turn of events for what is still the preeminent social movement in South Africa. Many smaller NGOs and activist organizations have shut down completely. The crisis thus represents a profound challenge to the maintenance of current organizational forms of activism. It might also present an opportunity, though, for recalibrating both the strategic focus and the forms of institutional and financial dependence that characterize activism today.

The funding crisis in HIV has also brought the question of HIV funding into more direct relationship to funding needs for other health problems. Though the WHO's recent interest in the significant global burden of non-communicable diseases (NCD) had been developing before the global financial crisis (World Health Organization, 2010), the recent shrinking of health budgets and donor funding has directly raised the question of the balance of priorities between HIV and NCD funding. While some AIDS activists have experienced this as a direct challenge to the long-standing global prioritization of HIV funding, others have argued that the fight against NCDs has much to learn from the global HIV response (Rabkin & El-Sadr, 2011). Going forward, they will need to consider both how best to advocate for continued HIV-specific support as well as how to integrate their interests with those of other health activists in ways that reduce competition and promote more sustainable and systemic improvements in health.

The growth of public-sector ART programs in many places in the world has meant a shift in register from one emphasizing crisis to one focused on chronicity. The changes reviewed above in the world of global public health also, on their own terms, pose implicit and explicit challenges to the exceptionality of HIV and AIDS. Responding effectively to these changes in the narratives about HIV is one of the central challenges activists will face in the near future. Though the specter of the wasted and excluded body of the African AIDS sufferer no longer haunts health activists and medical professionals in the way it used to, this image is also less available now to do the rhetorical work it once did.

Images of death, especially needless, gruesome death, evoke emergency and elicit crisis response. But the miraculous "Lazarus effect" seen in those who gain access to ART while hovering at the edge of death is slowly being replaced by treatment-as-prevention initiatives that will erase this embodied transition from "near death to new life" (Robins, 2006). While this clearly represents one of the most dramatic successes of AIDS activism, at the same time it also represents the next big question activists will have to answer in the era of treatment—how to maintain focus, generate outrage, and struggle against the new and continuing challenges of an epidemic that remains far from over, even as its most acute forms transform into something new.

## BIBLIOGRAPHY

Abdool Karim, Q., Abdool Karim, S. S., Frohlich, J. A., Grobler, A. C., Baxter, C., & Mansoor, L. E. (2010). Effectiveness and safety of tenofovir gel, an antiretroviral microbicide, for the prevention of HIV infection in women. *Science, 329*(5996), 1168–1174.

AVAC: Global Advocacy for Prevention (2010). *Making medical male circumcision work for women: South Africa country report.* New York City: AVAC: Global Advocacy for Prevention.

Berger, J. M. (2002). Tripping over patents: AIDS, access to treatment and the manufacturing of scarcity. *Conn J Int Law, 17*(2), 157–248.

Berridge, V. (1996). *AIDS in the UK: The making of a policy, 1981–1994.* Oxford; New York: Oxford University Press.

Boulle, A., Van Cutsem, G., Hilderbrand, K., Cragg, C., Abrahams, M., Mathee, S., . . . Maartens, G. (2010). Seven-year experience of a primary care antiretroviral treatment programme in Khayelitsha, South Africa. *AIDS, 24*(4), 563–572. doi: 10.1097/QAD.0b013e328333bfb7

Broder, S. (2010). The development of antiretroviral therapy and its impact on the HIV-1/AIDS pandemic. [Review.] *Antiviral Res, 85*(1), 1–18.

Centers for Disease Control and Prevention (1983). Prevention of acquired immune deficiency syndrome (AIDS): Report of inter-agency recommendations. *MMWR, 32*(8), 101–103.

Colvin, C. J. (2011). HIV/AIDS, chronic diseases and globalisation. *Global Health, 7,* 31. doi: 10.1186/1744-8603-7-31

Colvin, C. J., & Robins, S. (2009). Social movements and HIV/AIDS in South Africa. In P. Rohleder, L. Swartz, S. Kalichman & L. Simbayi (eds.), *HIV/AIDS in South Africa 25 Years On: Psychosocial perspectives.* New York: Springer.

Comaroff, J., & Comaroff, J. L. (2011). *Theory from the south, or, How Euro-America is evolving toward Africa.* Boulder, CO: Paradigm Publishers.

Cullinan, K., & Thom, A. (2009). *The virus, vitamins and vegetables: The South African HIV/AIDS mystery.* Auckland Park, South Africa: Jacana.

Department of Health (2004). *National antiretroviral treatment guidelines.* Pretoria, South Africa.

Engel, J. (2006). *The epidemic: A global history of AIDS.* New York: Smithsonian Books/Collins.

Epstein, S. (1996). *Impure science: AIDS, activism, and the politics of knowledge.* Berkeley: University of California Press.

Fee, E., & Fox, D. M. (1992). *AIDS: The making of a chronic disease.* Berkeley: University of California Press.

Friedman, S., & Mottiar, S. (2005). A rewarding engagement? The Treatment Action Campaign and the politics of HIV/AIDS. *Politics & Society, 33*(4), 511–565.

Garrett, L. (2007). The challenge of global health. *Foreign Affairs, 86*(1), 14–38.

Geffen, N. (2010). *Debunking delusions: The inside story of the Treatment Action Campaign.* Auckland Park, South Africa: Jacana Media.

Gillett, J. (2003). The challenges of institutionalization for AIDS media activism. *Media, Culture and Society, 25*(5), 607–624.

Harrison, A., Newell, M. L., Imrie, J., & Hoddinott, G. (2010). HIV prevention for South African youth: Which interventions work? A systematic review of current evidence. [Research Support, Non-U.S. Gov't.] *BMC Public Health, 10,* 102. doi: 10.1186/1471-2458-10-102

Hill, P. S., Dodd, R., Brown, S., & Haffeld, J. (2012). Development cooperation for health: Reviewing a dynamic concept in a complex global aid environment. *Global Health, 8*(1), 5. doi: 10.1186/1744-8603-8-5

Igumbor, J. O., Scheepers, E., Ebrahim, R., Jason, A., & Grimwood, A. (2011). An evaluation of the impact of a community-based adherence support programme on ART outcomes in selected government HIV treatment sites in South Africa. *AIDS Care, 23*(2), 231–236.

Kalichman, S. C. (2009). *Denying AIDS: Conspiracy theories, pseudoscience, and human tragedy.* New York: Copernicus Books.

Kelly, K. J., & Birdsall, K. (2010). The effects of national and international HIV/ AIDS funding and governance mechanisms on the development of civil-society responses to HIV/AIDS in East and Southern Africa. [Research Support, Non-U.S. Gov't.] *AIDS Care, 22 Suppl 2,* 1580–1587. doi: 10.1080/09540121. 2010.524191

Levine, R., & Oomman, N. (2009). Global HIV/AIDS funding and health systems: Searching for the win-win. *J Acquir Immune Defic Syndr, 52 Suppl 1,* S3–5.

Mandell, B. (2010). HIV: Just another chronic disease. *Cleveland Clinic Journal of Medicine, 77*(8), 489.

Mauchlin, K. (2009). Official government justifications and public ARV provision: A comparison of Brazil, Thailand and South Africa. *AIDS 2031 Working Paper.* Centre for Social Science Research: University of Cape Town.

McEnery, R. (2011). Oral tenofovir arm of VOICE trial discontinued early. *IAVI Rep, 15*(5), 21.

Nattrass, N. (2004). *The moral economy of AIDS in South Africa.* Cambridge: Cambridge University Press.

Nattrass, N. (2007). *Mortal combat: AIDS denialism and the struggle for antiretrovirals in South Africa.* Scottsville, South Africa: University of KwaZulu-Natal Press.

Neocosmos, M. (2010). *From "foreign natives" to "native foreigners": Explaining xenophobia in post-apartheid South Africa: Citizenship and nationalism, identity and politics* (2nd ed.). Dakar, Senegal: CODESRIA.

People's Health Movement, Medact, & Global Equity Gauge Alliance (2011). Global health watch: An alternative world health report (p. v.). London; Pretoria: Zed UNISA Press.

Philpott, S., Slevin, K. W., Shapiro, K., & Heise, L. (2010). Impact of donor-imposed requirements and restrictions on standards of prevention and access to care and treatment in HIV prevention trials. *Public Health Ethics, 3*(3), 220–228.

Rabkin, M., & El-Sadr, W. M. (2011). Why reinvent the wheel? Leveraging the lessons of HIV scale-up to confront non-communicable diseases. *Glob Public Health, 6*(3), 247–256.

Ravishankar, N., Gubbins, P., Cooley, R. J., Leach-Kemon, K., Michaud, C. M., Jamison, D. T., & Murray, C. J. (2009). Financing of global health: Tracking development assistance for health from 1990 to 2007. *Lancet, 373*(9681), 2113–2124.

Rehle, T. M., Setswe, G., Pillay, V., Metcalf, C., Jooste, S., Rispel, L., & Sekhobo, J. P. (2006). Assessing the impact of HIV and AIDS prevention and care programmes in South Africa. Pretoria, South Africa: Human Sciences Research Council.

Robins, S. (2005). From "medical miracles" to normal(ised) medicine: AIDS treatment, activism and citizenship in the UK and South Africa. *IDS Working Papers.* Brighton: Sussex University.

Robins, S. (2006). From "Rights" to "Ritual": AIDS activism in South Africa. *American Anthropologist, 108*(2), 312–323.

Robins, S. (2009). Humanitarian aid beyond "bare survival": Social movement responses to xenophobic violence in South Africa. *American Ethnologist, 36*(4), 637–650.

Savigny, D., & Adam, T. (2009). Systems thinking for health systems strengthening. Geneva: Alliance for Health Policy and Systems Research.

Schneider, H., & McIntyre, J. (2003). Scaling up the use of antiretrovirals in the public sector: What are the challenges? *Southern African Journal of HIV Medicine, 4*(3), 19–23.

Schneider, K., & Garrett, L. (2009). The end of the era of generosity? Global health amid economic crisis. [Editorial.] *Philos Ethics Humanit Med, 4,* 1. doi: 10.1186/1747-5341-4-1

Seale, A., Lazarus, J. V., Grubb, I., Fakoya, A., & Atun, R. (2011). HPTN 052 and the future of HIV treatment and prevention. *Lancet, 378*(9787), 226.

Shilts, R. (1988). *And the band played on: Politics, people, and the AIDS epidemic.* New York: Penguin Books.

Shisana, O., Rehle, T., Simbayi, L., Zuma, K., Jooste, S., Pillay-van Wyk, V., . . . SABSSM III Implementation Team (2009). *South African national HIV prevalence, incidence, behaviour and communication survey, 2008 a turning tide among teenagers?* Cape Town: HSRC Press.

Siegfried, N., Muller, M., Deeks, J. J., & Volmink, J. (2009). Male circumcision for prevention of heterosexual acquisition of HIV in men. *Cochrane Database Syst Rev*(2), CD003362.

Treichler, P. A. (1999). *How to have theory in an epidemic: Cultural chronicles of AIDS.* Durham: Duke University Press.

UNAIDS (2010). *UNAIDS report on the global AIDS epidemic.* Geneva: UNAIDS.

Vliet, V. v. d. (2001). AIDS: Losing "the new struggle"? *Daedalus, 130*(1), 151–184.

World Health Organization (2010). Global status report on NCDs. Geneva: World Health Organization.

Zachariah, R., Van Damme, W., Arendt, V., Schmit, J. C., & Harries, A. D. (2011). The HIV/AIDS epidemic in sub-Saharan Africa: Thinking ahead on programmatic tasks and related operational research. *J Int AIDS Soc, 14 Suppl 1,* S7. doi: 10.1186/1758-2652-14-S1-S7

# 11

# AIDS Mobilization in Zambia: Agency versus Structural Challenges

*Amy S. Patterson*

## AIDS MOBILIZATION IN AFRICA

The literatures on AIDS mobilization and African politics provide several clues about the factors that influence advocacy. I first highlight how factors within organizations such as the agency of group participants and leaders may push mobilization. I define agency as the ability of individuals or groups to shape political, economic, and social outcomes that affect them, either at the community or national level. I then turn to broader structural factors that affect activism. I use South Africa's Treatment Action Campaign (TAC) and Uganda's The AIDS Support Organization (TASO) to illustrate these theoretical points. Formed in 1998, TAC has utilized mass protests, lawsuits, media campaigns, and formal and informal lobbying to force the South African government to develop AIDS policies such as provision of nevirapine for prevention of mother-to-child transmission and free access to antiretroviral treatment (ART) for all South Africans who need it (Patterson, 2006; Mbali, 2004; Johnson, 2004). TASO began in 1987 to provide care to people living with and affected by HIV and AIDS; it has advocated for the rights of PLHAs at the local, national, and international levels (Muriisa, 2010).

## Internal Factors, Agency, and Mobilization

I divide internal factors into four categories: collective identity, members' sense of efficacy, leadership, and internal group structures. Collective identity is the sense of unity and solidarity that fuels participation to achieve a common goal (Snow, 2001). In the case of HIV, such identity stems from one's personal and often intense experiences with the disease (Robins, 2006). Knowledge about HIV/AIDS among group members and a sense of ownership over the AIDS problem can influence identity (Campbell, Gibbs, Maimane, Nair, & Sibiya, 2009). PLHIV groups provide a safe arena in which people can disclose their status and receive information about the disease, thus fueling identity creation and individual ownership of the disease. Yet stigma, fear, and denial can limit that identity and ownership and hamper activism. Through its community AIDS education programs, TAC promotes knowledge about the disease and combats stigma. It seeks to transform the AIDS stigma into a "badge of pride" that is publicly displayed on "HIV-positive" T-shirts at funerals, workshops, and demonstrations (Robins, 2006).

A sense of confidence (or efficacy) that one can positively affect one's situation also influences activism. In situations with high levels of poverty and political marginalization, individuals may feel paralyzed to respond, they may exhibit fatalism, or they may merely wait for external assistance (Campbell, Gibbs, Maimane, Nair, & Sibiya, 2009; Beckman & Bujra, 2010). A collective HIV identity can combat this lack of efficacy, because it constitutes a basis for a new form of citizenship. For example, in South Africa and Mozambique PLHIV groups have increasingly mobilized to demand protection of basic socioeconomic rights by the state. TAC has been particularly adept at using a rights-based approach in its advocacy, in order to create a new citizenship identity (Robins, 2006; Fenio, 2011; Mbali, 2004).

While the social movement literature has paid limited attention to leadership (Morris & Staggenborg, 2004), leadership is a crucial determinant of mobilization. Leaders can frame issues in ways that urge participation, challenge structural variables such as exclusive political systems or gender-based cultural norms, and urge new forms of collective identity (Warren, 2001). Leadership is particularly crucial when there are few precedents about how to respond to an issue or when issues are ill-defined (Trice & Beyer, 1991). For local organizations, leaders act as intermediaries between local constituencies and external resource providers such as advocacy groups or nongovernmental organizations (NGOs). In the case of TAC, the charismatic leader Zackie Achmat framed AIDS as a human rights issue, bringing a moral call to the organization's demands for ART. Emerging at a time when the AIDS policy realm was murky and state reactions were slow, TAC leaders capitalized on their experiences in the antiapartheid struggle and built ties to the global AIDS movement (Mbali, 2004; Friedman & Mottair, 2004).

Finally, an organization's internal structure may shape activism. Authoritarian group leaders who centralize power or limit transparency may cause groups to lose legitimacy. If members are disgruntled or leave the organization, it is more difficult for it to advocate for policy changes. Hierarchical structures that limit members' ability to voice concerns or develop innovative programs may also squash advocacy efforts. To prevent these problems, TAC devolved power to provincial bodies and ensured that representatives from local chapters participated in decisions made at the national level (Friedman & Mottair, 2004).

## Larger Structural Determinants of Mobilization

Factors outside the control of local organizations, such as political, economic, and social structures, also influence mobilization. Political transitions can provide openings for mobilization (Tarrow, 1989; Tilly, 1978), as was the case with TAC and TASO. TAC emerged in a new postapartheid democratic space during the tenure of the African National Congress government, a regime that had only begun to seriously grapple with AIDS in the late 1990s (Furlong & Ball, 2005). TASO was formed at the end of the Ugandan civil war, when the newly installed President Yoweri Museveni wanted to address AIDS. South Africa's liberal constitution, independent judiciary, and open society provided political openings for activism, and while Uganda is not as democratic as South Africa, the Museveni regime has provided space for civil society, including PLHIV groups (Patterson, 2006).

African states are characterized by neopatrimonialism, or rule through personal networks. While neopatrimonialism varies across the continent, the general pattern is that state officials centralize power and use patronage to reward their supporters and buy off potential opponents. Because decision making often lacks transparency, leaders may use state resources for personal gain (van de Walle, 2001). Neopatrimonial networks exclude some in society, such as women, the poor, and migrants, because the regime neither needs their support nor feels threatened by them. Fenio (2011) finds that high levels of power centralization and patronage networks hampered PLHIV advocacy in Swaziland and Mozambique.

Because people involved in politics do not want to limit patronage opportunities by confronting power brokers, neopatrimonialism has often meant that policymaking in Africa has tended to be rooted in consensus building, not confrontation. While TAC has directly confronted the state, many other African PLHIV groups have not. Instead, they have sought to educate government officials about HIV, to gain representation on national AIDS policymaking committees, and to build strong connections to political decision makers (Zambian government official, personal communication, August 14, 2007; Ghanaian NGO official, personal communication, September 2, 2008). TASO, for example, asserts that its positive relations with government have led to its successes (TASO, 2011).

Poverty and economic desperation drive citizens' attention from AIDS, a disease whose devastating effects may not be felt for years. Despite high HIV rates throughout southern Africa, populations in those countries have not tended to view the disease to be politically salient; instead they prioritize food security and job creation. Because AIDS is pushed off the political agenda, broad-based mobilization is more difficult (Justesen, 2011). But it is not just poverty that may hamper mobilization, since it is not solely poor individuals who are HIV-positive. In Zambia, for example, men and women with higher levels of education were at greater risk of HIV infection than those with little or no education (Ministry of Health, National AIDS Council, & Joint United Nations Programme on HIV/AIDS [UNAIDS], 2011, p. 28). The challenge is that wealthier, more educated individuals do not need the material support that PLHIV organizations often provide to low-income members, and thus they have little incentive to mobilize. TAC also has struggled with issues of cross-class participation: Its leadership remains predominantly educated and professional in contrast to its rank-and-file membership (Friedman & Mottair, 2004).

Cultural attitudes about political participation, AIDS, and gender may influence activism. Despite relatively high levels of voter turnout, participation in civil society remains relatively weak in Africa, with religious organizations being the most popular avenue for involvement (Patterson, 2011). The AIDS stigma may prevent participation in any AIDS-related activities, since individuals do not want to be identified with the disease. Gender norms shape mobilization since, as Michel Sidibé, executive director of UNAIDS, said, "This epidemic unfortunately remains an epidemic of women" (UN News Centre, 2010). While women tend to be the majority of PLHIV group members, they are underrepresented in broader political and economic structures: They hold only about 19 percent of Africa's legislative seats and they lag behind men in education and formal employment (Yoon, 2004). Religious teachings and expectations about motherhood and household work limit women's public role (Geiser, 2006). These gendered trends are evident in TAC and TASO. TAC's founding members were not African women (though by 2008, women led the organization), but gay men (Friedman & Mottair, 2004). TASO's founders were women, but TASO's initial role was somewhat gendered, since it sought to provide care for the sick, dying, and orphaned (TASO, 2011).

Finally, African PLHIV organizations are set within a global context, in which the international AIDS movement has advocated for greater donor attention to AIDS, Africa PLHIV groups have formed regional organizations, and bilateral donors and international NGOs have devoted large sums of money to AIDS in Africa (Smith & Siplon, 2006; Patterson, 2011). In the new millennium, local African activists have used global connections to access resources and moral support and to legitimate their claims (Keck & Sikkink, 1998). While only a minority of groups have these ties, those that do have benefited from global publicity, resources for local development efforts, and access to timely information and training (Campbell, Gibbs, Maimane, Nair, & Sibiya, 2009). But external resources also may hamper mobilization, if these material assets become a type of patronage that local elites utilize to stay in power. Recipients who rely on such resources may not engage in activism, because they do not want to challenge patronage-dispersing local decision makers. In Tanzania, for example, this pattern led PLHIV groups to play a minor role in policymaking, rarely challenging the state (Beckmann & Bujra, 2010).

## THE ZAMBIA CASE AND RESEARCH METHODOLOGY

Zambia has been greatly affected by AIDS, with an estimated 14 percent of 15–49-year-olds being HIV positive in 2009. Sixty percent of Zambians infected with HIV are women. As of 2009, free ART and massive distribution efforts meant that approximately 68 percent of Zambians needing ART could access it (Ministry of Health, National AIDS Council, & UNAIDS, 2010). The country has many active and well-established AIDS groups, with the oldest and biggest being the Network of Zambian People Living with HIV and AIDS (NZP+). As a national network with groups in all of Zambia's 72 districts, NZP+ has lobbied the national government to devote more attention to AIDS and to provide free ART. Since the emergence of democracy after the Kenneth Kaunda era, the number of civil society organizations has greatly increased in Zambia, and groups like NZP+ have capitalized on this open political space. Civil society formation, particularly in the context of social service delivery, also has been fueled by millions in donor funds that have come into the country. In 2006 alone, $207 million was spent on HIV and AIDS, with 78 percent of that amount coming from external donors (Ministry of Health, National AIDS Council, & UNAIDS, 2010).

Zambia is relatively homogeneous in terms of religion, with 85 percent of citizens identifying themselves as Christian. While minority religious groups such as Muslims, Hindus, and Baha'is exist, there has not been religiously based violence in the country. Interfaith cooperation on HIV and AIDS has occurred through the Zambia Interfaith Networking Group on HIV/AIDS, and NZP+ groups involve individuals from all Christian denominations and some minority religions (NZP+ national leadership, personal communication, March 7, 2011). While the country has over 70 recognized ethnic groups (many with their own language), ethnic violence has been rare. Thus, ethnic or religious identities do not limit mobilization within NZP+ groups (NZP+ member, personal communication, March 22, 2011), though religious identification has made collaboration between NZP+ and church-based PLHIV groups more difficult (Patterson & Stephens, n.d.).

Zambia's underdevelopment allows for an investigation of how poverty shapes mobilization. The country's GDP per capita is $1,500, and its Human Development Index ranking of 164 out of 187 makes it one of the world's most underdeveloped countries. Income inequality also is quite high. The country relies heavily on copper exports and agriculture, and official development assistance comprises roughly 27 percent of Zambia's GDP (United Nations Development Programme [UNDP], 2011). Zambia is also one of Africa's most urbanized countries, due to migration to the Copperbelt and the capital, Lusaka. Seventy percent of Lusaka's residents live in shantytown compounds where overcrowding, poor sanitation, and crime are common. In such compounds, the informal sector comprises 70 percent of employment, and unemployment rates can reach 80 percent (Resnick, 2011). Zambia also has high levels of gender inequality, another factor that may shape PLHIV mobilization. The country is situated in the bottom 20 in the world in terms of its gender equality index, and only 11 percent of legislators are women (Inter-Parliamentary Union, 2011; UNDP, 2011).

I examined local-level advocacy efforts among NZP+ groups in urban Zambia. I chose NZP+ because of its long history, wide reach, and national-level advocacy efforts. I employed data from 34 focus group interviews with NZP+ community groups and 20 interviews with NZP+ leaders. To verify data from NZP+ members, I also interviewed individual PLHAs, donor and NGO officials, and community elites. Research was conducted during 2011 in Lusaka and four other urban centers. Interview and focus group questions investigated group activities, as well as interactions between PLHIV groups and community leaders, donors, and NGO officials. All interviewees were assured that they would remain anonymous in any publications.

## MOBILIZATION EFFORTS IN ZAMBIAN URBAN COMMUNITIES

Of the 34 NZP+ groups I studied, only five advocated for local programs or policies to benefit their members. To be clear, even though the other 29 groups did not engage in public advocacy, they did actively participate in community AIDS education efforts, HIV testing and counseling campaigns, income-generating projects, and home-based care programs. Below I describe the mobilization efforts of the five groups and explore the factors that made this activism possible.

### Cases of Community Activism

Led by a woman, Group A met at a government clinic in a Lusaka compound. For several years, the overcrowded clinic did not have a separate wing for people who needed an HIV test, PLHAs who were ill, or more recently, PLHAs who needed to obtain ART medications. The group organized before the 2006 election and demanded that candidates for the local council and the parliamentary constituency promise to build an AIDS wing at the clinic. The group attended campaign rallies to voice its demands, exhibiting some of the same activist traits that TAC has used. After the election, it continued to pressure officials until the clinic addition was built. Although it was unclear whether the government or donors actually financed the construction, the NZP+ group claimed that its advocacy led to this outcome (NZP+ member, personal communication, March 24, 2011).

Groups B and C, both located in urban areas outside of Lusaka, successfully advocated to their local government authorities to get land on which to build community schools for orphans and vulnerable children. To advocate, they wrote proposals, informally and formally met with local officials, and attended council meetings. They did not utilize confrontational tactics, instead patiently enduring the rather long and bureaucratic process that accompanies land requests (NZP+ member, personal interview, June 25, 2011; NZP+ member, personal interview, April 18, 2011). A woman headed Group B, while a man led Group C.

Led by a man, Group D was situated on a military base that was 30 kilometers outside of Lusaka. The organization lobbied for the free provision of ART at the camp's medical clinic. While the group contained a few military recruits and officers, its members were mostly from surrounding communities who used the clinic. Before ART provision at the clinic, they had to travel great distances to Lusaka for medication. Advocacy involved discussions with the camp's commanding officer, who then worked with "higher ups" in the military to get the medications (NZP+ member, personal communication, May 9, 2011).

Located in a peri-urban area two hundred kilometers outside of Lusaka, Group E convinced local government officials and religious leaders to discuss AIDS at public meetings and during religious services. PLHAs faced high levels of stigma in this particular community, and local leaders were viewed as essential in stopping discrimination (NZP+ district coordinator, personal communication, April 15, 2011). Advocacy included public and private negotiations with local leaders, as well as HIV education campaigns (NZP+ member, personal communication, April 15, 2011). A man served as the group's leader.

## Factors Contributing to Community Mobilization

Members of most of the 34 NZP+ groups had strong collective identities, AIDS knowledge, and a sense of issue ownership. Members often referred to their peers as "family" because they cared for and loved co-members. NZP+ members developed a collective identity after being stigmatized by family and neighbors, who sometimes referred to them as "the dead moving bodies" (NZP+ member, personal communication, March 24, 2011) or "useless, sick people" (NZP+ member, personal communication, March 23, 2011). One woman said about identity: "Because we are HIV-positive, whatever we make [as a decision], it becomes solid. Meaning, we know we are all committed, because we are all with this virus" (NZP+ member, personal communication, March 24, 2011). Collective identity fueled peer education, care programs, and HIV testing efforts. While a necessary condition for advocacy, it alone was insufficient for mobilization.

Similarly, many NZP+ members had extensive knowledge about HIV/AIDS and felt strong ownership of the issue, often because they served as peer educators and counselors at local clinics. NZP+ groups provided a safe space for knowledge acquisition and identity formation. Members echoed themes such as: "This group is a place where I can be free" or "This group is where I don't have to worry about hiding my status" (NZP+ member, personal communication, March 24, 2011; NZP+ member, personal communication, April 15, 2011). For many participants, identity, knowledge, and ownership helped them fight stigma and denial in society (NZP+ member, personal communication, April 11, 2011).

While collective identity, AIDS knowledge, and issue ownership were common factors among most NZP+ groups, a strong sense of efficacy among members and leaders who urged community advocacy was not. The five groups that advocated illustrated a certain amount of initiative, arguing that if they wanted to succeed they had to look to their own skills. A Group C member said, "We are progressing, progressing … through our own contributions we have been able to work hard" (NZP+ member, personal communication, June 25, 2011). The five groups did not wait for donors or NGOs to bring them resources. Instead, they began income-generating projects, asked government officials for land, and sought local NGO officials who could provide them with advice, if not resources. While these groups had experienced challenges, they continued to be quite hopeful. One participant said members felt like role models in the community, since they showed others what could be done when community members commit to a goal (NZP+ member, personal communication, April 18, 2011).

The leaders of the five groups recognized that to achieve their goals of children's education, stigma reduction, and better health facilities, they needed to engage local policymakers (NZP+ member, personal communication, April 15, 2011). These leaders tended to have more education than rank-and-file members, and several leaders had connections to decision-making elites and NGOs in their communities. For example, the leaders of Group D were military personnel, while those for Group E were village headmen.

These five groups faced the same economic, political, and social structures that other NZP+ groups did. They were situated in Zambia's neopatrimonial political context, and the vast majority of their members worked in the informal economy, if they had employment at all. Food insecurity and lack of money for rent and children's school fees were common problems. Gender inequality affected all NZP+ groups, even Groups A and B, which had female leaders. In these two groups, male members dominated the focus group discussions and appeared to be the most connected to local power brokers, local NGO officials, and NZP+ district officers (NZP+ focus group, personal observation, June 25, 2011; NZP+ focus group, personal observation, April 18, 2011).

But the five groups differed from other NZP+ groups because they had forged relationships with external actors, such as traditional and religious leaders, political officials, and NGO officials. A member of Group A was on staff at the NZP+ district office, which allowed him to connect with the national NZP+ secretariat and various NGOs. Groups B and C also had close relationships with district NZP+ officials, who often directed NGO projects and funding to them. Group D leaders included military officials, who could represent group interests to military commanders. Because

Group E leaders included village chiefs and traditional authorities, they could connect with other local elites in their stigma reduction campaign.

In summary, the internal factors of members' efficacy and leadership fostered a sense of agency in advocacy, while the structural variable of external linkages to NGOs and community elites helped ensure that these groups' views would be heard. Agency and structure were intertwined: Groups with visionary leaders and a strong sense of efficacy were more likely to attract the attention of external officials. One NZP+ staff member explained: "Some groups are very motivated and some are not. You want to work with those that are motivated" (NZP+ district coordinator, personal communication, June 25, 2011). Once a group gained a positive reputation, external actors tended to continue their support through capacity-building programs, advocacy training, and financial resources. These resources made it possible for groups to continue to meet their objectives, a pattern that increased members' efficacy and fueled their participation (NZP+ district official, personal communication, March 30, 2011).

## OBSTACLES TO COMMUNITY MOBILIZATION IN ZAMBIA

While the five groups had visionary leaders, high efficacy, and linkages to external supporters, many NZP+ organizations did not have these characteristics. In this section, I examine how the internal organization of NZP+ and the external economic, political, and cultural structures made grassroots advocacy more difficult for most groups.

### The Organizational Structure of NZP+

NZP+ leaders and organizational bylaws stressed that local PLHIV groups were supposed to be small, with between five and 15 members (NZP+, n.d.; NZP+ national leadership, personal communication, March 7, 2011; NZP+ district leader, personal communication, March 21, 2011). While this small size facilitated intragroup trust and accountability, it also limited the public voice of PLHAs in the community. Social movements are more likely to be successful when they can mobilize large numbers of followers (Snow, Soule, & Kriesi, 2004), and community organizations in Zambia that have achieved political goals have recognized this fact. For example, an urban-based church-related poverty reduction and AIDS campaign mobilized pastors and congregants in over 30 churches to successfully lobby local officials for better schools and clinics (Zambian pastor, personal communication, May 20, 2011). Local government officials,

NGOs, and donors were less likely to pay attention to groups with few members, merely because the payback in project results or election votes could be quite small. Perhaps in recognition of this fact, three of the five NZP+ groups that advocated ignored organizational rules and had at least 50 members (NZP+ member, personal communication, June 25, 2011; NZP+ member, personal communication, April 15, 2011; NZP+ member, personal communication, May 10, 2011).

According to the NZP+ Handbook, only the National Secretariat is tasked with developing a national advocacy strategy and representing NZP+ members in policymaking. District-level NZP+ boards, secretariats, and coordinators are not given an explicit advocacy role. Instead, they channel resources and technical information to community groups and monitor and evaluate local PLHIV programs (NZP+ n.d.; NZP+ district coordinator, personal communication, April 18, 2011). Because National Secretariat members were paid (while district staff members were not), local and district-level leaders tended to look to the National Secretariat to play this advocacy role. Zambia's hierarchical culture reinforced this trend (AIDS expert, personal communication, May 31, 2011). Because grass-roots PLHIV organizations expected the National Secretariat to advocate for them, many local demands for particularistic benefits were not voiced.

## Economic Structures and Donor Programs

Zambia's high level of poverty led one-third of NZP+ groups to say their members often faced food insecurity and almost half of the groups to report that their members needed income-generating opportunities. NZP+ participants wanted material benefits, and their expectations intertwined with the experiences that PLHIV groups had when the government and donors scaled up ART access in 2005. Donors provided food supplements to individuals who tested HIV positive, and this resource was often channeled through community-level PLHIV groups. In the process, donors shaped the expectations some members had of group participation, and they influenced members' sense of efficacy. One NZP+ district officer (personal communication, March 21, 2011) explained:

> Initially you know what it used to be? Someone is tested and they are put on a program, maybe nutritional supplements, being given food supplements. The church groups are giving them rations, maybe those under home-based care are getting a package of soap and some foodstuffs. So they have now attuned their minds to free handouts of everything.

The NZP+ officer then described how things changed:

> Eventually those institutions [international donors and NGOs] started pulling away, saying, "Let these people since they are now fit, they are on ARVs, take care of themselves. They are now productive." ... But the recipients, they still have this mindset, saying, "Since I'm HIV-positive, I need everything for me for free." People were questioning where they would get their support; some were even [contemplating] suicide.

When some members discovered there were few material benefits in these PLHIV groups, they quit the organizations. Other potential members refused to join groups. One woman explained: "Three-fourths of the group has left. There was information we would receive assistance [from an NGO that helped to start the group], but in the long run, we didn't. So people decided to scatter" (NZP+ member, personal communication, March 30, 2011). This suboptimal level of participation affected the groups' ability to accomplish their goals, including advocacy (NZP+ member, personal interview, April 18, 2011). Poverty and dependence on donors colored participants' hopes for group involvement.

Additional economic structures shaped activism. Since work in the informal economy was unstable and unpredictable, members sometimes had to miss group activities because employment opportunities arose (NZP+ member, personal communication, March 24, 2011). Members sometimes moved to new compounds in search of better markets in which to sell their labors or lower-priced housing. The large gap between Zambia's wealthy and poor citizens also affected mobilization. Because PLHAs in professional positions did not need the material benefits PLHIV groups could provide, they did not join PLHIV groups. Stigma remained quite high among Zambians of higher socioeconomic status. One professional explained: "[As a wealthy person] you don't have anyone to share [your status with]. There you are driving a good car, you're living well, and then what will people think of you? The bottom line is that [high-status] people are not willing to come out in the open because of what the next person might do or say" (high-status PLHIV, personal communication, May 10, 2011). This interviewee then explained that it "wouldn't be possible" for lower- and upper-status HIV-positive Zambians to be in the same PLHIV group. Higher-status HIV-positive individuals would be too afraid that their lower-status counterparts would divulge their HIV status (high-status PLHIV, personal communication, May 10, 2011). The lack of cross-class interaction hinders activism because high-status PLHAs have the political connections, education, and efficacy to engage in advocacy. More broadly, the lack of cross-class collaboration prevents Zambian PLHAs from building networks of trust and reciprocity, values that could contribute to a broad-based AIDS movement (Putnam, 1992).

## Political Structures That Limit Mobilization

Political centralization and neopatrimonialism affect local mobilization. Despite legislation to decentralize state power after Zambia's return to multiparty democracy in 1991, municipal councils have few resources and little power to pass and implement policies to benefit community members. Because local officials have tended to belong to the then opposition Patriotic Front, the former ruling party (the Movement for Multiparty Democracy [MMD]) did not want to give these officials resources with which to design pro-poor policies. The MMD feared that urban voters then would reward the Patriotic Front in national elections (Resnick, 2011). (In 2011, the MMD lost national elections and the Patriotic Front took control of the presidency and the national legislature. Urban voters supported the opposition in large numbers, despite the MMD's strategy to weaken local party leaders on municipal councils.) Many PLHIV groups may have recognized that local councils were somewhat impotent and that advocacy to community leaders would yield limited benefits. However, local councils did have the ability to grant land, to fight the AIDS stigma, and to lobby members of parliament and civil servants for resources for their communities. The five advocating groups sought to capitalize on those powers of local councils.

Neopatrimonial networks and their potential for creating opportunities for corruption shaped NZP+ advocacy. In terms of resource access, NZP+ relied heavily on money that was channeled through the Zambia National AIDS Network (ZNAN), a principal recipient of grants from the Global Fund to Fight AIDS, Tuberculosis and Malaria (the Global Fund). Since 2003, ZNAN has been awarded grants of over $60 million (Global Fund, 2012). In 2009, Global Fund auditors discovered that ZNAN had mismanaged over $10 million, purchasing cars for staff members' personal use, awarding exorbitant salaries, and disbursing funds to subrecipients who could not provide auditors with financial records. One of the more egregious examples was a grant that lacked supporting documents to the Maureen Mwanawasa Community Initiative, which was headed by Zambia's former first lady (Plus News, 2011). In the urban communities, rumors flew about how ZNAN set up "shadow organizations" through which it channeled money to ruling party officials (NZP+ member, personal communication, March 24, 2011). Because of the auditor reports, Global Fund grants were suspended to ZNAN, and new funding policies were put into place. Several community PLHIV groups (including NZP+ organizations) lost resources, and NZP+ district-level staff lost funding for capacity building, advocacy efforts, and community education (NZP+ member, personal communication, March 22, 2011; NZP+ member, personal communication, March 30, 2011). By 2011, PLHAs in several groups, including NZP+, demanded that another entity take over ZNAN's role as a principal recipient. The centralized nature of power in ZNAN's leadership and its alleged neopatrimonal relations with the MMD weakened NZP+'s access to the resources it needed to empower local members and leaders for advocacy (multilateral donor, personal communication, February 23, 2011).

In terms of representation, most community NZP+ groups were not part of neopatrimonial networks between state officials and local patrons. As patrons who rewarded loyalty with spiritual and material help and built followings among marginalized individuals, religious officials are some of the more powerful local elites (religious official, personal communication, February 17, 2011; Ellis & ter Haar, 2004). Afrobarometer (2009) found that 46 percent of Zambians said they had contacted a religious leader for help with a problem at least one time during the last year, compared to 18 percent who had contacted a local councilor and 8 percent who had contacted a member of parliament. Because many NZP+ groups had not forged ties to local patrons, their members remained outside this neopatrimonial network. As a result, the voice of many NZP+ groups was sidelined in decision making. Sometimes this exclusion reflected stigma and elitism, while at other times it reflected the desire of local patrons to access resources for their own followers (NZP+ district official, personal communication, March 21, 2011; religious leader, personal communication, March 30, 2011). At the national level, NZP+ often had a weak voice in policymaking because, unlike pastors from mega-churches and representatives from the mission-based hospitals, it lacked long-standing and close ties to government officials (donor official, personal communication, February 23, 2011; religious leader, personal communication, March 30, 2011; Key Correspondents, 2011).

## Social and Cultural Values

Beliefs about the state-citizen relationship, political participation, gender, and AIDS presented structural challenges for mobilization. On the one hand, public opinion surveys indicate that individuals are not opposed to collective action, with 35 percent reporting in 2009 that they had attended community meetings and 25 percent saying they had gotten together with others to raise an issue to local leaders. While these percentages are relatively small, they do present an increase from 1999. On the other hand, attitudes of hierarchy and dependence limit advocacy. In 2009, 65 percent of respondents agreed that "people are like children and government should take care of citizens like a parent." In contrast, 32 percent said that "people should control government" (Afrobarometer, 2010).

Levels of self-reported citizen participation also are quite low. Seventy-one percent of Zambians said that they had never contacted a local official about a problem, though 44 percent think they could convince community leaders to listen to a grievance. Participation remains quite low in civil society organizations that are not religiously based; only 20 percent of individuals report being in a voluntary group compared to 58 percent for membership in a religious group (Afrobarometer, 2009). One NZP+ interviewee echoed this theme of nonparticipation when he said that there were "many, many" individuals who were HIV-positive but who did not join NZP+ groups (NZP+ member, personal communication, April 12, 2011). In one Lusaka neighborhood, an ART clinic had roughly 20,000 HIV-positive individuals enrolled in its programs. Of those 20,000, only about 200 (or 1 percent of all ART recipients) were in the clinic's PLHIV group (Lusaka clinic, personal observation, June 7, 2011). The larger political culture of limited participation in civil society organizations contributed to this outcome.

Low levels of political participation and belief in hierarchy may partly reflect Zambia's experience with one-party rule between 1972 and 1991. President Kenneth Kaunda used patronage, cooptation, and intimidation to limit challenges to his rule and to build an ideology of unity that discouraged public criticism. Even after the introduction of multiparty democracy, some of these practices have continued, with the goal of weakening civil society leaders and journalists who have criticized the state (Bauer & Taylor, 2005). Either because they fear violence or communal ostracism, Zambians report they are relatively hesitant to speak about politics. In 2009, 62 percent agreed that people need to always or often be careful about what they say about politics (Afrobarometer, 2009). Fear that political involvement might bring negative ramifications may hamper NZP+ advocacy efforts (community leader, personal communication, May 22, 2011).

Gender norms in Zambia prevent advocacy, particularly since over 80 percent of NZP+ members were women (NZP+ district officer, personal communication, March 21, 2011). Practices such as domestic violence, property grabbing, and sexual cleansing rituals for widows make women vulnerable to HIV infection and increase their economic marginalization (Frank, 2009). In 2002, over half of women who had ever been married reported that they had been beaten by a husband. In the same survey, a large majority (85 percent of women and 69 percent of men) believed a husband was justified in beating his wife (Human Rights Watch, 2007). Numerous female PLHAs told stories of domestic violence and family ostracism after their HIV status was discovered. One woman said that her group's biggest challenge was the fact that "we are just widows" (NZP+ member, personal communication, March 24, 2011); another woman said that, since widows lack political and economic voice, "We can do nothing" (NZP+ member, personal communication, March 23, 2011).

Finally, the AIDS stigma interacted with dependence on and fears of the state, limited participation, low political efficacy, and gender inequality to further limit PLHIV mobilization. When potential NZP+ members did not join groups because of stigma, they limited the numerical power and voice of NZP+ advocacy, both at the national and local levels. Stigma made individuals feel that they were "less than human beings," a belief that eroded confidence (NZP+ member, personal communication, May 5, 2011). Stigma meant that PLHAs were not given a chance to play leadership roles in their communities. One man explained that he was never chosen to serve as an elder or deacon in his church, "because they [church members] just say I am going to die soon" (PLHIV, personal communication, March 9, 2011). Another said that the community simply ignores her NZP+ group, because "they say we are like matches. We are burning bright right now, but will soon burn out" (NZP+ member, personal communication, March 24, 2011). Stigma excluded PLHAs from decision-making arenas and decreased efficacy, causing some NZP+ groups to depend on outsiders and to doubt their abilities to generate solutions to their problems.

## CONCLUSION

PLHIV mobilization in urban Zambian communities exhibits the tension between agency and structure often seen in the social movement literature (Snow, Soule, & Kriesi, 2004). A small number of local PLHIV groups capitalized on members' efficacy and leaders' visions and connections to external actors to advocate for programs or policies to benefit PLHAs and their family members. But the vast majority of urban PLHIV organizations in this study faced numerous challenges, from gender norms that limited women's voice in the public realm to neopatrimonial structures. Zambia's political culture of limited citizen participation and an underdeveloped civil society, as well as the country's high poverty rates, made mobilization among PLHAs difficult. Stigma prevented wealthier, more educated Zambians with HIV who had political skills and linkages from joining a broad PLHIV movement.

Specific policy concerns about AIDS mobilization in countries with weak norms of participation and high levels of poverty emerge from this article. The five NZP+ groups illustrate that mobilization to meet local needs is possible, particularly if leaders devise clear goals and work with external actors to achieve those objectives. AIDS activists and policymakers who seek to promote AIDS advocacy should support more leadership training and help facilitate connections between leaders and external NGOs, donors, and elites. Similarly, policymakers should urge decentralization in organizations, so that a culture of advocacy develops at all levels, not just among national secretariats. To urge greater efficacy, policymakers and activists must consider how donor programs may create attitudes of dependence and may discourage local populations from voicing concerns or forging ties to community decision makers. But the fact that structural challenges create large obstacles for PLHIV advocacy should give activists and policymakers reason to pause, particularly since one goal of multilateral donors such as UNAIDS and the global AIDS movement is to promote advocacy efforts by PLHAs. Thus, efforts to promote AIDS mobilization cannot be divorced from the larger questions of political and economic development in poor countries like Zambia. To promote the voice of PLHAs, long-term programs that combat poverty, gender inequality, and hierarchical political cultures must be supported within a comprehensive approach to AIDS in Africa.

## ACKNOWLEDGMENTS

I wish to thank the U.S. Fulbright Africa Scholars Research Program and Calvin College for support for fieldwork for this study. Additionally, I am grateful to Nikki Vander Meulen and Brad Wassink, two Calvin College students, for assistance with transcribing interviews. Helpful comments from a reviewer and the editor improved the chapter.

## BIBLIOGRAPHY

Afrobarometer (2009). Summary of results, round 4 Afrobarometer survey in Zambia [Database]. Retrieved from http://www.afrobarometer.org/index .php?option=com_content&view=category&layout=blog&id=27&Itemid=103

Afrobarometer. (2010). Zambian citizens, democracy and political participation. *Afrobarometer briefing paper, 80.* Retrieved from http://www.afrobarometer .org/index.php?option=com_content&view=category&layout=blog&id=27& Itemid=103

Bauer, G., & Taylor, S. (2005). *Politics in Southern Africa.* Boulder, CO: Lynne Rienner.

Beckman, N., & Bujra, J. (2010). The "politics of the queue": The politicization of people living with HIV/AIDS in Tanzania. *Development and Change, 41* (6), 1041–1064.

Campbell, C., Gibbs, A., Maimane, S., Nair, Y., & Sibiya, Z. (2009). Youth participation in the fight against AIDS in South Africa: From policy to practice. *Journal of Youth Studies, 12* (1), 93–109.

Ellis, S., & ter Haar, G. (2004). *Worlds of power: Religious thought and political practice in Africa.* New York: Oxford University Press.

Fenio, K. (2011). Tactics of resistance and the evolution of identity from subjects to citizens: The AIDS political movement in Southern Africa. *International Studies Quarterly, 55* (3), 717–735.

Frank, E. (2009). Shifting paradigms and the politics of AIDS in Zambia. *African Studies Review, 52* (3), 33–53.

Friedman, S., & Mottair, S. (2004). A moral to the tale: The Treatment Action Campaign and the politics of HIV/AIDS. *Paper for the Centre for Policy Studies.* Durban, South Africa: University of KwaZulu-Natal.

Furlong, P., & Ball, K. (2005). The more things change: AIDS and the state in South Africa. In A. Patterson (ed.), *The African state and the AIDS crisis* (pp. 127–155). Aldershot, UK: Ashgate.

Geiser, G. (2006). A second liberation of lobbying for women's political representation in Zambia, Botswana, and Namibia. *Journal of Southern Africa Studies, 32* (1), 69–84.

Global Fund to Fight AIDS, Tuberculosis and Malaria (2012). Grant portfolio— Zambia [Database]. Retrieved from http://portfolio.theglobalfund.org/en/ Grant/List/ZAM

Human Rights Watch (2007). Hidden in the mealie meal: Gender-based abuses and women's HIV treatment in Zambia. *Report, 19.* Retrieved from http:// www.hrw.org/sites/default/files/reports/zambia1207web.pdf

Inter-Parliamentary Union (2011). Women in national parliaments [Database]. Retrieved from http://www.ipu.org/wmn-e/classif.htm

Johnson, K. (2004). The politics of AIDS policy development and implementation in postapartheid South Africa. *Africa Today, 51* (2), 107–128.

Justesen, M. K. (2011). Too poor to care? The salience of AIDS in Africa. *Afrobarometer working paper, 133.* Retrieved from http://www.afrobarometer .org/index.php?option=com_docman&Itemid=39

Keck, M., & Sikkink, K. (1998). *Activists beyond borders: Advocacy networks in international politics.* Ithaca, NY: Cornell University Press.

Key Correspondents (2011, January 28). Zambian campaigners petition Minister of Health [Web comment]. Retrieved from http://www.keycorrespondents .org/2011/01/28/zambian-plhiv-petition-minister-of-health/

Mbali, M. (2004). The Treatment Action Campaign and the history of rights-based, patient-driven HIV/AIDS activism in South Africa. *Research Report, 29.* Durban: University of KwaZulu-Natal.

Ministry of Health, National AIDS Council, & UNAIDS (2010). *Zambia country progress report: UNGASS 2010 reporting.* Retrieved from http://www.unaids .org/en/dataanalysis/monitoringcountryprogress/2010progressreportssubmit tedbycountries/zambia_2010_country_progress_report_en.pdf

Morris, A., & Staggenborg, S. (2004). Leadership in social movements. In D. Snow, S. Soule, & H. Kriesi (eds.), *The Blackwell companion to social movements* (pp. 171–196). London: Blackwell.

Muriisa, R. (2010). The role of NGOs in addressing gender inequality and HIV/AIDS in Uganda. *Canadian Journal of African Studies, 44* (3), 605–623.

NZP+. (n.d.). *Network of Zambian People Living with HIV/AIDS (NZP+) management handbook.* Lusaka: USAID.

Patterson, A. (2006). *The politics of AIDS in Africa.* Boulder, CO: Lynne Rienner.

Patterson, A. (2011). *The church and AIDS in Africa: The politics of ambiguity.* Boulder, CO: First Forum Press.

Patterson, A., & Stephens, D. (n.d.). AIDS mobilisation in Zambia and Vietnam: Explaining the differences. (Unpublished paper)

Plus News (2011, March 14). Zambia: Corruption scandal rocks ARV programme [News release]. Retrieved from http://www.plusnews.org/PrintReport .aspx?ReportID=92191

Putnam, R. (1992). *Making democracy work.* Princeton, NJ: Princeton University Press.

Resnick, D. (2011). In the shadow of the city: Africa's urban poor in opposition strongholds. *Journal of Modern African Studies, 49* (1), 141–166.

Robins, S. (2006). From "rights" to "ritual": AIDS activism in South Africa. *American Anthropologist, 108* (2), 312–323.

Smith, R., & Siplon, P. (2006). *Drugs into bodies: Global AIDS treatment activism.* Westport, CT: Praeger.

Snow, D. (2001). Collective identity and expressive forms. In N. J. Smelser & P. B. Baltes (eds.), *International encyclopaedia of the social and behavioural sciences* (pp. 196–254). London: Elsevier Science.

Snow, D., Soule, S., & Kriesi, H. (eds.). (2004). *The Blackwell companion to social movements.* London: Blackwell.

Tarrow, S. (1989). *Democracy and disorder: Protest and politics in Italy 1965–1975.* Oxford: Clarendon Press.

TASO (2011). Background information [Data file]. Retrieved from http:// www.tasouganda.org/index.php?option=com_content&view=article&id=56& Itemid=67

Tilly, C. (1978). *From mobilization to revolution.* New York: Random House.

Trice, H., & Beyer, J. (1991). Cultural leadership in organizations. *Organizational Science, 2,* 149–169.

UNDP (2011). Zambia country profile: Human development indicators [Data file]. Retrieved from http://hdrstats.undp.org/en/countries/profiles/ZMB.html

UN News Centre (2010, June 9). Noting progress to date, Ban urges greater efforts against HIV/AIDS [News release]. Retrieved from http://www.un.org/apps/news/story.asp?NewsID=34977&Cr=aids&Cr1

Van de Walle, N. (2001). *African economies and the politics of permanent crisis.* New York: Cambridge University Press.

Warren, M. (2001). *Dry bones rattling: Community building to revitalize American democracy.* Princeton, NJ: Princeton University Press.

Yoon, M. (2004). Explaining women's legislative representation in sub-Saharan Africa. *Legislative Studies Quarterly, 29* (3), 447–510.

# 12
# From Dissidence to Partnership and Back to Confrontation Again? The Current Predicament of Brazilian HIV/AIDS Activism

*Carlos Guilherme do Valle*

After fifteen years of military rule, political liberalization started in Brazil in the late 1970s, when social pressure forced the reinstatement of civil rights. This social reorganization intensified in the following years and traditional political actors were joined by newly emerging social movements, such as feminism and homosexual politics. However, improvements in the political climate were not matched by the economy. The public health system was also sharply affected by these economic crises. The decay in the health services and an endemic lack of resources led to the mobilization of health professionals and to protests among sectors of the population, coinciding with the period of political reform. However, these expressions of social dissatisfaction did not result in substantive improvements in public health. On the contrary, health institutions occupied a crucial position in the ways that Brazilians perceived their sense of moral plight. *Crisis* would be the defining theme of the 1980s. AIDS also emerged as a social problem and should be inserted into a wider framework of crises that erupted in Brazil.

The AIDS epidemic started to affect Brazil at the beginning of the 1980s. By the middle of the decade, Brazil had become one of the four countries with the highest prevalence of AIDS cases in the world and the highest in Latin America. Until 2011 there were 608,230 reported cases (1980–2011): 397,662 men and 210,538 women. Each year, 35,000 new cases are reported (Brasil, Ministério da Saúde, 2012a). Although associated with homosexuality, the epidemic also affected heterosexuals since the beginning. Women, for example, have been mostly infected by heterosexual transmission (Guimarães, 2001). In 1984, the male/female ratio of HIV infection was 44.5/1, but it reduced to 1.6/1 in 2009, that is, 16 men for 10 women (Brasil, 2012a). In 2011, 30.5 percent of all male cases were linked to a heterosexual context; 20.1 percent of male cases were linked to a homosexual context; 11.5 percent to bisexual contexts; 17.2 percent to intravenous drug use. For female cases, 87.5 percent were linked to heterosexual transmission; 7.3 percent to intravenous drug use. In terms of cumulative deaths (1980/2010), there were 241,469 cases (Brasil, 2012a). Therefore one of the characteristics in the Brazilian profile of the AIDS epidemic would be the social diversity in HIV transmission (Parker, 1990). While characterized mostly by sexual transmission, the epidemic affects a heterogeneous group of people.

The first forms of social mobilization started to take place around 1983. The few existing gay groups distributed HIV information materials to the local population, but the impact was limited. In 1985, the Ministry of Health held a meeting to discuss the epidemic and the National Division of STD and AIDS was set up. In fact, public health decisions occurred with extreme delay and with no rigorous epidemiological control policy. As a result, the rapidly increasing number of AIDS cases had a significant social impact. In short, the first years of the epidemic in Brazil were marked by the limited scope of social mobilization and the relative absence of actions by the Ministry of Health.

Since 1984 the Brazilian media has regularly reported on AIDS. Therefore, an examination of the cultural history of AIDS in Brazil will reveal the emergence of a cornucopia of identity categories referring to people with HIV/AIDS. In the mid-1980s a term was coined that became the most used category by the media to identify someone living with HIV/AIDS: *aidético*. This was a real shift in the understandings both of the epidemic and of those individuals who would be infected. *Aidético* suggested a broader identity that categorized and encompassed people of the most diverse trajectories. The cultural meanings of *aidético* were crucial for defining the social identity of an HIV-positive person (Valle, 2002). It was essentially generic and could identify anyone who was infected by HIV. The category also implied the symbolic violence (Bourdieu, 1990) of the meanings of illness and death, associated with bodily devastation and an impending, unwanted finitude.

## A POLITICS OF SOLIDARITY?

In 1985, the first Brazilian and Latin American HIV/AIDS NGO was created in São Paulo: the *Grupo de Apoio à Prevenção à AIDS* (GAPA-SP).

The first HIV/AIDS NGOs positioned themselves critically against the state of structural decay, scarcity of resources, and stigmatization against HIV-positive people and led to political statements to the media, which began to characterize the public image of NGOs. To understand the trajectory of Brazilian HIV/AIDS NGOs, it is necessary to look at their links with gay activism.

In the 1980s the Brazilian "homosexual movement" was unorganized. Nevertheless, the first initiatives for civil mobilization against the epidemic were found among gay organizations and antedated responses from the government. But the fear of "AIDS ghettoization" was discernible, and many gay activists at the time realized the need to divert attention around AIDS from homosexuality (Terto, 1996). Therefore, many gay men decided to set up HIV/AIDS NGOs marked by general criteria of membership, that is, organizations that were not based on particularism, especially of sexual orientation and gender. On the contrary, gay men wanted to participate in NGOs that were broadly committed against the epidemic and favored general values of citizenship. They aspired to the possibilities of collective action around AIDS without being only concerned with sexual politics. In 1987 these NGOs achieved public visibility through the media and showed their political strength in this emerging social field by becoming the agencies that would mediate and represent civil society in relation to HIV/AIDS.

The meanings of "HIV/AIDS activism" overlay and contrasted with ideas of a "homosexual militancy." In fact, this militancy was framed by a historical context in which an antiauthoritarian ideology was prominent. With the rise of HIV/AIDS activism, different perspectives and practices were created. Although a criticism of Brazilian government endured after the new civilian regime, activists were not looking to engage in a fight for "democracy," but rather for citizenship and the guarantee of human rights. Brazilian HIV/AIDS activism was related to a particular social field and particular issues, health-defined, even if crossed by ideas of citizenship. In short, LGBT activism suffered from a lack of political strength in the social field of struggles for citizenship in Brazil. One of the ways to contest AIDS stigmatization was to disassociate the epidemic from homosexuality. However, gay men and lesbians comprised most of the founding members of the NGOs. In fact, discourses on homosexuality and a rather camp ethos were both present in many NGOs. These aspects influenced some groups, becoming a crucial point in facilitating or hindering the affiliation to HIV/AIDS NGOs. As soon as it was noticed that LGBT activism was not incompatible with HIV/AIDS politics, a new activism began to bloom in the 1990s (La Dehesa, 2010). Many LGBT groups began to develop HIV prevention work with a close relationship to the new scenario of international funding motivated by AIDS.

HIV/AIDS NGOs were also influenced by previous civil associations. They gathered people who had a political perspective and questioned the military government. Related to these NGOs, the *Associação Brasileira Interdisciplinar de AIDS* (ABIA; Brazilian Interdisciplinary AIDS Association), created in 1986, and *Grupo Pela Vidda* (GPV; Group for LIFE— "Vidda is a Portuguese acronym representing enhancement, integration and dignity of people living with HIV/AIDS"; Daniel & Parker, 1993; Valle, 2000) were founded in Rio de Janeiro by people who had political trajectories. They became leaders of national importance in the epidemic. This was the case with Herbert de Souza (Betinho), who was also HIV-positive and hemophiliac. He gathered people with public credibility to set up ABIA, such as Herbert Daniel, a writer who had been a political refugee until 1981, and a sexual politics activist. Although other NGOs, such as the numerous GAPAs found widely all over the country, were also important, ABIA and GPV are ideally placed here to give us an understanding of how certain leftist trajectories influenced the social world of AIDS. This phenomenon seemed to be particularly related to Rio de Janeiro, linked to the political centrality of the city in Brazil. However, ABIA and GPV should not be seen as the paradigmatic model to understand the diversity in the Brazilian responses to AIDS. Since the mid-1980s many HIV/AIDS NGOs have been created throughout the country. They illustrate the manifold social demands that have not been adequately addressed by public health policies and authorities.

HIV/AIDS NGOs such as ABIA, GPV, and GAPA had a central role to provide another source of symbolic resources and cultural discourses on the epidemic. These NGOs emphasized the need to generate solidarity (*solidariedade*) in the predicament of AIDS stigmatization. The political and symbolic meanings of *solidariedade* represented a central ideological "weapon" to counterattack the disempowerment caused by stigmatization. These meanings were further developed in a coherent discourse by some of the first NGO leaders, especially Betinho and Herbert Daniel, who synthesized the position defended by ABIA and GPV. Betinho denounced the "clandestine" life imposed on HIV-positive people (Souza, 1994). Herbert Daniel asserted a political attitude against what he called "civil death," the predicament lived by HIV-positive people pressed by prejudice, stigma, and secrecy (Daniel, 1994). They emphasized the need for looking at AIDS as an issue of human rights.

In the context of the Global Program on AIDS of the World Health Organization, solidarity became central as an ethical principle in the protection of human rights. Jonathan Mann, the head of the GPA/WHO, emphasized the need for global collaboration against AIDS and echoed the importance given to the community-based organizations around the world. This resulted in the involvement of NGOs locally and globally and also in their widespread funding. A close collaboration and sociopolitical affinity between the GPA/WHO and the leaders of some Brazilian NGOs was manifest in 1988. As Galvão (2000) pointed out, Brazilian activists who attended the meeting Opportunities for Solidarity, before the Sixth World AIDS Conference (1989), decided to organize the first National NGO meeting (ENONG). Positioned at a strategic point between local and global levels, ABIA was one of the organizers of the first two Brazilian NGO meetings. In 1990 the idea of solidarity was definitively incorporated into the ideological agenda of the Brazilian NGOs. However, the political implications of solidarity would be more problematic. At both the national and global levels, solidarity as a principle was not ideologically contested by AIDS NGOs, but their political practices followed a different dynamic, linked to crucial disputes for hegemony and for resources at various different levels. At the Third Meeting of the Brazilian Network of Solidarity, AIDS NGOs were caught in this conflict (Galvão, 2000). At this event, a political struggle took place in relation to the legitimacy and hegemonic position that NGOs such as ABIA and GPV had attained at the national and global levels. Two antagonistic positions were represented by ABIA and GPV, on one side, and on the other side, the *Grupo Gay da Bahia* (GGB; Gay Group of Bahia), an activist group from northeastern Brazil that carried out HIV prevention work. From that occasion onward no other Brazilian AIDS/NGO meeting was organized with the aim of forming of a "network of solidarity."

## CREATING AND MAINTAINING BRAZILIAN HIV/AIDS NGOs

To provide a better understanding of the current dilemmas experienced by Brazilian activism, this section will focus on only a few HIV/AIDS NGOs, most of them located in Rio de Janeiro. ABIA and GPV can be singled out as the preeminent NGOs by national and global parameters. Highly professionalized activist organizations, sponsored by international funding agencies, they have been closely linked in the public eye. ABIA is known for its independent and oppositional stand in relation to Brazilian public health policy on AIDS (Galvão, 2000). Furthermore, it was set up to intervene nationally with a clear emphasis on a *Brazilian* response to AIDS in contrast to locally or regionally circumscribed work. In 1989, the first Brazilian mutual-help group was also created: the *Grupo Pela Vidda* (GPV). Founded by a leading ABIA member, Herbert Daniel, GPV has maintained a unique trajectory as an HIV/AIDS NGO. It has been intimately connected with political activism and HIV-positive volunteer work. GPV antedated the creation of another important NGO, the *Grupo de Incentivo à Vida* (GIV; Group for Life Incentive), which was set up in São Paulo. GIV is mainly characterized by contributing to the empowerment of HIV-positive people.

GPV organized the first public protest of "people living with HIV and AIDS" in Brazil, informed by ideas of a common global struggle against the pandemic. It has privileged a direct contact to social demands and, therefore, legitimacy in responding to AIDS. Since 1991, GPV has organized the National Meeting of People Living with HIV and AIDS (also called *Vivendo*) in Rio de Janeiro. However, it became a biennial event in the 2000s, when the congress expanded beyond the NGO's capabilities of organization and fund raising.

GPV activism has been a model for many Brazilian AIDS NGOs. Although members have joined this NGO for political and personal motivations, they also shouldered the dilemmas and responsibilities of professionalization, a central theme for most NGOs in the 2000s. They have had to deal with the challenge of surviving as organizations that are both expensive and nonprofit. Management rationalization and a clearer definition of functional roles have become prevalent concerns and have had an impact on affiliation in many NGOs. In 22 years of HIV/AIDS activism the changes at GPV have been a result of various factors, which include changes in affiliation as a result of epidemiological trends, new patterns of institutional funding, and new directions in political and social intervention. Class hierarchy marked by differences in educational background also affected changes in roles within Brazilian NGOs. Middle-class members tended to move up from earlier volunteer work into specialized managerial roles and were replaced by lower-income volunteer members, while drop-in socializing activities became less important.

## Singularizations and Counterexamples

The 1990s saw a strong expansion of HIV/AIDS NGOs across Brazil. This was a period of intense social and political mobilization (Galvão, 2000). Some NGOs played a major role at the local and regional levels, such as the numerous different organizations named GAPA, which were set up throughout the country. Organizations were increasingly founded in countryside towns. Also, NGOs began to work with specific groups and needs, such as attending to HIV-positive children. In addition, organizations not previously connected to the epidemic started to carry out intervention projects. For instance, the first Brazilian groups of transgendered people were created and started to be funded through HIV prevention projects. All of them benefited from an influx of resources from transnational funding agencies. Furthermore, a contrast was made between the service-based NGOs and the ones with a more activist agenda. In the 1990s, this differentiation became prominent among AIDS NGOs, but it took on an intense rivalry in Rio de Janeiro. The competition and the political opposition between NGOs affected not only the ways in which a particular social world was formed, but also the ways by which the local authorities and the NGOs responded to the epidemic.

Many organizations were based on an ideology of work and social support that prioritized direct intervention toward HIV-positive people. Less concerned with political activism, they aimed to provide services. They occupied a social niche of health/social provision that was not offered by the public health services: hostels, nursing homes, and hospices to HIV-positive people. Sometimes adopting a religious approach, these NGOs were mostly motivated by ideals of charity and philanthropy. According to Biehl, these "pastoral spaces of health care" had to "bear the medical and social burden of the AIDS crisis among the poorest" (2007: 63). As health services were supposed to be maintained by the government, the idea of AIDS NGOs as health providers was not widely accepted in Brazil. The criticism against service-based organization helped to consolidate HIV/AIDS activism, which was invoked by NGOs such as ABIA, GPV, and GAPA. They were concerned with the guarantee of human rights and citizenship to HIV-positive people. This became an ideological principle of their social practices and helped to define and motivate a particular meaning of HIV/AIDS activism.

In addition, disputes between Brazilian HIV/AIDS NGOs were strongly conditioned by their access to economic resources. Most of the activist-oriented NGOs received funding from international agencies, which allowed them to develop activities at an advantage and more successfully. They were set up in the 1980s, when international funding for AIDS community-based organizations was beginning to become more available. The presence of highly professional staff members facilitated their contacts at the global level. Greater professional competence and control of financial resources explain the leading role some NGOs took. Also, the political-ideological agenda of these organizations became dominant in the country. Those NGOs that specialized in service-based activities had to be content to intervene in a smaller and nonhegemonic niche of the AIDS world.

However, this cleavage between service-based organizations and politically engaged activism should not be emphasized. Some of the service-based NGOs also received an influx of resources and hired professionals to manage their activities. They had their own ideological principles and political aims, but shared other principles with the AIDS activist groups, such as solidarity, although associated with ideas of *help* and *hope.* Furthermore, they were not alien to the political struggles in the social arena where AIDS was being fought. According to Galvão (2000), the difference between HIV/AIDS activism and service is a false dualism. Service-based HIV/AIDS NGOs can also be politicized and those more politically defined NGOs can be involved with practices of assistance. More recently, HIV/AIDS activism became very much blended with service.

## Local/Global Intercessions

Brazilian NGOs must be connected with global forces, either politically or economically. There was an enormous increase in funding aimed against AIDS, which became plentiful in the 1990s, mainly through a global financing structure. Global agencies also encouraged communitarian responses to AIDS. For several years, the Brazilian government response was low level, unsystematic, and belated, and it was the NGOs that eventually brought about an AIDS policy embedded within the Global AIDS Strategy developed by the GPA/WHO. This fact can explain the tense relationship between the AIDS National Program and many of the leading Brazilian HIV/AIDS NGOs (Galvão, 2000). This conflict between governmental policy and civil mobilization lasted several years.

In 1994, Brazil signed an agreement with the World Bank through the Ministry of Health, which allowed the gradual funding of Brazilian HIV/AIDS NGOs. Later, in 1998, a second agreement was signed, which lasted until 2002 and emphasized once again HIV prevention projects (Galvão, 2000). Therefore, *partnership* became a central idea to legitimize these institutional practices between the government and the NGOs, which began to compete for resources available through projects submitted to the Brazilian AIDS Program. An NGO Articulation Sector (*Setor de Articulação com ONG*) was created around this time (1993–1994) which indicated a significant change in the relationship between the Ministry of

Health and the Brazilian activism (Galvão, 2000; Valle, 2000). Partnership was stimulated through institutional practices, which did not question the major political aim of joint work against the epidemic. Since the agreement with the World Bank, the Brazilian AIDS Program became one of the main sources of funding to many Brazilian NGOs. However, financial support became more specific in scope and aims. It was not directed to cover daily expenses, but, on the contrary, particular target "projects." In other words, Brazilian HIV/AIDS NGOs became more and more concerned with the process of fund raising. The aspect that perhaps most characterizes this period was a substantial change in some of the aims and social composition, and a sharper definition of what professional work and socialization meant to AIDS NGOs. In short, Brazilian activism had to adjust the political antagonism, which had historically defined their practices, to a relative dependency on external trends of international funding. When Brazilian NGOs achieved better means of institutional maintenance, they also became concerned with their political autonomy in relation to the Brazilian AIDS Program and the implications of their partnership. This was not, however, a real concern for the majority of HIV/AIDS NGOs, but only for the leading activist organizations in the late 1990s.

Another important issue has been the Ministry of Health's policy in relation to AIDS drugs. While the conventional treatments were available through the public health system, importing drugs and distributing freely was the result of a long struggle by HIV/AIDS NGOs, by deputies and politicians, and by the negotiation of the Brazilian AIDS Program with the WHO and the World Bank. In 1991, AZT started to be distributed through the public health system. Not until 1996 under President Fernando Henrique Cardoso was a new law passed that asserted free access and distribution of AIDS drugs to everyone infected in Brazil. However, HIV-positive people have been concerned both with delays in distributing the AIDS drugs and with the continuation of legal guarantees of the right.

Furthermore, health structures have still been dogged by serious problems in services, care, and material resources. Public clinics and hospitals are routinely overloaded with an increasing demand for AIDS treatments. Lately, more people have tested for HIV and as a result enrolled in AIDS services, which have been shaken by recent waves of new HIV-positive patients. Although AIDS has resulted in increased resources targeted at the public sector, this input has been directed to institutional structures that respond to Brazilian citizens in general, regardless of their HIV status. Paradoxically, however, this higher influx of resources has been counterbalanced by a continuing lack of institutional support in public hospitals for both AIDS patients and the wider population. As a result, health services continue to be generally rudimentary. It is very difficult to give a thorough diagnosis of problems that may be traced to gaps between legal reform, policymaking, and the implementation of health services, but might also be caused by the societal dynamics of Brazilian health institutions, which tend to be bureaucratic, inefficient, and overcrowded. In short, contradictions and gaps have historically characterized the public sector. In the last 30 years, the actual conditions of Brazilian public health services generally have been considered by health professionals, patients, and HIV/AIDS activists as a hindrance to their work and to the well-being of the Brazilian population.

With regard to HIV testing, a system was slowly introduced in Brazil after 1985 in a rather haphazard way, depending on the laboratory services maintained by each Brazilian federal state. Until the early 1990s, which was a period of still limited alternatives of AIDS treatment, HIV testing was considered with extreme caution by Brazilian activists, who questioned the public position in favor of large-scale, mandatory testing. Informed by North American activism, HIV/AIDS NGOs defended HIV testing only as a personal, free-choice decision. HIV testing became more systematized only with the political changes that occurred in the Brazilian AIDS Program since 1992, when it was included in the guidelines of the AIDS public health policy (Biehl, Coutinho, & Outeiro, 2001). As a matter of fact, since testing has a crucial role for knowing one's serologic status, it has been encouraged as a strategic technical procedure in public health policy for HIV prevention in Brazil (Valle, 2002). Since 2006, rapid HIV testing campaigns have been implemented across the country. HIV/AIDS activists have also asserted the importance of knowing earlier one's serologic status in order to start AIDS treatment as early as possible, in agreement with the guidelines of the Brazilian AIDS Program. During the 2000s, HIV testing has been strongly recommended by HIV/AIDS activism and LGBT organizations, such as *Arco Íris* (Rainbow), a group from Rio de Janeiro. They have conducted regular campaigns in favor of rapid testing for HIV and other sexually transmitted diseases. Therefore, many people have gone through the process of testing, and HIV-tested Brazilians have incorporated the social meanings implicated in knowing their biological identity as an HIV-positive or an HIV-negative individual (Valle, 2002; Biehl, Coutinho, & Outeiro, 2001).

Biomedical testing categories, such as *soropositivo* (seropositive) and *soronegativo* (seronegative), became pervasive in clinical settings, such as hospitals and laboratories, but they would also be widely circulated in AIDS NGOs, where activists preferred their clinical meanings rather than culturally loaded terms, such as *aidético*. *Soropositivo* and *soronegativo* soon became social identities by which people and individuals were labeled and culturally represented in social life. These categories have been used frequently to help in the construction of the self as well as the social experience of being HIV-positive. Actually, these categories depend on the combination of different social and cultural orders. First, we should consider the ideas and practices of health professionals, who are grounded in biomedical criteria (Rabinow, 1992). However, the social experiences of people affected and infected by HIV/AIDS have to be properly addressed if we want to understand the rise of clinical identities, such as *soropositivo* or *soronegativo* (Valle, 2000, 2002). In addition, the dissemination of these identities was compounded by a more intense circulation of sexual identities, which in many ways reflected the concurrent making of Brazilian LBGT activism.

## A BRAZILIAN WAY OF "PEOPLE LIVING WITH HIV/AIDS"?

Among the first Brazilians to disclose publicly their HIV-positive status, Herbert Daniel, ABIA and GPV leader, could be credited for motivating a discursive sphere of "living with HIV and AIDS" (Daniel, 1994). He rejected the label *aidético,* popularized by the media, and asserted that to be alive was a "political act." Ideas on citizenship, democracy, human rights were to be found side by side with discussions on illness and HIV-positive status. These ideas highlighted a defense of life considered in a broad existential dimension. In 1989, chosen to be the candidate for the Green Party in the first presidential elections in 30 years, Daniel identified himself on TV as homosexual and HIV-positive. At this stage, his actions were publicized to the whole nation.

Idealized by Daniel, the *Grupo Pela Vidda* was based on solidarity as a social and political premise obtained through the collective struggle for human rights, citizenship, and democracy. Therefore it aimed to involve Brazilians in an attempt at raising "political awareness" of the AIDS epidemic. Notably, solidarity was to be invoked by "people living with HIV and AIDS," considered by the GPV as a broad social label, which includes HIV-positive people and their "friends, relatives, lovers and anyone who feels that his everyday life has been affected by the epidemic." Therefore this NGO has been opened to everyone, regardless of their HIV status. This organizational model was resounding and competed with GAPA as a model for Brazilian NGOs. After Rio de Janeiro, an additional seven

NGOs named GPV were set up in different Brazilian cities. In the 1990s, the creation of HIV/AIDS NGOs and mutual-help groups composed by "people living with HIV and AIDS" was an important shift in HIV/AIDS mobilization in the country. Therefore, identity politics was minimized in relation to the politics of solidarity in Brazil. But conflict also occurred around HIV serologic status in other settings, such as GPV. Broadly, this kind of conflict reflected the contrast between the ideological models encamped in different forms of AIDS organizations.

The GPV category "people living with AIDS" was not similar to the label PWA as it is normally found on a global level. First, "people living with AIDS" (PWA) was a political category used in Anglo-Saxon countries (Altman, 1995). When AIDS was associated with gay men, the idea of "people living with AIDS" was effective for political reasons at contradicting assumptions of death and exclusive HIV infection among gay men. Besides, PWA implies a communitarian aim, whose politics has resonated at a global level, from international meetings to transnational arenas of funding, policymaking, and justice.

Located in São Paulo, the *Grupo de Incentivo à Vida* (GIV) claims similar ideas of HIV-positive experience and identity as those found in a global PWA perspective. For reasons that had less to do with political antagonism than with ideological differences about the meanings of "living with AIDS," activists from GIV and GPV had distinct perspectives that caused mutual suspicion and criticism until the late 1990s. For GPV, the idea of "living life positively" implied a generic attitude toward life, which included the political sense of self-making as HIV/AIDS activists. GPV attached importance to the personal and political impact caused by AIDS, but was opened to anyone, regardless of HIV status. GIV, on the other hand, emphasized HIV-positive identity and the personal experiences of "living with AIDS." It offered activities based on reflexive-discursive practices (discussion groups) or aimed at individual expression, such as meditation, body therapies, and art workshops, but made them accessible only to HIV-positive people.

In the mid-1990s, identity became a highly political issue in the AIDS world. In some NGOs, "positive" members accused "negative" staff members of trying to control economic resources. It also addressed a criticism of the bureaucratization and professionalism affecting HIV/AIDS NGOs. In fact, NGOs' conflicts around identity need to be identified with broad ideological disputes and the coexistence of different models of AIDS organization. The crucial moment was exemplified by the creation of the National Network of People Living with HIV and AIDS, also known as RNP+. If the public visibility of a discourse of "living with HIV and AIDS" was made apparent by GPV, it was later on that HIV-positive people became noticeable as a political agent. In 1995, the RNP+ was set up and composed of individual HIV-positive members in contrast to NGOs, but similar to HIV-positive networks, such as the Global Network of People Living with HIV (GNP+) and the International Community of Women Living with HIV/AIDS (ICW). The RNP+ has prioritized HIV-positive identity politics and empowerment related to global PWA politics. These networks were widely spread in Brazil and have developed more recently into other forms, such as the *Movimento Nacional de Cidadãs Posithivas,* a network of Brazilian HIV-positive women, created in 2004, which is now found in most states in the country. A National Network of young HIV-positive people represents yet another level of social and political mobilization, focusing on a specific category of people defined by serologic status and age. Considered a "vulnerable group" for HIV/AIDS infection, "young people" have been targeted in Brazilian HIV prevention campaigns, and age-specific projects have been developed by HIV/AIDS NGOs, supported by UNAIDS guidelines and global funding to promote changes in HIV risk-behavior. These are some new developments in the past 12 years, which have produced social unity as well as fragmentation.

Therefore persistent tensions between models of identity construction have operated in Brazil since the early 1990s (Valle, 2000) and have shown a culturally particular way of dealing with ideas of solidarity and agency. The creation of RNP+ and its ideological dispute with AIDS NGOs, such as GPV, showed the social effects of a broad process of identity formation in relation to HIV/AIDS. These disputes related to the social organization, identity formation, and political representation of HIV-positive people were associated with the connections between Brazilian NGOs and global HIV/AIDS activism. In the 2000s, the conflicts caused by identity politics and the differences between models of "living with HIV and AIDS" have apparently weakened. Even so, two different events called National Meeting of People Living with HIV/AIDS have been organized, one called *Vivendo,* organized by GPV since 1991, another organized by RNP+ since 2005. Other national and regional events aimed at women and young people have multiplied since the early 2000s.

## Spaces of Participation, Partnership, and Conflict: Forums, Meetings, and Committees

In the late 1980s, the emerging Brazilian HIV/AIDS NGOs established the first collective initiative to enable political discussions and negotiations between activist groups with the intent of guaranteeing improvements in AIDS policy. Public events were created to consolidate the social movement around the fight against AIDS. ABIA designed the networks of solidarity, while GPV-Rio was the main force behind *Vivendo*. In 1989 the first National Meeting of AIDS NGOs, ENONG, was also organized. At the beginning, ENONG expressed a clear confrontation against the Brazilian government, reflecting the context of the late 1980s and early 1990s. At that time AIDS NGOs insisted upon a systematic and qualified response by the Ministry of Health in relation to AIDS. ENONG defended a political perspective against the purely technical approach of the governmental response to the epidemic, but this perspective was marked by internal differences based on the specific political ideas and practices of each AIDS NGO. Therefore ENONG as a political arena was in fact very heterogeneous, pervaded by the ideological divisions discussed earlier in this chapter. However, civil organizations attempted to reach a collective position in regard to the epidemic.

During the 1990s, *Vivendo* and the ENONGs were the most important collective political events of Brazilian HIV/AIDS activism. In 1997, the ENONG became a biennial event. However there was an open increase in the number of political events in response to the new scenario of projects and partnerships motivated by the changes in AIDS policy and the relations between HIV/AIDS NGOs and networks and the Brazilian government. Some of these events were regional in character, such as the Regional Meetings of AIDS NGOS, called ERONGs; others had a state-level circumscription, gathering NGOs and networks from individual Brazilian states, the so-called EEONGs. This development marked the last decade and reflected attempts to decentralize the social movement against AIDS.

After 1996, AIDS NGO forums also appeared in Brazilian states such as São Paulo, Rio de Janeiro, Rio Grande do Sul, and Ceará. They can be seen as institutional spaces of political articulation between HIV/AIDS NGOs and governmental agencies. They also allowed a higher level of organization of HIV/AIDS activism, which would enable direct demands to health authorities at the state and city levels. Parallel to the expansion of HIV-positive networks in the country, these forums were conceived to implement a new model of negotiation between different AIDS organizations, which previously had been conducted in a haphazard and isolated way. Each Brazilian state now has its own forum, although some of them, like the state of São Paulo, have more than one, reflecting a local history of social mobilization. In their regular meetings, HIV/AIDS activists discuss questions related to the epidemic, to funding, and to other problems affecting the NGOs. These spaces of articulation have enabled practices of mediation and collective action through debate and negotiation between NGOs and networks, although disputes always occurred. When funding and AIDS drugs became more accessible in Brazil, the AIDS NGO forums allowed the discussion among organizations of strategies regarding their main political demands. Work groups and temporary committees were created to debate and find common standing on such themes as human rights and justice for HIV-positive people, the organization of common activities at World AIDS Day, and issues concerning children and young people with HIV/AIDS. Again, the idea of partnership has been put into action through the forums, when NGOs and governmental agencies have to deliberate about common propositions and work. It explains how the forums play a strategic role in the relation between the social movement and the government.

When we consider all these events, we can see how an articulated political dynamic has been constructed through all these different spaces of participation in Brazilian activism, which has brought about a much more cohesive political mobilization of AIDS NGOs and HIV networks, starting at the state level and going up to higher levels of decision making, such as regional and national levels. These spaces of participation have been important occasions for the election of delegates to represent the HIV/AIDS social movement in different committees of pluri-institutional representation, such as the National Health Council (CNS), the National AIDS Committee (CNA), the National AIDS Vaccines Committee, and the UNAIDS Working Group (GT UNAIDS). These various activist meetings and the HIV/AIDS forums constitute spaces of political articulation that permit mediation between the civil society, HIV/AIDS activism, and the governmental agencies regarding public health policy. And this partnership with the government had been a top political priority for the activists, as they had struggled for effective ways of participating in government policy decisions regarding HIV/AIDS since the early 1990s.

Brazilian HIV/AIDS activists have always defended *controle social,* a Portuguese expression meaning roughly social accountability, in relation to public policies. This idea goes back to the early days of the Brazilian social mobilization movements in favor of better public health, which culminated in the structural reorganization of the SUS—*Sistema único de Saúde* (Unified Health System)—in the early 1990s. Therefore relations between government and society in general, enhanced by social agents, including HIV/AIDS NGOs, have been considered crucial to health policy. Quite different but related to partnership, direct participation has been singled out by activists as their major goal, as essential for the improvement of health standards in Brazil. Effective activist participation at all different institutional levels and arenas related to Brazilian HIV/AIDS policy comprises direct formulation, proper monitoring, and evaluation of these policies. And for many activists the initially tense relationship between government and HIV/AIDS NGOs was bound to change when their partnership in AIDS policy started to be stimulated in the mid-1990s. This situation was contemporary to the positive effects generated by public health policy in late 1990s, when the Brazilian AIDS Program was considered a successful model for HIV prevention and treatment by UNAIDS/WHO. Therefore, activist meetings and the AIDS forums became privileged social spaces for NGOs and HIV-positive networks to assert collective positions.

In the last two years, however, some NGOs such as ABIA, GPV, and GIV have positioned a much more oppositional discourse toward governmental decisions and policies. There is renewed criticism of the increasing negligence of activist participation on the part of the government in all these committees and spaces of political decision related to the epidemic. In 2012 activists also criticized the last-minute changes in the HIV prevention campaign directed to gay men, which was to be launched by the National AIDS Program during the Brazilian Carnival. They accused the Ministry of Health and the Brazilian government of giving in to pressure from politically conservative and religious groups. In fact, a resurgent opposition has taken a much more combative profile, which brings to mind the antagonism that existed between Brazilian AIDS activism and the government in the late 1980s and early 1990s.

## BREAKING AIDS DRUGS PATENTS

Since 1996, AIDS drugs have been accessible and distributed for free for all Brazilians who need to start treatment. Through the years, there was a significant increase of people who sought access to combination therapies, which obliged the Ministry of Health to import drugs at a high cost. Since Brazil is an important and profitable market, the pharmaceutical industry has profited by selling antiretroviral drugs to the country since the 1990s (Galvão, 2002). According to official data, there are estimates that more than 215,676 Brazilians used AIDS drugs in 2011 (Brasil, 2012b). Although some antiretroviral drugs have been produced domestically, others still have to be imported at a high cost. Therefore, the Brazilian government has to negotiate with pharmaceutical companies to reduce prices of AIDS drugs. However, this has not been an easy task, since the drug companies are dealing with a profitable product in an increasing and competitive market. In fact, research has shown how the costs of drugs have been escalating in Brazil, and AIDS drugs have a great impact on it (Grangeiro, Teixeira, Bastos, & Teixeira, 2006).

Relations between Brazil and the pharmaceutical companies have become bitter and tense in the last 10 years. Even the former Brazilian president, Luis Lula da Silva, questioned the intransigent and "unethical" position of the drug companies. On several occasions, the Brazilian government threatened to break AIDS drug patents in direct opposition to the prices charged by the drug companies. Breaking an AIDS drug patent was a political decision greeted with great satisfaction by HIV/AIDS activists, both in Brazil and abroad, since the official Brazilian decision could be replicated in other developing countries. Since 2005 AIDS drugs such as Kaletra, Efavirenz, and Tenofovir were the subject of negotiation and conflict by the Brazilian government, which threatened companies with the compulsory licensing of antiretrovirals. Each drug represented a complex set of negotiations in which not only the government, but also the Brazilian judiciary and the activists participated. AIDS drugs patents became a central political issue for Brazilian NGOs, which explains why it has been discussed in several activist meetings, such as ENONG. In fact, AIDS drugs have been part of the political agenda and praxis of HIV activists since the late 1980s when AZT was made available to treat AIDS (Epstein, 1996). Global connections between AIDS activists from different contexts and countries have encouraged their political action in relation to AIDS drugs research, license, and industrial production (Smith & Siplon, 2006: 70). Also, vaccines research has been given close attention in the political practices of Brazilian activists (Bastos, 1999). HIV/AIDS NGOs and networks have organized several events around new scientific research, in addition to their participation in the National AIDS Vaccines Committee.

In 2003, the creation of the *Grupo de Trabalho sobre Propriedade Intelectual* (GTPI; Work Group on Intellectual Propriety), associated with a network of NGOs, social movements, and professional corporations, called REBRIP, enabled plain conditions for activist debate on the politics of AIDS drugs. GTPI gathered some of the most important Brazilian AIDS NGOs. Notably, this Work Group is engaged in advocacy and providing updated information on AIDS drugs. Considered a central topic in public health, *accessibility* to AIDS drugs is the key focus for GTPI. They also propose legal actions in favour of compulsory licensing of drugs, such as Kaletra, initiated in December 2005. These HIV/AIDS activists are not only being critical of pharmaceutical companies and their extensive commodification of drugs, but they also demand a vigorous position by the Brazilian government in favor of compulsory licensing of AIDS drugs. Therefore, we can see how AIDS drugs became a political problem by which NGOs, the government, and the drug companies have attempted to impose their opinions as well as their social and/or economic interests. Examining a new issue such as AIDS drugs patents and the possibility of compulsory licensing, we observe how different social groups and agencies have positioned themselves in relation to one another, including the Brazilian AIDS NGOs. Patents and intellectual property discussions can be seen as a course by which Brazilian activism has aimed to renew itself through critical political action.

## THE CRIMINALIZATION OF HIV TRANSMISSION: STIGMA, MORALITY, AND POLITICS

In the 2000s HIV/AIDS activists have pointed out that stigmatization still occurs in Brazil. One example is the recent trend in legal actions to criminalize HIV transmission, an expanding phenomenon crossing national boundaries and jurisdictions (Weait, 2007; Cameron, Burris, & Clayton, 2008). This issue has been highlighted by some of the leading HIV/AIDS NGOs and discussed in spaces such as AIDS NGO forums. Since 2007 events and seminars have been organized by activists to expose and openly criticize these legal attempts to prosecute people for HIV transmission.

In the 1990s accusations of responsibility in HIV transmission explored by the news media dealt mostly with the heterosexual context. Condemned among activists, these accusations point to how HIV risk could be understood in many different and ambiguous ways. Moral meanings play an important role in these accusations, concerning the primary responsibility of HIV-positive people in the "protection" of their sexual partners. In fact, sexuality has been the main axis of these moral accusations related to risk and the definition of blame (Douglas, 1992). In the 2000s this question has been magnified not only by interpersonal accusations and the "moral panic" created in the media, but has been dealt with through legal prosecution.

Since the early 2000s, solicitors and politicians have fought for legal reform and the passing of a criminal law devoted specifically to HIV transmission. They argue that someone who knows his or her own illness should be responsible for what they do to others. A number of HIV-positive people have been prosecuted since the 1990s, although most cases remain unknown. However, some cases became public through the media.

Activists admit that these may be only a small part of the cases that have been enforced by law. Since 2009 this issue has been focused on much more attentively by AIDS NGOs.

AIDS activists started to thoroughly research courts to evaluate the number of criminal prosecutions carried on by Brazilian jurisdiction that led to legal condemnation (Guimarães, 2011). In fact, criminalization of HIV transmission has been the central issue debated in seminars held in São Paulo and Rio de Janeiro. These events were associated with a larger political agenda concerning the epidemic. Therefore, some central ideas, such as solidarity, the guarantee of human rights, and the denial of stigmatization have been conveyed through a positioned perspective against the risks of the criminalization of HIV transmission. An ideological agenda has been recovered and has prompted a renewed critical position by activists. They have asked support from barristers and obtained direct assistance from the Ministry of Health, which endorsed their position against criminalization of HIV transmission through official documents. Therefore partnership is still an important practice between HIV/AIDS NGOs and the government, which can be also renewed, even if criticism by NGOs has been surfaced with strength lately. Nonetheless criminal prosecution of HIV-positive people is still a challenge for HIV/AIDS activism.

## HIV/AIDS ACTIVISM, SOCIAL INCLUSION, AND SUSTAINABILITY

Forged as an idea with global resonance, *sustainability* properly describes the current challenges to the Brazilian model of free access to HIV/AIDS drugs. However, sustainability means another dilemma for Brazilian activism. In the 2000s, some HIV/AIDS NGOs have endured for an unexpectedly long period of time, sometimes more than 20 years, although many of them have been closed down, including some GAPAs and GPVs in different cities. As a result of the end of the agreement between Brazil and the World Bank, there is limited funding available to Brazilian NGOs. Lately they have competed with LGBT groups for funding of HIV-prevention projects. There was also a gradual reduction of professional personnel, in part because many other career opportunities were opened to activists within the government and transnational agencies. But NGOs have gathered members with incomplete formal education, which revealed class differences that crossed activist spaces. When these changes became clear to activists, "social inclusion" emerged as a central issue to be dealt with together with the NGOs' sustainability.

For many years, finding and keeping a job was a struggle for HIV-positive people, since illness often impaired their work routine. Government retirement benefits made available for AIDS patients in Brazil at that time were a way to reduce the financial strain. As Brazil was under economic strain until the 1990s, work opportunities created by NGOs constituted another relative social advantage. In the 2000s, however, these opportunities have become more rare. Social benefits were also cut back when HIV-positive people showed improvement in their health conditions and life expectancy. This has forced people to search for work after years without proper employment. Furthermore, due to limited education resulting from social inequality in Brazil, many low-income HIV-positive people previously engaged in activist groups have found their chances of finding work further reduced when employers know their HIV serologic status.

As inclusion also became a major issue to manage, many NGOs have embraced activities to provide their HIV-positive members with skills training that could improve their chances to work. Sometimes, particular groups and people have been prioritized to receive training, including transgendered people, youth, and people with low incomes. They are targeted as groups with the need of "social inclusion" and associated with "vulnerability." Some groups are selected according to new directions of funding. Therefore, they become the focus of intervention and activism. Again NGOs have to confront an old dilemma: political activism or service-based activities?

HIV/AIDS NGOs have been faced more and more with fragile and impoverished conditions of institutional maintenance, in marked contrast with the past, when these organizations were consolidated and funding was more readily available. Some organizations have closed down, and the leading Brazilian NGOs that remain active have also seen a reduction of their activities. In recent years at national AIDS NGOs meetings, sustainability has been a key issue in the discussions, and it has also been present in public statements and documents. A gloomy mood has been manifest and is considered as a sign of a wider crisis. Activists perceive this situation as a consequence of having lost political space in institutional arenas related to HIV/AIDS policy, indicated by reduced participation in the last two years. They criticize the Brazilian government for minimizing their role in the fight against the AIDS epidemic. For activists, the present context is particularly disappointing because of the electoral and political support given by Brazilian social movements to the election of presidents Luiz Inácio Lula da Silva and Dilma Rouseff, both from the PT—*Partido dos Trabalhadores* (Worker's Party)—in the last decade. President Rouseff has been openly criticized by HIV/AIDS activists for her current authoritarian policy in relation to the epidemic. Activists have been increasingly vocal in their criticism in public events as well as to the press. In the XIX International AIDS Conference in Washington, D.C., current HIV/AIDS policy by the Ministry of Health was publicly denounced by Brazilian activists.

## An Activist Politics of Memory

Beyond political antagonism, Brazilian activism has given a persistent importance to historical trajectory and memory. Particularly in Rio de Janeiro and São Paulo, various events have been held by long-running HIV/AIDS NGOs such as ABIA, GIV, and GPV, marking 20 to 25 years of activism. These events have revealed an emotional dimension of time, memory, and politics, as a focus on the past creates a historical and social evaluation of the NGOs. This evaluation was also present in the past at such collective events as the *Vivendo* and the ENONGs. However, this particular concern with social memory involves strong emotional meanings and adds a more sensitive element to their social and political engagement as activists begin to reclaim the historical trajectory of HIV/AIDS networks and NGOs.

In the past, emotions played an important role in Brazilian HIV/AIDS activism and helped construct the meanings behind volunteer work and activist engagement to an AIDS organization, similar to what happened with ACT UP in the North American context (Gould, 2009). In the 2000s, this sort of emotional work has been explored in a more collective configuration through social activities and cultural production that aspire to reconfigure memory and history through ritualized celebrations of political activism related to illness. They celebrate the long period of time in which NGOs have endured in their work against the AIDS epidemic. Some deceased leaders such as Herbert Daniel and Betinho, connected to GPV and ABIA, have been remembered as iconic figures whose ideas became a genuine legacy in the fight against AIDS. Documentaries and texts that were produced combine political intentions with cultural and symbolic meanings. HIV/AIDS activism has been reconsidered from a different perspective that harmonizes social events and political actions in favor of a collective project. Therefore the idea of solidarity and the refusal of civil death, formulated by the first Brazilian activists, have been reinforced in the fight against AIDS stigmatization. A politics of memory has been constructed along with a historical reassessment of the epidemic.

This cultural elaboration of a heroic past gives strong support to Brazilian activism today.

Illness, politics, and memory have been deeply articulated to explain the activist mobilization against AIDS. This expresses the emotional aspect through which people as well as facts have been treated. A sense of continuity is elaborated through a politics of memory of personal and social suffering (Das, 2007), engagement and political action associated with HIV/AIDS activism. It can be said that an idealized understanding of the past arises from the events organized by the NGOs, as a process of selective memory incorporates or ignores some facts and/or people rather than others. Even so, these events reveal a powerful concern with time and memory, stimulated by collective work conducted through HIV/AIDS activism.

## CONCLUSION

This chapter has given a brief and condensed presentation of Brazilian HIV/AIDS activism considered through an anthropological perspective. Brazilian AIDS NGOs and HIV-positive networks have described AIDS as a problem of personal, collective and public health dimensions. Brazilian activists have also differed in their forms of social and political intervention, according to their ideological framework and the economic resources available to implement their projects. In fact, Brazilian NGOs reached public recognition with the consolidation of AIDS policy at local and national levels. However, the AIDS epidemic has not been controlled successfully in the country. Perhaps this explains how a political criticism has resurfaced, caused by the limitations of the Brazilian health policy to control the epidemic. According to HIV/AIDS activists, the National Program on HIV/AIDS cannot be regarded as a "model" for other countries while old structural problems remain to be solved, such as the deteriorating conditions of public hospitals. Further, many Brazilian federal states suffer from the irregular availability of antiretrovirals and routine exams, such as viral load and genotyping tests. Therefore, AIDS activists have positioned against the contradictory limitations of the National AIDS Program.

Since the 1980s, Brazilian HIV/AIDS NGOs and HIV-positive networks have been motivated by a range of very complex personal and social interests. Some of them involve personal engagement, caused by HIV awareness and the experience of illness, which explains the motivations to be a member of HIV/AIDS activist organizations and networks. In addition, these various communitarian organizations and spaces have been historically defined by social and political actions characterizing a social field of struggles and disputes undertaken by very different Brazilian agencies and institutions throughout the last three decades in Brazil. HIV/AIDS organizations, public agencies, and HIV-positive people have been related to each other by an interconnection of social levels (local, national, and global). This social field has shown the permanence of historical relations that have led to both conflict and negotiation. Some ideological models guided different forms of social organization in the AIDS world, such as political or service-based activism, and HIV-positive networks. They have been sensitive to different conceptions of community work, activism, and identity politics. Normally, they coexisted and conflicted simultaneously. It should be emphasized that early activist ideas and perspectives have been reassembled and reconsidered in a new social context. Despite some new meanings ascribed to these ideas, we see an intricate social field in which relations have been undertaken through negotiation, partnership, and clear antagonism.

## BIBLIOGRAPHY

Altman, D. (1995). Political sexualities. Meanings and identities in the time of AIDS. In R. Parker & J. Gagnon (eds.), *Conceiving Sexuality* (pp. 97–108). London: Routledge.

Bastos, C. (1999). *Global responses to AIDS.* Bloomington, Indiana: Indiana University Press.

Biehl, J. (2007). *Will to live: AIDS therapies and the politics of survival.* Princeton: Princeton University Press.

Biehl, J., Coutinho, D., & Outeiro, A. (2001). Technology and affect: HIV/AIDS testing in Brazil. *Culture, Medicine and Psychiatry, 25,* 87–129.

Bourdieu, P. (1990). *In other words. Essays towards a reflexive sociology.* Cambridge: Polity Press.

Brasil, Ministério da Saúde (2012a). *Boletim epidemiológico. Ano VIII,* n. 1. Brasília, DF: Departamento de DST, AIDS e Hepatites Virais.

Brasil, Ministério da Saúde (2012b). *Relatório de progresso da resposta brasileira ao HIV/AIDS (2010–2011).* Brasília, DF: Departamento de DST, AIDS e Hepatites Virais.

Cameron, E., Burris, S., & Clayton, M. (2008). HIV is a virus, not a crime. *HIV/AIDS Policy & Law Review, 13*(2/3), 64–68.

Daniel, H. (1994). *Vida antes da morte/life before death.* ABIA: Rio de Janeiro.

Daniel, H., & Parker, R. (1993). *Sexuality, politics and AIDS in Brazil.* London: The Falmer Press.

Das, V. (2007). *Life and words: Violence and the descent into the ordinary.* Berkeley: University of California Press.

Douglas, M. (1992). *Risk and blame: Essays in cultural theory.* London: Routledge.

Epstein, S. (1996). *Impure science: AIDS, activism, and the politics of knowledge.* Berkeley: University of California Press.

Galvão, J. (2000). *AIDS no Brasil.* Rio de Janeiro: ABIA/Editora 34.

Galvão, J. (2002, November 5). Access to antiretroviral drugs in Brazil. *The Lancet,* 1–4. Retrieved from http://image.thelancet.com/extras/01art9038web.pdf

Gould, D. (2009). *Moving politics: Emotion and ACT UP's fight against AIDS.* Chicago: University of Chicago Press.

Grangeiro, A., Teixeira, L., Bastos, F. I., & Teixeira, P. (2006). Sustentabilidade da política de medicamentos anti-retrovirais no Brasil. *Revista de Saúde Pública, 40* (Supl). 60–9.

Guimarães, C. D. (2001). *AIDS no feminino: Por que a cada dia mais mulheres contraem AIDS no Brasil?* Rio de Janeiro: Editora da UFRJ.

Guimarães, M. (2011). HIV/AIDS não é sentença de morte. *Coleção ABIA, 3.* Rio de Janeiro.

La Dehesa, R. De (2010). *Queering the public sphere in Mexico and Brazil.* Durham: Duke University Press.

Parker, R. (1990). Responding to AIDS in Brazil. In B. Misztal & D. Moss (eds.), *Action on AIDS: National policies in comparative perspective* (pp. 51–79). Westport, CT: Greenwood Press.

Rabinow, P. (1992). Artificiality and enlightenment: From sociobiology to biosociality. In J. Crary & S. Kwinter (eds.), *Zone 6: Incorporations* (pp. 234–252). Cambridge: MIT Press.

Smith, R. A., & Siplon, P. (2006). *Drugs into bodies: Global AIDS treatment activism.* Westport, CT: Praeger.

Souza, H. (1994). *A cura da AIDS.* Rio de Janeiro: Relume Dumará/ABIA.

Terto, V. (1996). Homossexuais soropositivos e soropositivos homossexuais. In R. Parker & R. Barbosa (eds.), *Sexualidades Brasileiras* (pp. 90–104). Rio de Janeiro: Relume Dumará.

Valle, C. G. (2000). *The making of people living with HIV and AIDS: Identities, illness and social organization in Rio de Janeiro, Brazil* (unpublished doctoral dissertation). University of London. London.

Valle, C. G. (2002). Identidades, doença e organização social: Um estudo das "pessoas vivendo com HIV e AIDS." *Horizontes Antropológicos,* 17. Porto Alegre, 179–210.

Weait, M. (2007). *Intimacy and responsibility: The criminalization of HIV transmission.* Abingdon: Routledge/Cavendish.

# 13

# The NGO-ization of HIV/AIDS Activism in Mexico: Not So Scandalous After All?

*Antonio Torres-Ruiz*

This chapter offers some reflections on the effects that the process of professionalization or NGO-ization of civil society groups with work on HIV/AIDS is having and could potentially have on the public sphere. These reflections are mostly based on my own research on the political economy of HIV/AIDS in Mexico, which has led me to contend that this phenomenon has had some concrete positive effects. At the same time, however, I also point to some ongoing challenges, such as the need for activists and other stakeholders to maintain a certain degree of autonomy vis-à-vis government institutions, while consolidating and furthering their successes. Although some prospective analysis is offered, I must express some of my own misgivings about any attempt to predict future challenges. Thus, subscribing to a Benjaminian understanding of time and history, I prefer to put the emphasis on the past and present states of the struggle against the epidemic, which show that, in fact, there are still ongoing issues that will likely remain at the center of the struggle for the foreseeable future (Barglow, 1998). Similarly, as will be outlined below, I argue that a critical analysis of NGO-ization has to be inscribed within the dynamics of the process of globalization. As such, the main purpose of my work, including this chapter, is to contribute to a better understanding of the effects that NGO-ization has had and can potentially have on the official response to the epidemic, and more generally on the public sphere and the democratization process.

## GLOBALIZATION AND CIVIL SOCIETY NGO-IZATION

The worldwide emergence and proliferation of nongovernmental organizations (NGOs) is not exclusive to civil society's mobilization around HIV/AIDS.

In fact, this process of NGO-ization is very much associated with the phenomenon known as *globalization,* defined here as the long-term process of universal and multifaceted cultural, economic, political, social, and technological interconnectedness that characterizes the world (see Giddens, 1990; Held, McGrew, Goldblatt, & Perraton, 1997; Held, 1999). What is characteristic of this phenomenon's current phase, though, which Castells (1996) calls the age of the network, is that the localization of polity has paralleled with the globalization of some issues. In other words, we are witnessing the simultaneous participation of civil society groups, among other actors, locally and globally. As such, I make a clear distinction between globalization and *neoliberal globalism,* or the ideology of neo-classical economic prescriptions associated with the Washington Consensus. Defining neoliberal globalism as a political agenda helps us recognize the undercurrent of ideological commitment to market sovereignty that infuses the discourse generated by such leading international financial and economic institutions as the International Monetary Fund (IMF), the World Bank, the United States (U.S.) Treasury, the World Trade Organization (WTO), and other powerful global actors, most particularly trans-national corporations (TNCs) (see Howse & Nicolaidis, 2003).

Although I conceive of the international arena as a heterogeneous constellation of interwoven political, cultural, and economic interests, I take it as established that the globalist agenda has steered the phenomenon of globalization for the past three decades. This most recent phase of globalization is further characterized by the growing NGO-ization of civil society groups, both at the domestic and the international levels. In this relatively new context, NGO-ization represents not just the spontaneous proliferation of NGOs (with specialized staff, structured funding, and salaries) but also the active promotion of their formalization by governments, international institutions, and donors (Ryfman, 2004). In fact, and in line with the neoliberal globalist agenda, the preferred NGOs are expected to be rhetorically restrained, politically collaborative, and technically proficient in their practices. Under these circumstances, most critics have pointed to the detrimental impact of this phenomenon on the autonomy of social movements vis-à-vis the state. As a good example of the increasing attention paid to this phenomenon in Latin America, George Yúdice, in *The Expediency of Culture* (2003), states:

> NGOization is not scandalous, but nevertheless contributes to the weakening of the public sphere, precisely the opposite of the intent of the social movements. That institutionalization resulted in activism

giving way to bureaucratic administration. Those movements have been permeated by international discourses on cultural citizenship, where identity is the lynchpin of rights claims. To be sure, how identity is deployed depends on the performative possibilities holding in different societies. In such contexts, there is little to be gained by deploying identity or disidentity if there is no juridical or other institutional uptake to transform rights claims into material changes. This question of uptake is crucial and it has confounded many a study that has presumed the receptivity to identity rights claims on the basis of experiences in other contexts. (pp. 77–78)

As stressed by Yúdice, it is undeniable that in most instances institutional channeling tempers activism and can favor the assertion, in public, of certain identities and not others. This can force social movements to dovetail with the agendas set by governments and funders, whereby funding patterns often lead to a shift away from the construction of ideological or transformational alternatives to project-based and often limited developmental activities. Furthermore, some weaker groups or smaller organizations, which ultimately depend on the same pull of grant providers, risk their continuing existence due to the lack of professional means to sell their projects and activities like their bigger sisters. For their part, some of those more "successful" NGOs end up becoming social service providers to governments, global institutions, and even businesses, thereby undermining their autonomy and social activism. Ultimately, there is often less room for organizations to be actively engaged in the ideological construction and promotion of alternative forms of global political organization, wider social inclusion, and democracy. Nevertheless, and despite those warnings, the actual effects of professionalization have been positively surprising in some cases, with great effectiveness shown in engaging with the state and international institutions while maintaining a significant degree of autonomy. Thus, it is based on the analysis of various networks of HIV/AIDS and sexual minorities or lesbian, gay, bisexual, and transgendered/transsexual (LGBT) activists in Latin America that I argue that the effects of NGO-ization are more nuanced.

In the following pages, I will engage in a twofold exercise. On the one hand, I contend that the adoption of a human rights discourse by various HIV/AIDS NGOs, within the process of democratization in Mexico, has served as a strong discursive and political tool for the emancipation of previously excluded and marginalized groups. In fact, the creation of HIV/AIDS NGOs and the corresponding policy networks (permeable clusters of interdependent organizations and individual actors [public and private], with frequent interactions and a common interest, connected to one another by resource dependencies, with a core and a periphery, whose members participate in the formulation and implementation of a set of policies) has allowed civil society actors to engage in some transformational practices that take place at several points in those networks, which has made social action possible. On the other hand, however, I will also argue that although this process of professionalization has resulted in their growing visibility, positioning, and influence on the policymaking process, there are some concrete challenges regarding the continuity, the scope, and the broadening of their agenda.

## HIV/AIDS AND NGO-IZATION IN MEXICO: SUCCESSES AND CHALLENGES

As will be shown below, HIV/AIDS activism in Mexico has had some concrete and positive effects on the visibility and empowerment of traditionally marginalized and vulnerable social groups, especially sexual minorities. Through their NGO-ization and active participation in the creation of what I refer to as HIV/AIDS policy networks (see Torres-Ruiz, 2006, 2011), activists have made specific gains in terms of public policy-making and implementation, as well as in transforming and expanding the public sphere (see also De la Dehesa, 2010). The increasing engagement of civil society actors in Mexico is also partly explained by the fact that, in the 1990s, major donors broadened their focus on NGOs and began funding a more diverse set of civil society groups. As a consequence, an important number of HIV/AIDS NGOs were created and received a steady stream of funding from international agencies. Yet, as pointed out above, this increasing interest in the promotion of NGO activities responded also to one of the central tenets of the globalist agenda: the insistence on less government and reduced public budgets.

Once again, observers of NGO-ization have warned about the consequences this phenomenon can have on the weakening of social movements' autonomy and their causes (Álvarez, Dagnino, & Escobar, 1998). However, an overview of the history of the struggle around HIV/AIDS in Mexico will allow us to understand the extent to which civil society's mobilization has had a significant and positive impact on the current state of public policies. Furthermore, and along the lines of Marsiaj's (2010) analysis of the case of Brazil, I will also show how such mobilization and NGO-ization facilitated the visibility, acceptance, and ultimately access to the agenda-setting process of public policy and implementation by those marginalized groups. This access resulted in some concrete policy effects, such as the conformation and reformulation of the juridical framework pertaining to HIV/AIDS.

## CIVIL SOCIETY'S MOBILIZATION
## AND HIV/AIDS PUBLIC POLICIES

In Mexico, as in other parts of the world, at the end of the 1970s and the early 1980s, various individual actors and groups began getting organized around the increasing demand for visibility and acceptance of sexual minorities. This mobilization took place before the emergence of HIV/AIDS and resulted in the formalization of many of those groups, allowing them to have the structures in place that would turn out to be useful in confronting the new challenges posed by the epidemic. It would be impossible to list here all of those actors and groups, but some deserve a special mention due to their impact and longstanding presence in the struggle against HIV/AIDS.

The mobilization and organization of sexual minority groups took place throughout the country, albeit mostly in big urban centers. In Mexico City, for example, among some of the key groups were the Movimiento de Liberación Homosexual de México (Homosexual Liberation Movement, 1971), led by well-known artist, public intellectual, and activist Nancy Cárdenas; the Frente Homosexual de Acción Revolucionaria (FHAR, Homosexual Front of Revolutionary Action, 1978); the Grupo Lambda de Liberación Homosexual (Lambda Group of Homosexual Liberation, 1978); the lesbian organizations Grupo Lesbos (1977) and Oikabeth (1978), and Colectivo Sol (1981) (see Brito-Lemus, 2003). There were other organizations founded in the early 1980s in other parts of the country, such as in the northern border cities of Tijuana and Ciudad Juárez. In the former, there was the Frente Internacional para las Garantías Humanas Tijuana (FIGHT, International Front for Human Guarantees), whose founders, Emilio Velásquez and Max Mejía, also created the influential newspaper *Frontera Gay*. In Ciudad Juárez, there was the Federación Mexicana de Asociaciones Privadas de Planificación Familiar (FEMAP), which suffered a split and led to the creation of the still running Proyecto Compañeros (Project Companions), with support from the Asociación Fronteriza Mexicana Estadounidense de Salud (The Mexican-U.S. Border Association for Health), with headquarters in El Paso, Texas. As we will see below, some of these organizations continued with their work throughout the 1990s and beyond, but it was mostly reoriented toward

HIV/AIDS once the disease began affecting their members and the population at large.

As the country was experiencing a significant social transformation and increasing demands for democratization, the detection of the first cases of AIDS in Mexico occurred in March 1983. The first victims, who were mostly gay men, confronted the denial of access to housing and funeral services, as well as forced testing, firing from their workplaces, and general neglect by public authorities and local communities. Thus the essential role played by civil society organizations in addressing such urgent challenges and in filling the apparent governmental vacuum. As evidenced in Monsiváis's (1996) account of the official response throughout the 1980s, this was purely epidemiological, neglecting social, economic, cultural, and educational factors. In fact, the federal government of Miguel de la Madrid (1982–1988), which faced a major economic and external debt-related financial crisis, opted for hiding information around the epidemic, in spite of the fact that health protection was recognized in the Constitution as a fundamental right in 1983, which then led to the formulation of the Ley General de Salud (General Health Law) of 1984. In 1986, however, and partly as a consequence of the pressures to make the first antiretroviral (ARV), known as azidothymidine (AZT), available to all patients, and as a response to the World Health Organization's (WHO) calls to take more proactive actions, the Mexican government created the National Committee for the Prevention of AIDS (Comité Nacional para la Investigación y el Control del Sida), which was the first official effort to respond to the epidemic at the national level (Sepúlveda, Bronfman, Ruiz Palacios, Stanislawski, & Valdespino, 1989). This took place under Guillermo Soberón Acevedo's supervision (President Miguel de la Madrid's secretary of health), and the following year they launched the telephone service TELSIDA, in order to make a phone line available to those in need of some concrete information about the new disease and the available services. On August 24, 1988, before leaving office, de la Madrid decreed a new and higher status for the committee, transforming it into the National Board for the Prevention and Control of AIDS (Consejo Nacional para la Prevención y Control del Sida, CONASIDA), which continued to function mainly with international funding until 1992 when public authorities committed to provide the board with an official budget. Interestingly, 13 years later, Guillermo Soberón Acevedo (secretary of health during de la Madrid's government) co-authored an assessment of the situation in a short article entitled "El Sida a 13 años de su aparición en México" (1996). In it, Soberón describes the governmental actions around the epidemic in an attempt to shed some light on the way the government had dealt with public health, human rights, discrimination, and equity in social relations during those first years. What is surprising in that piece is the lack of assumed responsibility, especially by Soberón himself. In contrast, years earlier, HIV/AIDS and human rights activist Francisco Galván (1988) published a critical assessment of the role of the government in denying the right to health protection and against discrimination during that same period.

In short, throughout that first decade, the official public position was characterized by a lack of interest in and neglect of sexual minorities' needs, as well as by pressures from conservative groups and the Catholic Church to refrain from campaigns such as the promotion of the use of condoms, especially from the Comité Nacional Provida (Prolife National Committee), which sued CONASIDA for promoting promiscuity and perverting underage children. Although those charges were not sustainable, they were effective in silencing some of the first official prevention campaigns (García-Murcia et al., 2010, p. 89). As stated above, this lack of appropriate governmental response generated a direct reaction to the epidemic by civil society, with some of the older organizations reorienting their work while other groups launched new organizations. In the city of Guadalajara, for instance, a circle of gay men created the Comité Humanitario de Esfuerzos Compartidos Contra el Sida, A.C. (CHECCOS, Humanitarian Committee of Joint Efforts against AIDS). In the southern city of Mérida, there was the Asociación Regional del Sureste contra el Sida, A.C. (ARSCS, Regional Association of the Southeast against AIDS, 1989). In Mexico City, in 1987, the Fundación Mexicana de Lucha contra el Sida, A.C. (Mexican Foundation against AIDS) was created by Luis González de Alba, and in 1989, human rights activist Arturo Díaz Betancourt first formed Cálamo, Espacios y Alternativas Comunitarias, A.C., and later on, together with Francisco Galván, created the network Mexicanos contra el Sida (Mexicans against AIDS). The latter was supported by the technical assistance of the Dutch Humanist Institute for Cooperation with Developing Countries (HIVOS). Mexicanos contra el Sida included different projects, such as information and education, provision of services, helping other groups to develop, and network building. Together with their older LGBT sisters, these HIV/AIDS NGOs and some of their members would become central actors in forcing a proper governmental response. Their efforts were also aided by the active involvement of journalists and intellectuals, such as Alejandro Brito Lemus and Carlos Monsiváis, who together with Arturo Díaz Betancourt created *Letra S: Salud, Sexualidad y Sida,* a monthly insert in the influential national newspaper *La Jornada*. *Letra S* represented an effort to rescue and in a way continue a previous editorial project named *Sociedad y Sida,* directed by Francisco Galván, which had been published before in the newspaper *El Nacional.* The coordinated efforts of all these groups led to the formation of a strong national HIV/AIDS policy network that helped rethink the role of the state and the responsibilities of the different levels of government concerning HIV/AIDS. A fundamental component of such efforts was the focus on a human rights discourse, which was put forward at the first meeting of the International Council of AIDS Service Organizations (ICASO) in 1989 in Paris, when Francisco Galván and others triggered an intense debate around HIV/AIDS and human rights, political participation, and citizenship (García-Murcia et al., 2010, p. 160).

The most evident impact of the engagement strategy observed in Mexico was the radical change in the makeup of the body in charge of formulating HIV/AIDS public policies, which went from being completely exclusionary in 1986 to becoming much more inclusive from the late 1990s onward, incorporating NGOs into the core of the policy network and the policy-making process. In the eyes of most observers, though, these changes were long in coming and very slow. Even under Carlos Salinas de Gortari's administration (1988–1994), and despite the fact that CONASIDA received more federal resources due to its new status, most of its operations continued to be carried out with international financing from various international organizations, including the WHO's Global Program on AIDS (Saavedra, Izazola, Prottas, & Shepard, 1999). As pointed out before, in its early years, CONASIDA did not incorporate or consult any civil society actors and thus was not responsive to the actual needs and human rights demands of those affected by the disease. In contrast, under Salinas de Gortari's administration, human rights increasingly became a major focus. This was due in part to the North American Free Trade Agreement (NAFTA) negotiations and some human rights–related concerns in the two northern neighbors. Despite Mexico's 1981 ratification of the main international and regional human rights treaties, the country had a reputation of impunity regarding their violations. Thus, increasing domestic and external pressures led the Mexican government to create the National Human Rights Commission (Comisión Nacional de Derechos Humanos, or CNDH) in 1990, based on article 102 of the Federal Constitution. The CNDH, however, has played a limited role in reducing the number of human rights violations, primarily because it is not vested with the power to prosecute violators, and most recommendations handed down by the commission have been only partially implemented. In this context, concerns about HIV/AIDS-related violations became the point of increasing pressure from the HIV/AIDS policy network, which together with international pressures led to the reformulation and conformation of the juridical framework around HIV/AIDS at the end of Salinas de Gortari's administration. At that point, the federal government began discussions on the Norma Oficial Mexicana para la Prevención y el Control de la Infección por VIH: NOM-010-SSA2-1993 (Official Mexican Regulation for the Prevention and Control of Infection by the Human Immunodeficiency Virus). This process involved the direct participation and input of some of the aforementioned civil society organizations, such as Mexicanos contra el Sida, Fundación Mexicana para la Lucha contra el Sida, Amigos contra el Sida, Proyecto Compañeros, and Colectivo Sol, among a total of 19 NGOs. It resulted in wide governmental legal commitments for attention to and prevention of AIDS and represented the culmination of civil society actors' efforts to imbue HIV/AIDS policies with a strong human rights discourse. The questioning of Carlos Salinas de Gortari's election and the widespread accusations of electoral fraud might have contributed to the inclusion of civil society's demands as a way to get some legitimacy (Aguayo-Quezada & Parra-Rosales, 1997). This forward-looking legislation (NOM-010-SSA2-1993) was published and went into effect on January 17, 1995, under the new administration of President Ernesto Zedillo Ponce de León (1994–2000) (Torres-Ruiz, 2011, pp. 43–44). This law represented a concerted effort by Mexican authorities at different levels to address the HIV/AIDS epidemic within the parameters of the right-to-health guarantees enshrined in Mexico's Constitution (González-Martin, 1996).

What we saw in the second half of the 1990s was the strengthening of the national HIV/AIDS policy network with an increasing emphasis on human rights and the explicit concern for the health and well-being of men who have sex with men (MSM). This was accompanied by a more active promotion of condom use and the public discussion of sexual diversity and sexual work. In addition, as was the case for activists around the world, the introduction of a new generation of ARVs at the 1996 AIDS Conference in Vancouver represented a turning point for the renewed collaboration among civil society groups in Mexico. This led to the creation of the Front for Persons Affected by HIV/AIDS (Frente de Personas Afectadas por el VIH/SIDA, Frenpavih, 1996) and was followed by a major protest in Mexico City during a conference of epidemiologists in 1997.

These events marked the beginning of an effective universal drug-access advocacy campaign, thus revitalizing the movement and creating a cooperative spirit (Frasca, 2005). Although the National Social Security

Institute (IMSS) committed to the provision of ARVs to its members at the beginning of the 1990s, in October 1997, the Front for Persons Affected by HIV/AIDS (Frenpavih) appeared before the Health Commission of the Chamber of Deputies to complain that the IMSS was not in fact keeping its commitment to make the medicines available. This led to the temporary creation of a special fund (FONSIDA), which was not very successful in its attempt to attract public and private donations for the provision of medications for all. That same year (1997), Zedillo strengthened CONASIDA by giving it the status of a deconcentrated body of the Ministry of Health. Later, and as part of Zedillo's decentralization reforms in the health sector, state-level councils were also created (Consejos Estatales para la Prevención del SIDA, or COESIDAS) and significant reforms to the Official Regulations (NOM-010-SSA2-1993) were introduced in 1999 and published on June 21, 2000, in order to make it mandatory for all public institutions to provide full services to all HIV/AIDS patients. Since Zedillo's final year in office—and the last year of the consecutive seven-decade federal rule by the Partido Revolucionario Institucional (PRI)—reforms to the HIV/AIDS program have increasingly reflected the emergence and strong positioning of the policy network. In the early 2000s the highly active antiretroviral therapy (HAART) became available for use throughout the world, which served as an additional catalyst for policy network members' coordination.

A stronger human rights discourse, a less confrontational style of civic activism, and the relative decline of the PRI seem to have united forces (personal interview with Alejandro Brito, director of *Letra S,* December 5, 2001), giving a further impulse to the consolidation and influence of the HIV/AIDS policy network. Drawing lessons from the Brazilian case (see De la Dehesa, 2010; Torres-Ruiz, 2011), between 1999 and 2000, for instance, a major World Bank loan with a substantial HIV/AIDS component was negotiated with the direct involvement of civil society organizations. Silvia Panebianco (of the HIV/AIDS NGO MEXSIDA), José Antonio Izazola (of SIDALAC), and Díaz Betancourt (of *Letra S* and Mexicanos contra el Sida) worked together on the proposal for the HIV/AIDS content of the loan. This important step in the greater inclusion of civil society actors in policymaking was part of the democratization process and a sign of the increasing strength of the HIV/AIDS policy network. All of these are part of a larger group of national HIV/AIDS NGOs that have benefited from domestic and international funding for their continuing work in favor of sexual and human rights for HIV/AIDS affected groups (see Torres-Ruiz, 2006, 2011).

More recently, a significant restructuring of the national program further strengthened the network's participation. In July 2003, under President Vicente Fox Quezada (2000–2006, of the right-of-center Partido Acción Nacional or PAN), CONASIDA became the collegiate body of coordination (*órgano colegiado de coordinación*) formed by the secretaries of Health and Education, the directors of the two main social security institutions (Instituto Mexicano del Seguro Social [IMSS], the Instituto de Seguridad y Servicios Sociales de los Trabajadores del Estado [ISSSTE]), and the National Institute for Nutrition and Medical Sciences (Instituto Nacional de la Nutrición). Its new mandate is to strengthen cooperation and coordination among public entities for the prevention and control of HIV/AIDS and other sexually transmitted diseases. According to these reforms, the functions previously assigned to CONASIDA are now the responsibility of CENSIDA. Thus, CENSIDA not only continues to perform the same functions assigned to CONASIDA before; its director general also functions as technical secretary of CONASIDA (as established in article 46 of the respective decree). The appointment of Dr. Jorge Saavedra as CENSIDA's new director in September 2003 was of major significance for strengthening the HIV/AIDS policy network. As an openly gay health professional, activist, and public official living with HIV, with long experience in HIV/AIDS work with a special focus on MSM issues, as well as former manager of the previously mentioned 1999/2000 World Bank's loan, Saavedra's appointment was the result of consultation with the broader policy community. In the eyes of most members of the policy network, he had the expertise and legitimacy required for the position, which resulted in their full support for his designation. After the presidential election of August 2006, in which PAN's Felipe Calderón Hinojosa entered office, Saavedra was confirmed in his position and remained as head of the program until 2009. Under Saavedra's CENSIDA they created the Centros Ambulatorios de Prevención y Atención en Sida e ITS (CAPASITS, Ambulatory Centers for AIDS and STDs Prevention and Attention), which are key to the materialization of universal access. That same year, in February, he was replaced by José Antonio Izazola, who was also involved in negotiating the World Bank's loan and had joined the secretary of health in 1985. As an expert in public health and also openly gay, from the beginning Izazola worked hard to convince decision makers to pay attention to the epidemic, in what he described as a "macho government structure" that made it hard to convince authorities to act against a disease that affected MSM (Frasca, 2005). Among some of these recent appointments, Carlos García de León, of the NGO Ave de México, took his new position as CENSIDA's director of prevention and social participation. García de León had worked with Díaz Betancourt and CENSIDA authorities to create the Department for NGOs, putting together for the first time a national database of all civil society organizations working on this issue. As such, Ave de México, MEXSIDA, Mexicanos contra el Sida, and others found themselves, together with CENSIDA, at the core of the domestic network. This has allowed them to play a central role in the strengthening and functioning of the network as a whole and in the definition and implementation of recent policies, such as prevention campaigns among MSM, campaigns for access to treatment, and campaigns against homophobia. For its part, *Letra S,* under the direction of journalist and LGBT activist Alejandro Brito, has also played a central role in consolidating a freer press that pushes for increased transparency and government responsiveness.

Another positive and significant step has been the relatively slow but steady increase in the public budget devoted to treatment and prevention (see Torres-Ruiz, 2011). As late as 1994, the federal government had vowed "zero funding" for AIDS treatment. For Mexico, in contrast to Brazil, NAFTA meant that the generic solution was out of the question (see Torres-Ruiz & Clarkson, 2009). Yet because of persistent pressure from members of the HIV/AIDS policy network and a more receptive secretary of health (Dr. Julio Frenk), Fox's government committed to universal treatment coverage for all HIV/AIDS patients by the year 2006, reaching the goal—in terms of resources available for the implementation of such program—three years earlier. This was possible through the creation of the Fund for Catastrophic Health Expenses (which was part of the corresponding reforms to the General Health Law). In addition, and as a result of global pressure on the pharmaceutical industry, there was a reduction in ARVs prices; Merck Sharp and Dohme, for example, lowered the price of one of its AIDS drugs by 82 percent. This contributed to a decrease in the cost of individual treatment per year from US$9,000 in 2000 to about US$5,000 in 2003 (online Mexican news agency *Notiese,* June 25, 2004). Yet there are still concerns regarding the persistently high prices of medications in Mexico, which in some cases are up to 30 times higher than in other countries with a similar level of per capita GDP (Mexican newspaper *La Jornada,* June 17, 2008).

Although the aim is to reach all those who need and want to be treated, to this day, not all patients have access to treatment. Because of lack of a proper health infrastructure and distribution problems, of the 90,043 registered cases of AIDS, only 28,600 have access to ARV treatment. Of those, IMSS treats 13,303 patients, while the secretary of health treats around

8,304 and ISSSTE about 2,388 (the remainder are treated privately). Even in the case of IMSS and ISSSTE, which are committed to providing treatment to all their respective affiliates, there are reports of lack of availability of ARVs and other drugs needed to treat HIV/AIDS patients. In fact, most cases of HIV/AIDS, up to 2009, were concentrated in the Federal District (DF) and the states of Baja California, Morelos, Nayarit, and Yucatán. The number of cases is registered and regularly updated by the Secretariat of Health on its website (http://www.ssa.gob.mx). These figures must be taken with some caution, since there is an underregistration of cases and the government privileges the registration of AIDS over HIV cases.

Another central element of an effective response to HIV/AIDS is the adoption of domestic legislative measures to guarantee individuals and communities access to effective judicial or other appropriate remedies in the face of human rights violations concerning their sexual health and sexuality or sexual identity. However, in Mexico, persistent problems in the administration of justice and the impunity of violators confirm the often-argued disconnect between the law and its observance (Panebianco, 2000; Reding, 1995). It must be acknowledged, however, that with increasing social pressure, some gains have been made in improving the country's legal framework for combating discrimination based on sexual identity or orientation and HIV status, especially at the federal level and in the Federal District (Mexico City). These include the aforementioned creation of the Human Rights Commission and the National Council to Prevent Discrimination (CONAPRED) on July 11, 2003, with the appointment of long-time activist and respected political figure Gilberto Rincón Gallardo as president until his recent death.

The pressures from various human rights groups and the HIV/AIDS policy network have also resulted in new legislation, such as the 2003 Federal Law to Prevent and Eliminate Discrimination (Ley Federal para Prevenir y Eliminar la Discriminación). For its part, and as a response to a concerted civil society lobbying campaign, the government of Mexico City (from the left-of-center Partido de la Revolución Democrática, PRD) introduced sexual orientation among the issues addressed in the July 2006 Law to Prevent and Eliminate Discrimination in the Federal District (Ley para Prevenir y Erradicar la Discriminación en el Distrito Federal), as well as created the Council for the Prevention and Elimination of Discrimination in the Federal District (Consejo para Prevenir y Erradicar la Discriminación en el Distrito Federal) in October 2006.

Related to these positive changes, first, in November 2006, the Federal District adopted the Law on Domestic Partnerships (Ley de Sociedades de Convivencia), which, though limited in its scope, allowed for legally recognized unions between same-sex partners (online Mexican news agency *Notiese,* 2006). A similar and more ambitious law was approved three months later by the legislature in the state of Coahuila (Del Collado, 2007). More recently though, the Federal District's local assembly voted 39–20 (on December 21, 2009) in favor of same-sex marriage, including the right to adopt, representing a major success for the advancement of equal rights for sexual minorities.

As we can see, and in spite of some of the risks associated with the close collaboration required between governmental and nongovernmental actors around the epidemic, there have been some positive outcomes. In particular, we have witnessed successful initiatives around human rights issues being brought forward, some of which go well beyond the more narrowly defined goals of HIV/AIDS and health-related policies. In fact, some NGOs and individuals (part of the HIV/AIDS policy network) have been able to strategically engage with the state, both at the federal and the state levels, and mobilize resources, while prioritizing their own agendas and retaining their character, advocating for the legal recognition and enforcement of more broadly defined sexual minorities' rights. The LGBT community elaborated a human rights discourse based on the notion of sexual health as a basic human right and built on the idea of legal entitlements of individuals before the state, other individuals, and institutions, which has been supported by the United Nations (UN) system. This discourse has been reinforced by the 2006 Yogyakarta principles on the application of international human rights legislation around sexual orientation and gender identity issues (see the 2006 Yogyakarta principles on the application of human rights to sexual orientation and sexual identity: http://www.yogyakartaprinciples.org/index.html). Furthermore, in the process of redefining the discursive field by adopting the human rights framework, civil society actors realized the need to establish direct relations with the official structures of the state, given that in the modern world, the enforcement of those rights (or the right to have rights) lies within the sphere of the state's protection (see Arendt, 1965).

## SOME ONGOING CHALLENGES

Although the emphasis so far has been on the specific accomplishments, we also need to point to some ongoing challenges. In fact, and not unlike other cases, in Mexico we can observe certain limitations to what NGOs can actually do, explained by what could be termed as the multidimensional axes of marginalization and the ongoing religious and conservative opposition to certain HIV/AIDS-related policies (for the case of Brazil, see Marsiaj, 2010). These limitations are also explained by the lack of state capacity in some areas and the aforementioned threats to movement autonomy, all of which, of course, are interconnected.

Unfortunately, as shown by Luis Manuel Arellano (2008) in his analysis of the ongoing stigma and discrimination associated with HIV/AIDS and nonheteronormative sexual identities and behaviors, and despite the official commitment against homophobia-driven crimes by public authorities, there are growing concerns regarding impunity. It must be stressed that the judicial system remains permissive and neglectful. Even though the creation and strengthening of the CNDH represented an important step, its investigations are mostly based on desk work, the responses are too lengthy, and there is a lack of legal tools to make its recommendations obligatory. For their part, the National Council to Prevent Discrimination (CONAPRED) confronts the challenge to create a network of offices at the regional and state levels, while the Secretariat of Education needs to do more in terms of incorporating sex education, human rights, gender equity, and antidiscriminatory content into the official curricula. All these factors contribute to explain the ongoing marginalization of a significant proportion of the affected population.

Discriminatory attitudes against HIV/AIDS patients and homophobic crimes have been extensively documented (González-Ruiz, 2002; Del Collado, 2007; Panebianco, 2000). For instance, according to statistics from the CNDH, more than 570 HIV/AIDS-related complaints were lodged with the commission between 1992 and 2006. The complaints centered on issues associated with homophobia and stigma, such as the alleged denial of adequate health services or medication for HIV/AIDS patients, acts of discrimination or negligence by medical personnel, and violations of confidentiality. Subsequently, the CNDH issued several recommendations to state and federal institutions, including hospitals, prisons, and educational facilities, requesting that they improve services for persons with HIV/AIDS. Most of the victims of human rights violations were MSM. Thus a civil society response to this reality was the creation of the Citizens' Commission against Homophobic Hate Crimes (La Comisión Ciudadana contra los Crímenes de Odio por Homofobia, or CCCCOH), on May 6, 1998 (Del Collado, 2007).

For the most part, there has been a lack of reliable statistical information on the level of discrimination against homosexuals in Mexico. However, in August 2005, CONAPRED presented a survey prepared jointly with the federal secretary for social development (SEDESOL). The study was based on 1,482 interviews with members of the general public and 200 self-identified homosexuals. According to the study, 94.7 percent of Mexican homosexuals face some degree of discrimination. Díaz Betancourt, who at the time was coordinator of programs on discrimination based on sexual orientation at CONAPRED (also involved in the negotiations of the World Bank loan), noted that negative public attitudes against homosexuals and HIV/AIDS patients persist, particularly in smaller urban centers and in rural areas (personal interview with Arturo Díaz Betancourt, Mexico City, September 10, 2002).

As a response to CONAPRED's survey results and the coordinated efforts of the HIV/AIDS policy network, the right-of-center federal government of Fox launched a national radio campaign against homophobia in 2005. The campaign, which was very explicit and challenged traditional conceptions, was organized by CONAPRED and CENSIDA with full support from the national Secretariat of Health and financial support from the Pan-American Health Organization and UNAIDS (Mexican newspaper *La Jornada,* March 23, 2005; for a transcript of the actual campaign see Saavedra, 2007a; Torres-Ruiz, 2011). The very launch of the campaign points to the surprising effectiveness of the policy network to work within a PAN administration, given that, in the case of Mexico, sexual minorities seem to have traditionally benefited from their alliance to and participation in a more progressive political front (De la Dehesa, 2007). However, religious and conservative opposition remains strong, as seen in the most recent campaign on the use of condoms, "Un condón es más confinable que el destino" (A condom is more reliable than fate), and the aggressive response of conservative groups against it (see E-consulta.com, July 16, 2012).

When it comes to state capacity and accessibility to services and treatment, one of the main challenges faced by health authorities is the detection of the virus, given that, as pointed out recently at the 2012 AIDS Conference in Washington, to this day in Mexico as in other parts of the world, most of those infected ignore that they are HIV carriers. Additionally, in order to make HAART available for treatment and as a prevention measure, the capacity of the CENSIDA's Ambulatory Centers (CAPASITS) mentioned above must be improved (see also Julio Montaner's op-ed in the Canadian newspaper *The Globe and Mail,* "The end of SIDA? We have the tools," of July 30, 2012, available online: http://www.theglobeandmail .com/commentary/the-end-of-aids-we-have-the-tools/article4445109/). Although they do have the technical expertise to fulfill their task, they are presently functional in only 10 states, and they lack the required sensibility training to attract and retain the target populations. Similarly, the state-level AIDS programs (COESIDAS) present serious limitations, both in terms of budgets and regarding the appointment of officials who do not have the necessary knowledge and experience. Another major challenge, when it comes to the necessary financial resources to cover for universal access to treatment, lies in the funding mechanism in place. As stated above, the money comes from the Federal Fund for Catastrophic Health Expenses, which is meant to cover all sorts of other emergency expenses. Thus, the funding for ARVs is not yet completely guaranteed, suggesting the need to create an AIDS-specific budget.

Last, some concerns have been raised about the preferential treatment to some NGOs, hinting again at the risk of some form of corporatism and pointing to the lack of clear accountability mechanisms. The most recent scandal involved the Circuito de la Diversidad Sexual (Cidisex, Sexual Diversity Circuit), whose leadership has been accused by fellow activists of misappropriation of public funds (see *Notiese,* July 25, 2012: http://www .notiese.org/notiese.php?ctn_id=5823). This could also result in NGOs losing some autonomy and taking unfair advantages from their own positioning. Thus, the need at the CENSIDA level to put in place mechanisms that could lead to greater transparency in the relations with the civil society side of the HIV/AIDS policy network and some evaluation mechanisms for the performance of governmental actions. These improvements could help shed light on the processes of recognition or exclusion of concrete NGOs and other civil society groups.

## CONCLUSIONS: NOT SO SCANDALOUS AFTER ALL?

In assessing the challenges faced for the foreseeable future, and based on the analysis of the recent history of civil society's involvement in the process of HIV/AIDS public policymaking in Mexico, it is possible to reach different conclusions about the process of NGO-ization. On the one hand, it could be argued that we have seen a successful push for a more democratic policymaking process, which has been a consequence of the effective organization and professionalization of social movements. On the other, there might be some observers who will continue to warn us about the detrimental impact on the autonomy of civil society and consider this process of NGO-ization as nothing more than a new way of corporatization or cooptation. Without taking sides and acknowledging the soundness of some of those critiques, it must be recognized that some of the key and positive developments witnessed in recent years could not be explained without the active participation of those NGO-ized actors, and we would not do them justice by trying to obscure their positive and constructive role. Having said that, it is also important to recognize that risks do exist and that attempts to silence critical views by cooptation and other means will continue to represent a challenge to the autonomy of social groups vis-à-vis government authorities.

Based on the evidence, I would also argue that the opening of the policymaking process can hardly be characterized as a top-down one. In fact, with the victory of a right-of-center government at the federal level, most observers predicted an ideological rejection of the previous HIV/AIDS-related policies by PAN's presidents Vicente Fox and Felipe Calderón. However, and against such predictions, members of the HIV/AIDS policy network managed to work at the federal level with PAN and at the state level with the other two main political parties (PRI and PRD). Thus, the recent history of HIV/AIDS policies in Mexico shows how some observers often underestimate the capacity of civil society actors to keep a healthy distance from governments and successfully influence policy. In a way, and paraphrasing Alejandro Brito, the construction of the policy network and its collaboration with the government might be considered a sign of maturity and tolerance on all counts (Frasca, 2005).

Together with other recent analyses of HIV/AIDS at the global level, the Mexican case helps to confirm an early prediction made by Dennis Altman (2001), in the sense that the epidemic served as a catalyst for the visibility of LGBT groups with their subsequent participation in public policymaking (De la Dehesa, 2010; Torres-Ruiz, 2011). Moreover, the creation of domestic and international policy networks has led to some democratic openings and increasing representativeness, especially when contrasted with cliques dominating other health policy fields. In contrast, policy networks working on health care financing are characterized by being less inclusive, with a relatively small and tightly integrated group of policymakers, technical advisers, economists, and scholars who define the content and process of policy reform (Lee and Goodman, quoted. in Merson, Black, & Mills, 2001). In other words, the professionalization of HIV/AIDS activism and their reframing of HIV/AIDS-related policies within a human rights discourse represented a strategic move that has empowered civil society groups politically engaged in the fight against the epidemic and discrimination against sexual minorities. Ultimately, under a human rights approach, policy networks have made clear that becoming healthy and remaining so is not merely a medical, technical, or economic problem but also a question of social justice and concrete government obligations.

Although there is an ongoing contrast between de jure and de facto citizenship, as shown by the persistence of homophobic crimes, the gains made so far must be recognized for their concrete and symbolic importance, the consolidation of which will depend on the capacity and will of the state to make those reforms effective.

Further scrutiny of the increasing role of civil society organizations and their close engagement with state agencies represents an analytical challenge for those of us interested in better understanding the long-term effects of NGO-ization. In developing a prospective analysis, contemporary sociological considerations of politicized identities and their function in public life might help us in understanding HIV/AIDS and sexual minorities' activism. As argued by Bhambra and Magree (2010), among others, the politicized identities of some individuals or groups are social constructions that respond to the need to mobilize in order to overcome structural sociopolitical and economic barriers for full participation in the public sphere. One of the central goals of the assertion of those identities in the public sphere is the construction of more inclusive and democratic futures in conversation with other actors. They further argue that such identities tend to weaken when the conditions that originated their politicization disappear, which forces us to identify the ongoing circumstances that continue to justify the mobilization of HIV/AIDS and sexual minorities' organizations and their active engagement with the state. In this case, some individuals and groups were already politicized before, yet they went through a process of professionalization or NGO-ization, with a change of orientations or a broadening of their agendas once the epidemic hit. Others were created as a direct response to it. Here I want to point out that in analyzing their engagement with the state, it is useful to consider Judith Butler's (2002) contention that public institutions make us desire the state's desire, in the sense that for activists, as for most other citizens, it is often hard to resist the narrative of the state, with the risk of being fooled and suddenly finding themselves being caught up in the same game of neoliberal discourses and structures. Yet, as stated above for the case of Mexico, there seem to be some NGOs and individuals who work on HIV/AIDS who have been able to keep some distance from the state's narratives with a focus on their own strategic and long-term goals.

The challenge though, as Jessop (1990, p. 10) reminds us, for individuals and NGOs lies in finding ways to negotiate the terms of entry into public life, since a given type of state and regime will be more accessible to some according to the strategies they adopt. Thus, NGO-ization can be seen as a process equivalent to an attempt by social movements to participate as "free citizens" in the elaboration of alternative discourses. In the case of Mexico and HIV/AIDS-related policies, the fact that some offices within government have been created and penetrated by some civil society organizations and activists might serve as evidence of how the state itself is being reshaped or reconstituted (metamorphosed) by the ways in which governmental actors and activists interact in the process of government. This case can also help us recognize the fact that it is actual individuals who belong to some of these different organizations and who join and position themselves within certain key departments or public bodies, which makes it impossible for them not to bring other dimensions of their identities to their functions as officials, and in the process, help transform or reshape, even if only partially, the same state they end up being part of.

Seriously considering activists' protagonist role in the promotion of a new approach and a set of policies, together with the ongoing challenges, might allow us to draw more nuanced conclusions about the current state of, and prospects for, the struggles confronted by the HIV/AIDS community. Contrary to early warnings regarding their lack of autonomy, we have seen a kind of hybrid character of some of those HIV/AIDS and sexual minorities' NGOs, whereby they engage as both experts and critics of the status quo. Or as put by Colombian feminist and sociologist Magdalena León (as cited in Álvarez, 2009, p. 178), they have been mainstreamed and sidestreamed, spreading horizontally, becoming a veritable tangle of networks ("un enredo de redes")—both formal and informal, which in the case of HIV/AIDS allows them to keep what I would like to refer to as two different fronts or two pathways. Along these lines and in an honest revision of her own critical formulations on the NGO-ization of the feminist movement in Latin America, Sonia Álvarez (2009) has more recently acknowledged that the effects of civil society groups' professionalization are not so clear-cut. Thus, Álvarez acknowledges the hybrid character of many NGOs, arguing that although they have established a formal structure on paper, this does not always correspond with the continuing informal and flexible structures shown by many of them. So that often, what we have is a formal or a more bureaucratic structure side by side with another more "real" and flexible one of the social movement. Moreover, she asserts that the data and analysis generated by NGOs have provided vital foundations for more effective advocacy in a variety of settings, mobilizing ideas and not just people (Álvarez, 2009, p. 178), effectively promoting rights at the local level through the use of global resources.

Similarly, for the case of HIV/AIDS in Mexico, what we have is a tangle of international and domestic networks, with doctors and activists in key positions within CENSIDA, PAHO, the International Aids Society (IAS), and UNAIDS, some of which also work hand in hand with NGOs and social movements. They do engage with governments or the state in order to influence public policy, while at the same time some among them continue their support for social action and mobilization. Thus the image of two pathways or two fronts: one along expertise on sexual health and HIV/AIDS and the other along sexual minorities' rights. Although it could be argued that the engaged front is more "well-behaved" than the other one, which tends to be more confrontational or combative, both are joined by the human rights discourse. Also, these two pathways or fronts have simultaneously developed at both the national and the global levels. More concretely, we have witnessed the positioning of some gay activists within national and international bodies engaged in the fight against the epidemic, which resulted in the empowerment of the LGBT community at large. This is similar to what Keck and Sikkink (1998) have called the "boomerang effect," which is used to show how domestic and transnational social movements unite to bring pressure from above and from below on national governments to accomplish human rights change. This resulted in a set of HIV/AIDS policies that was more responsive to the demands of the most affected, which has been defined by increased budgets for prevention and universal coverage. These inroads in the public sphere then led to antidiscrimination legislation against homophobia and mistreatment of HIV/AIDS patients, even under two consecutive socially conservative PAN administrations in Mexico. Furthermore, they resulted in the passing of legislation in favor of same-sex marriage and adoption in Mexico City. Thus, it can be argued that the professionalization of some civil society groups has had some very concrete and positive effects, giving continuity to HIV/AIDS policies.

Obviously, some challenges remain. First of all, it is necessary to consider whether it will be possible to maintain those two fronts or pathways. In other words, will it be possible to consolidate the position, visibility, access, and influence achieved so far without neglecting the centrality of the concerns of the larger community or social groups that developed and adopted the politicized identities that allowed their mobilization in the first place? In this regard, the nature of the LGBT community as a minority makes it hard to think of a radical change in circumstances, so that it would be unnecessary to keep a united front, despite class issues and other differences. An emphasis on monitoring and contestation will also continue to be indispensable. The challenge will be to criticize the government and other institutions without risking funding and support. These activities are indispensable in order to secure the actual implementation of hard-won policy gains, which requires further public pressure, not only through policy monitoring but also aiming at deeper or broader changes in public opinion and attitudes toward sexual minorities. This might also require a stronger engagement with counter-hegemonic spaces, which may prompt some NGOs to move away from the project-centered logic fueled by NGO-ization and back toward a process-oriented logic, which is more fluid, open-ended, and continuous, though not linear, with the aim to reform legal and cultural codes.

So far, it might be argued that through being contentiously entangled with national and global struggles in favor of human rights associated with sexual and social justice, HIV/AIDS and sexual minorities' activists have in fact contributed to the knowledge production and discourse around the epidemic. As such, we might also be able to argue that their NGO-ization is not so scandalous after all. However, it is also clear that we must continue to investigate and problematize the genealogy and development of NGOs in order to offer sounder prospective analyses of the effects of their engagement with the state on the construction of a vibrant and more democratic public sphere.

## ACKNOWLEDGMENTS

I want to acknowledge the invaluable help of journalist and HIV/AIDS expert Gabriel García-Gutiérrez as a research assistant in Mexico.

## BIBLIOGRAPHY

Aguayo-Quezada, S., & Parra-Rosales, L. P. (1997). *Las organizaciones no gubernamentales de derechos humanos en México: Entre la democracia participativa y la electoral.* Mexico: Academia Mexicana de Derechos Humanos.

Altman, D. (2001). *Global Sex.* Chicago: University of Chicago Press.

Álvarez, S. E. (2009). Beyond NGO-ization? Reflections from Latin America. *Development, 52* (2), 175–184.

Álvarez, S. E., Dagnino, E., & Escobar, A. (1998). *Cultures of Politics, Politics of Cultures: Re-Visioning Latin American Social Movements.* Boulder, CO: Westview Press.

Arellano, L. M. (2008). *Estigma y discriminación a personas con VIH.* Mexico: CONAPRED.

Arendt, H. (1965). *Eichmann in Jerusalem.* New York: Penguin Books.

Barglow, R. (1998). The Angel of History: Walter Benjamin's Vision of Hope and Despair. Tikkun Magazine; November.

Bhambra, G. K., & Margree, V. (2010, April 10). Identity Politics and the Need for a "Tomorrow." *Economic & Political Weekly,* xlv (15).

Brito-Lemus, A. (2003, June 5). Por el derecho a todos los derechos. Mexico: *Letra S.*

Butler, J. (2002). Is kinship always heterosexual? *Differences: A Journal of Feminist Cultural Studies,* 13(1), 14–44.

Castells, M. (1996). *The Rise of the Network Society.* London: Blackwell.

Dani, A. A.., & Varshney, A. (2012). *Citizenship, Governance, and Social Policy in the Developing World.* Washington, D.C.: World Bank.

De la Dehesa, R. (2010). *Queering the Public Sphere in Mexico and Brazil: Sexual Movements in Emerging Democracies.* Duke University Press.

Del Collado, F. (2007). *Homofobia: Odio, crimen y justicia, 1995–2005.* Mexico: Tusquets Editores.

Farmer, P. (2003). *Pathologies of Power: Health, Human Rights, and the New War on the Poor.* Berkeley: University of California Press.

Frasca, T. (2005). *AIDS in Latin America.* New York: Palgrave Macmillan.

Galván, F. (coord.) (1988). *El Sida en México: los efectos sociales.* Mexico: Ediciones de Cultura Popular, UAM Azcapotzalco.

García-Murcia, M., Andrade-Briseño, M., Maldonado-Arroyo, R., & Morales-Escobar, C. (2010). *Memoria de la Lucha contra el VIH en México.* México: Historiadores de las Ciencias y las Humanidades A.C., Consejo Nacional para Prevenir la Discriminación.

Giddens, A. (1990). *The Consequences of Modernity.* Cambridge, U.K.: Polity Press.

González-Martin, F. (1996). HIV/AIDS and Human Rights in Mexico. *Human Rights Brief,* 3(3), 16. Washington, D.C.: Center for Human Rights and Humanitarian Law at Washington College of Law, American University.

González Ruiz, E. (2002). *La sexualidad prohibida: Intolerancia, sexismo y represión.* Mexico City: Plaza y Janés.

Held, D. (1999). *Global Transformations: Politics, Economics and Culture.* Cambridge, U.K.: Polity Press.

Held, D., McGrew, A., Goldblatt, D., & J. Perraton, J. (1997). The Globalization of Economic Activity. *New Political Economy,* 2 (2), 2557–2577.

Hewitt de Alcántara, C. (1998). Uses and Abuses of the Concept of Governance. *International Social Science Journal,* 155, 105–114.

Howse, R., & Nicolaidis, K. (2003). Enhancing WTO Legitimacy: Constitutionalization or Global Subsidiarity. *Governance,* 16 (1): 73–94.

Jessop, B. (1990). *State Theory. Putting the Capitalist State in Its Place.* Cambridge: Polity Press.

Keck, M. E., & Sikkink, K. (1998). *Activists beyond Borders: Advocacy Networks in International Politics.* Ithaca, NY: Cornell University Press.

Marsiaj, J. P. (2010). NGOization of Civil Society and Social Movement Impact: The Case of the Lesbians, Gay, Bisexual and Travesti Movement in Brazil. Toronto, Canada: Paper prepared for delivery at the 2010 Meeting of the Latin American Studies Association (LASA, October 6–9).

Merson, M. H., Black, R. E., & Mills, A. J. (2001). *International Public Health: Diseases, Programs, Systems and Policies.* Gaithersburg, MD: Aspen.

Monsiváis, C. (1996). El Sida y el sentido de urgencia. In M. Platts, *Sida: Aproximaciones éticas.* Mexico: UNAM, IIF, FCE.

Panebianco, S. (2000). Salud y justicia: Hecha la ley, hecha la trampa—Respetos formales y violaciones reales de los derechos humanos en VIH/SIDA, en América Latina. *Fórum 2000:* 814.

Reding, A. (1995). *Democracy and Human Rights in Mexico.* New York: World Policy Institute.

Ryfman, P. (2004). Les ONG. Paris: La Découverte.

Saavedra, J. (2007a). Homofobia: Alcances y limitaciones en los servicios de salud. In C. & D. Soberón (eds.), *Homofobia y salud* (87–94). Mexico City: Comisión Nacional de Bioética, Secretaría de Salud.

Saavedra, J. (2007b). Mexico: Situation of Witnesses to Crime and Corruption, Women Victims of Violence and Victims of Discrimination Based on Sexual Orientation. *Issue Paper.* Mexico City: CONASIDA.

Saavedra, J., Izazola, J. A., Prottas, J., & Shepard, D. S. (1999). Costs and Expenditures for AIDS Medical Care in Mexico. Working Paper. Mexico City: SIDALAC.

Sepúlveda, J., Bronfman, M., Ruiz Palacios, G., Stanislawski, E., & Valdespino, J. L. (1989). *SIDA, ciencia y sociedad en México.* Mexico City: Secretaría de Salud, Instituto Nacional de Salud Pública, Fondo de Cultura Económica.

Soberón, G., & Izazola, J. A. (1996). El Sida a 13 años de su aparición en México. *Gaceta Médica de México,* 132(1). Mexico City: Instituto Nacional de Salud Pública.

Torres-Ruiz, A. (2006). Nuevos Retos y Oportunidades en un Mundo Globalizado: Análisis Político de la Respuesta al VIH/SIDA en México. *História, Ciencias, Saude,* 13(3). Manguinhos, Brazil.

Torres-Ruiz, A. (2011). HIV/AIDS and Sexual Minorities in Mexico: A Globalized Struggle for the Protection of Human Rights. *Latin American Research Review,* 46 (1).

Torres-Ruiz, A., & Clarkson, S. (2009). The Globalized Complexities of Transborder Governance in North America. In J. Ayres & L. Macdonald, (eds.), *Contentious Politics in North America: National Protest and Transnational Collaboration under Continental Integration* (pp. 155–176). New York: Palgrave Macmillan.

World Trade Organization (2001). Declaration on the TRIPS Agreement and Public Health. *Doha WTO Ministerial Conference,* Fourth Session, November 14, Geneva.

Yúdice, G. (2003). *The Expediency of Culture: Uses of Culture in the Global Era.* Durham, NC: Duke University Press.

# 14

# Children, HIV, Stigma, and Activism in the UK: Treading the Line between Innocence and Vulnerability, Vice and Virtue

*Richard Boulton*

In 2012 the UK charity Body and Soul started an advertising campaign, Life in My Shoes, aimed at reducing the stigma faced by young people with HIV (Body & Soul, 2011). The campaign comprises a series of high-profile celebrity portraits, initiated by the photographer Rankin, accompanied by a 30-minute short film, *Undefeated,* about the types of prejudice that young people with HIV have reportedly faced. An initial newspaper account about the campaign published in the *Guardian* was optimistic about the result this will have on public attitudes toward young people with HIV (Day, 2011). The stance of the article emphasizes the negative profile of HIV and the ensuing stigma that exists as a result, and then contrasts it against a backdrop of adolescent, teenage life that is presented as incompatible. The scene that is painted makes lucid some of the factors that compel adolescents to live and experience HIV adhering to strict confidentiality and secrecy. In terms of activism, children with HIV must negotiate a whole range of negative associations before being able to engage in an activist organization designed to bring about change in relation to HIV. Accordingly, beyond questions of visibility, profile, and latent ideas of innocence, the associations at work that adolescents and their families react to are implicated in the already outcast, foreign identity of patients (Mahajan et al., 2008). The majority of those with the condition in the UK are of African descent, which when added to connotations of HIV around illicit sex and drug abuse work against the ideals of family and childhood (CHIPS, 2011), but the example is relevant to other populations where HIV is present. The context of secrecy, shame, and confidentiality is the scenario that the Body & Soul campaign is launched into. This has many broad implications, but in this chapter I will question the tension between children's unwillingness to associate themselves to HIV and the resulting forms of activism that are present for young people with HIV, who must navigate dynamics of stigma, secrecy, and confidentiality. It will be argued that for this reason all forms of possible activism must be adapted to these accounts of negative stigma and take them as a central concern limiting the ways in which young people with HIV wish to engage in activism.

This chapter will contemplate ideas of stigma linked to examples of HIV organizations and popular representations of children with HIV to consider how it relates to patients engaging (or not) in activism and forming activist groups. The first section takes on ideas of stigma formed in classical sociology and develops it with the light use of the Actor Network Theory (hereafter referred to in the broader parent discipline of Science, Technology, and Society, STS), developed over recent years that emphasizes the emergence of reality through the semiotic-material associations between objects and agency. This investigation is framed around contemporary examples of HIV stigma and associations of childhood that contrast notions of innocence and vulnerability against those of vice and immorality. It is argued that this creates an antagonism in the concept of stigma and results in a dynamic not easily addressed within traditional models of activism. The second half of the chapter discusses this alternative activism engaged in by organizations on behalf of children and families that emphasizes the right of families to live out their HIV in confidentiality. The conclusion argues that the campaign of Body & Soul can be seen as a reaction to the dynamics of a community whose members have subverted visibility of their condition and find it necessary to prioritize their secrecy over their liberties.

## CHILDREN, HIV, AND STIGMA

Before discussing activism in relation to children with HIV it will be useful to identify what kinds of stigma are relevant to the condition of children with HIV in order to make it possible to link HIV stigma to activism. One of the most obvious examples of a medical condition suffering from negative stigma would probably be that of the Spastics Society and the strange interplay around changing the name to SCOPE in 1994. In the lead-up to this name change, the charity cited that the name *spastic* had long been associated with a negative stigma that was detrimental to the brand, causing volunteers, donors, and parents/children to disassociate from the brand (SCOPE, 2001). If we examine this case to see if there are any similarities with pediatric HIV, an anecdote comes to mind that professionals working in pediatric HIV would share with me during fieldwork. I was often told during research that children in the playground would taunt and tease each other with the word *spastic* and that children today no longer use the word *spastic* but say "you've got AIDS." It's hard to compare directly the stigma around the word *spastic* (or the resulting derogatory terms *spacker* or *spaz*) in the 1980s and 1990s with the stigma of HIV and AIDS today, but it is tempting to consider how this model of reducing stigma could prove to be prevalent to the question of how to reduce the stigma associated with HIV (see stigma scale, Berger et al., 2001). One effect the name change had was that the word *spastic* has been erased from popular English usage and has consequently reduced the visibility of the condition and made the use of the word unacceptable outside of a medical context. This ensured that future generations would not take the stigma further and that the figure once stigmatized was subjected to the past. It is not a giant leap of the imagination, therefore, to arrive at the question of whether or not it is possible to attempt the same thing with HIV. One of the self-professed aims of the director of the film *Life in My Shoes* is to address this stigma:

> It was important to counterbalance all the very dark images that came out a few years ago from films like *Philadelphia* and ads that showed people dying. The images that came out a few years ago were depressing, but when you meet the teens at Body & Soul, they're full of life, and we thought it was important to show that. We wanted to do something that challenged the stigma. (Tudor-Payne, cited in Day, 2011)

One glancing look highlights a precursory difference between *spasticity* and HIV, however. The term *spastic* seemed to be so loaded upon an imaginary figure that when official references to it disappeared from the high-street charity shop and were discouraged in the playground, the reference died down. What it was replaced with in the popular imagination was the more complicated and involuntary condition of cerebral palsy, which is more subdued and less prone to name-calling. In contrast, it would be difficult to imagine that if the name HIV were changed, it would have the same effect. Discussions exist around whether the term *AIDS* should be disassociated from HIV, which could arguably address stigma or promote advocacy

(Rintamaki, 2009). Or we can see a quite clear challenge to a stigmatizing term with the effacing of the term *gay-related immunodeficiency* (GRID). Therefore, the way the term is labeled has already been central to activist activities (see Rule & Vaughn, 2008). However, even if we acknowledge that there are important considerations in how HIV should be labeled, within HIV there has been a bombardment of imagery from the 1980s onward about all sorts of associated vice, not to mention that in terms of pediatric HIV the population in the UK is overwhelmingly of African descent that seems to give HIV a set of negative associations beyond its phraseology (79 percent were black African according to CHIPS summary data; CHIPS, 2011). Accounts from organizations such as Body & Soul have strived over successive years to counter and rationalize imaginations of HIV that make it into the public domain, but find it difficult to get away from negative connotations such as illicit sex, drug abuse, and immigration. Contrary to Tudor-Payne's idea of images of dying, there is a much more sinister set of associations connected to HIV stigma around choice and consequence, deservedness and culpability. Children with HIV are often seen as innocent victims of the disease who were unable to make HIV prevention choices to ensure that they would not become infected (Fassin, 2008). The inherent negative representations of sex, drugs, and immigration associated with HIV have their own well-tread history, and HIV activism in its various forms already has a long engagement with challenging these negative stereotypes as they come up. There is a prevailing trend in the analysis and theory of HIV that has taken as its subject these stereotypes and their relationship to politics and policy (Patton, 1991; Treichler, 1999). What is less developed, however, is how this stigma is altered when considering children with HIV. Discourses around children with HIV tend to bring into play associations of children being undeserving of the disease, not guilty of the act that would usually lead to the disease, or of child innocence obscuring the roots of activism among children themselves (Fassin, 2008). An example of these connotations of deservedness can be found in the British sitcom *Him & Her.* The situation unfolds as three of the principal characters are discussing money when waiting to watch an accumulated jackpot rollover draw in the national lottery. They have all bought tickets and anticipate winning, when the question is brought up: what would they spend the money on? Laura, whose character profile is painted as superficial and often conceited, replies:

> **Laura:** Me and Julie were saying that we're going to give some of our winnings to a charity.

**Shelly:** Oh yeah, if I could, I'd give all my money to the pandas.
**Laura:** Not me, I'd give mine to kids with AIDS.
**Shelly:** Oh, I love kids with AIDS.
**Laura:** I saw a thing about them, I mean they've got AIDS so I don't want to meet them, but it's not their fault if their mums are slags. (Laxton, 2011)

This example may be designed as satire and so caution must be placed as to how far these views can be projected to the wider world. The role of satire, however, is to ridicule the faults of engrained cultural attitudes; in this case what is highlighted is a dangerous public prejudice, that of nondeserving, nonculpability, and innocence between parents and children with HIV.

The identification of innocence around conceptions of childhood and chronic illness has already been the subject of a number of studies (see essays in Prout, 2000; Christensen, 2000; alternatively see Clark, 2003; Mayall, 1998). However, the setup encountered here, which mixes innocence with stigma, alters profoundly what both childhood innocence and stigma are considered to be (this has already been highlighted in studies documenting the overexposure of AIDS orphans in relation to families living with the disease; see Fassin, 2008; Henderson, 2006; Stephney & Deacon, 2007). If Goffman's (1968) famous categorization of stigma is brought into the discussion, a dilemma is highlighted that renders the application of conventional ideas of stigma more complicated. The premise that Goffman offers argues that stigma is an attribute that has been classified as undesirable, which results in individuals possessing the attribute to be associated with a negative, rejected stereotype rather than a normal, accepted one. As the interplay of stigma in relation to children with HIV is indirect and seems to relate to a large number of interrelations and extraneous factors (identity, ethnicity, sexuality, infection route), the chapter would rather like to invite a way of understanding stigma inspired by STS that invites analysis that expressly considers the interplay taking place between larger numbers of associations, such as those of innocence, vulnerability, vice, and virtue.

For the sociologically familiar reader, the argument would like to put forward the idea here that there is not one single version or mechanism that leads to stigma, but many possible associations that interact with each other differently to produce stigma. The classical way of approaching stigma stemming from Goffman seems to suggest that stigma is a sort of entity that exists between people and their relationship with the outside world.

Consider, however, that stigma is not something out there in the world, but rather it is part of the identity of a person and has a performative aspect that depends on what aspects of an individual are presented at a given time. Neither identity, stigma, nor their wider associations are categories that can be located outside of the contexts where they are referred to. Each one must be understood as performing together alongside the specificities of the situation that generates a stigma. Therefore, stigma is not one object over many situations, but has many different versions dependent upon the context of where it is performed (see Law, 1999).

Within the idea of stigma at work around children with HIV (or "kids with AIDS" as referred to in *Him & Her,* or a number of other manifestations we could pose), however, we can find elements of the stigma that would usually apply generally to HIV, but it is also displaced by the notion that children with the condition are *innocent victims,* or are not *responsible* for the lot they have been given, or don't *deserve* the condition they have been afflicted with (Fassin, 2008). The outcome is that when applied to childhood, the usual stigma of HIV is still present but it becomes altered by associations of innocence, resulting in a stigma that generates shame on the one hand and deservedness on the other. Therefore, stigma in this instance is not just the application of a negative stereotype but the interaction of a range of shifting associations and values. Consequently, the stigma faced by children with HIV is inherently different from the stigma faced by the Spastic Society and requires a different approach to confront it (see the specificities of stigma described by Melvin, 2007). The Body & Soul campaign is not neutral in relation to this, which can be seen in the quote of Tudor-Payne noted above. Regardless of whether or not the producers are conscious of these associations, in order to challenge preconceptions and stimulate activism, Body & Soul must attempt to offer an account that engages with connotations of stigma and innocence (Bhana & Epstein, 2007).

These undertones even extend to charities and the inception of charitable organizations. The Children with AIDS Charity (CWAC) was formed in 1992 around St. Mary's Specialist Paediatric HIV Service London, the first such specialist department in the UK, which was established shortly before in 1991. On the CWAC website under the description of CWAC history, the text describes how the charity was conceived by Rebecca Handel, whose daughter Bonnie was being cared for at St. Mary's.

> Together with the paediatric team of St. Mary's they decided to start a charity that could respond to the specific practical, emotional and

educational requirements of children and their families infected and affected by HIV. (CWAC, 2011)

In one plain passage in the text a clear reference to innocence is made:

Being white, middle-class and Jewish, Rebecca shattered all HIV-positive stereotypes, having become infected with HIV through a blood transfusion in her second pregnancy, before blood was screened for the virus. (CWAC, 2011)

The story had a far-reaching effect in British society; its newsworthiness was affirmed in 1996 when it became the subject of an ITV news documentary (Wilcox, 1996). Interlaced in the history of the charity is a connotation that children are innocent and do not deserve to have the disease that consequently spreads out to influence the basis and *raison d'être* of the whole organization. Among the charity's activities today it still lists a direct engagement with stigma and discrimination through the organization of an education program that arranges workshops for children in interested schools. Consequently, we can relate this to some of the associations that inspired the satire taken up in *Him & Her*.

This chapter does not wish to detract from the valuable work these organizations carry out, which also has a vital contribution to identifying and challenging HIV stigma. However, now that this element of deserving has been highlighted, it becomes possible to pose the question in relation to activism: what possibilities can be achieved through going down the path of deserving? When framing the need for benevolence for children with HIV, reasoning with associations of child culpability makes a contrast between innocent children on the one hand, and those who have acquired HIV in ways befitting the established stigma on the other. At one fell swoop it affirms the shamefulness of sexual transmission by distancing it from children who got the disease without engaging in what could be seen as a risky behavior, and it also places blame upon the mother who has *irresponsibly* conceived the child, assuming in the process that the mother contracted the disease conscious of the risk. When identified, the connotations found in this setup can be deemed to be reckless (as can also be seen from the exasperation of those trying to provide sex education to children at risk of HIV; Bhana, 2007; Campbell et al., 2009; Mitchell et al., 2004). This type of reasoning negates personal circumstance, casts unnecessary judgment, and most importantly sets families against one another by introducing an element of contention and blame between child and mother and often father and mother. Although the examples given here should be considered as nuanced and not wholly representative of attitudes toward children with HIV, we can see ways in which it feeds into a politics of blame and HIV criminalization (which is already an issue under heavy contestation; Shevory, 2004).

## IMPLICATIONS OF STIGMA ON ACTIVISM

The implications of how this stigma manifests in the lifestyle of families, practices in the clinic, the activities of HIV organizations, and activism are far-reaching. During research that I carried out in a pediatric clinic in north London at North Middlesex University Hospital (NMUH), it emerged that confidentiality was valued as one of the most important aspects of care, and as a result the organization of services and medicine would be carried out by practitioners to fulfil the requirement for secrecy (see Wiener et al., 2007, for disclosure techniques that rely on confidentiality). From an early age children with HIV are educated in the clinic about the disease and what information it is best not to share with others. In accordance with this, any medicines and services required in treating the virus are designed to be easily concealed. Children and parents would be recommended not to tell the school they attend of their status. If the question arose, parents would refer the principal to the pediatric consultant, who would confirm the need for medical attention without mentioning the condition HIV. Children with HIV are strongly advised not to let their friends know, and when telling siblings they are warned to display the utmost caution. Stigma is not only feared and prevented against in the clinic but can be seen as actively being a factor in decision-making processes and in adjusting the way HIV care is maintained for children. As presented in the Life in My Shoes campaign by Tudor-Payne, it is not just a question of image but is much more implicated in the ways that families and services act out HIV.

For many such families in the UK, the effect of HIV is only one among many other typecasts. Pediatric HIV in the UK has developed a particular profile associated with those coming from Africa in environments with high exposure to HIV and limited prevention and care resources (Swendeman et al., 2006) (CHIPS data designates the overwhelming majority of pediatric HIV cases, 79 percent, to be associated with African ethnicity). This raises a number of potential issues that immigrants must already face when arriving in the UK. For example, individuals may have complex personal reasons to want to emigrate, or an individual may be habituated to a different set of attitudes. Also, there is often a web of related people left behind or between borders, resulting in a protracted discourse between individuals and the UK Border Agency. Individuals may struggle to secure the necessities of life and may find it hard to integrate into new communities and navigate the uncertain gaze that wider society has toward recent migrants. Therefore, we can see that there are already a lot of factors that manifest themselves in the everyday activities of these populations before getting to specific considerations about HIV (see Melvin & Sherr, 1995; Hekster & Melvin, 2006 for a description of the London cohort). At NMUH during regular consultations the pediatric consultant would often have to write letters to the Border Agency, offer recommendations or advice, interpreters were often required, and the clinical specialist nurse would help with benefit claims. In addition to having an impact on care, these considerations make their way to the core of the activities of charities set up to help children and families dealing with HIV. Positive Parenting and Children (PPC) is a group set up in south London when there are, first, a high proportion of communities of African descent and, second, a community with a high rate of mother and child HIV (PPC, 2012a,b). The aims of PPC are to offer support to parents and children infected and affected by HIV. In essence, PPC organizes identified members into a community and arranges initiatives for children and parents to come together. For a number of weeks I visited the organization and witnessed some of the difficulties that PPC is structured to alleviate. One such reaction was the Family Project set up explicitly to offer

> a collaborative initiative that aims to reduce the impact of secrecy and stigma on families living with HIV, facilitate more comprehensive and earlier testing for undiagnosed children, improve family communication on HIV, sex and relationships and ensure that families receive support using the best possible practice models and methods.

This resulted in the development of

> a series of resources for communication and talking about HIV within families called "It's Good Talk.". Underpinned by research and evidence-based good practice, it has been shaped and informed by parents, young people and practitioners across the UK. (PPC, 2012a,b)

As already stated, what we can see from this is PPC's reaction to dealing with a number of different dynamics that stem from the particular demographics of its members. For PPC the services they aim to provide are modified when encountered by these difficulties and result in the condition becoming more difficult to organize. A striking example that the PPC team explained to me on more than one occasion was that it was a real struggle to organize a community due to the fact that parents wouldn't even touch anything inscribed with the words HIV (also see Lindau et al., 2006). Moreover, beyond the general refusal of taking anything away with the words HIV on it, some parents would refuse to take paraphernalia from the group at all (when thinking about this example it brings to mind Douglas's (1970) *Purity and Danger* and the processes of ordering hygiene, cleanliness, order, and disorder). Therefore, we must consider that parents becoming publicly open about HIV in any way offer even more possibilities to open themselves up to stigmatization.

In this context then, how is activism supposed to flourish, and with whom does the responsibility of organizing and pursuing activism rest? In both PPC and Body & Soul, the community and organizational structure of the group can be seen to be enacted from the top down. What is meant by this is that the task of organizing the group, defining who is included in the group, and what issues affect members is not necessarily done in open discussion with members but in more isolated forums, not because members are necessarily excluded or don't want the issues to be raised, but because members are afraid of jeopardizing their confidentiality (see the framework of Parker & Aggleton, 2003). Part of the job of propagating these groups is done in the clinic where consultants will refer patients to a group. This is contrasted against the patient groups of other conditions. A few years ago I held a research assistant position on a project investigating Batten disease (a rare, genetic, progressive neurodegenerative disease occurring in children). The position required integration into the Batten Disease Family Association (BDFA) and attendance at meetings. When looking back, one large difference between the groups is that the initiative of the BDFA came almost exclusively and at times exuberantly from the parents themselves. There are a lot of factors that account for this difference between Batten disease and HIV: the population is affected due to chance; there are none of the associations with sex, drugs, or immigration; and due to the circumstances of children losing the ability to communicate, parents must speak on behalf of their children (Scambler, 2005). However, there is something conspicuous about the lack of patient cohesion around children with HIV, so much so that when compared to other groups, HIV remains distinct.

If we look at the work of Callon (2003, 2004) and take the example of research with the *Association Réunionnaise Contre les Myopathies* (the Réunion Island muscular-dystrophy association) and the *Association Française Contra les Myopathies* (the French muscular-dystrophy association), what comes across is the range of possibilities of members of the group to outline their own forms of scientific knowledge and social identities. One of the possibilities evoked when patients come together is that groups gain the potential to alter care regimes and scientific/government agendas by not only altering the agendas presented but by forming new and more meaningful agendas for their collective position (Brashers et al., 2002). For charities this highlights two things: first, the dynamic of activism for children with HIV being acted out according to these associations of stigma, and second, the possibilities of identifying and engaging with the workings of this stigma. When considering these two possibilities in relation to the point raised earlier exemplified in *Him & Her* regarding the blame and culpability that place the innocent child on the one hand and the sinful mother on the other, the resulting consideration brings to light a standoff of responsibilities. The antagonism at the center of families dealing with HIV enacts blame between mother and child that negates the incentive for families to engage in activism and disrupts the unity between mother and child. If parents face public scorn and condemnation for passing HIV to their child, it becomes logical for them to keep it confidential for the sake of all family members (Michaud et al., 2009). Therefore, at some point all family members will question the prudence of making HIV visible for their family before feeling the freedom to engage in activism. Can it be assumed, therefore, that the mother feels the guilt and irresponsibility while wanting to keep the family together, the child/adolescent cares for the family and doesn't want to put those they love in the firing line, and fathers and siblings (perhaps not infected) don't want to burden mothers or children with dealing with any resulting pressure (see family dynamics of HIV-affected families described in Fassin, 2008)?

If we look back at the campaign of Body & Soul, we can see some interesting points emerge. The first is the aim of employing high-profile celebrities to increase the profile of the disease and disassociate it from some of its usual associations, and the second aim of the short film is to highlight prejudice. It has been deemed important to challenge these associations of death, sex, and immigration (which is especially important in accordance with the decline in mortality; Gibb, 2003). However, one more slightly hidden question becomes, does the campaign account for the internal blame and family member blame dynamics illuminated above? We will have to wait and see if attitudes will change, but an important step already taken by Body and Soul in their new campaign may be to ask others to place themselves in the shoes of others, as it is from there that it becomes possible to imagine how one would manage these associations in one's own life (also see the impetus behind Goertzel & Bluebond-Langner, 1991). Rather than making the condition less visible or altering the name of the condition, asking others to take on life from another perspective does not offer a full list of associations that can be taken up in regard to how life must be with HIV, but does highlight some of the daily factors involved and asks potential stigmatizers to place themselves on the other side of HIV and imagine their school and family life from the other perspective.

## DISCUSSION

What is activism, then, in this context? The way in which HIV activism is framed by those with the condition dictates what factors will go toward forming issues and how issues will be pushed. If groups that are focused on children with HIV are formed with the community choosing to engage together as a group in a capacity that portrays the importance for confidentiality and secrecy, these factors will become core factors in the ensuing activist group. In other HIV contexts activism is not necessarily the same as pediatric HIV and is categorized in ways that could be seen as polar opposites; as we know, HIV can be seen to have had an intense and vivid activist history (see Epstein, 1998). The worrying element comes when considering the rights of children and families with HIV, regulation, and government policy. It remains to be seen how families with HIV make their concerns bear on public policy and if there are any unresolved policy positions resulting from families feeling the need to live in secrecy. Tellingly absent from the websites of Body and Soul, CWAC, PPC, and CHIVA are the sorts of governmental, policy, or care debates that seem to identify other UK HIV charities such as Terrance Higgins Trust (THT) or Aidsmap (NAM). Two current examples that could be highlighted from THT and NAM is THT's campaign that protests about changes to benefit assessment structures that will assess HIV differently from the past (THT, 2012), or from NAM a piece on the effect that immigration regulations and removal centers have on HIV care (NAM, 2011). Both of these issues are potentially relevant to children and families living with HIV, and patients may be directly affected by these topics in unique ways. It may be very distressing to adolescents and children if they or people they know are affected by benefit or immigration assessments, and it could have big impacts upon their lives and care regimes. It is perhaps ironic, therefore, that this crippling burden of stigma around HIV is not pushed by potential activists to make its way higher on to government criterions of welfare and immigration (and others) when it is so acutely felt and dealt with by these groups of families (Bor et al., 2004). The question can be asked whether the stigma associated with HIV is as established in government rationality as the vulnerability and stigma reasoned with in terms of asylum seekers. The argument here is not that parents and children are excluded from these debates, or that THT, NAM, and even the National Society for the Protection of Children (NSPC) are seen as more appropriate forums for these discussions, but merely to raise the point that these types of discussions are almost entirely absent from the aforementioned child organizations and ask readers to speculate as to why this is the case.

This chapter has assessed how the dynamics of these discussions and patient groups are affected by ideas of innocence, culpability, and responsibility, and how these factors play their part alongside other associations, more generally of HIV. However, in the end, rather than imagining the dynamics of these elements of stigma, childhood, HIV, and activism as superficially linked, deliberation should be promoted on how these factors must be intricately elaborated at the base of each interaction. We can imagine that campaigners working in the field reason that it is not beneficial to pursue these issues under the guise of childhood and innocence, and, correspondingly, families must feel the need to uphold the secretive dynamic of life in the UK and HIV rather than grouping together (Spirig, 2002).

The associations active around childhood, HIV, and stigma cause patients to not want to organize in traditional forms of activism. Consequently, it becomes the major role of charities formed around the condition, including Body and Soul's campaign, to primarily address and combat stigma and discrimination rather than facilitating debate around liberties and activism. The focus for families is that which makes it possible to remain hidden and allow their HIV to remain invisible above the defense of other rights. The reasons for this are partly associated with the forums existing within other organizations like THT and NAM. However, as has been discussed throughout this chapter, the contradictory associations of stigma and of childhood innocence, vulnerability, vice, and virtue that render family members in opposed roles of *child victim* and *sinful parents* also play there part. In opposition to describing the defense of a patient's confidentiality outside the gambit of activism, however, it should rather be placed as forming a particular set of associations where the traditional spirit that in other contexts could be allied to activism is channeled by families into the right to deal with HIV in their own way in confidentiality and dignity. Upholding these privileges serves the interests of those infected by ensuring that individuals can continue to be accepted into their own African communities as well as the wider British society (U.K. Select Committee, 2011). However, it is still felt as regrettable by HIV organizations like Body & Soul and PPC that this spirit seems incompatible with debate in a public forum, as can be seen through the need, discussed in both organizations, to carry out campaigns designed to address stigma.

The examples given here and the consequent analysis have been very much focused on the UK. However, the universal aspects of the disease around stigma, immigration, and activism can be extended out to other contexts beyond the UK where some of the associations may be similar.

## BIBLIOGRAPHY

Bennett, J. (2010). *Vibrant Matter: A Political Ecology of Things.* Duke University Press.

Berger, B. E., Ferrans, C. E., & Lashley, F. R. (2001). Measuring Stigma in People with HIV: Psychometric Assessment of the HIV Stigma Scale. *Research in Nursing & Health,* 24(6), pp. 518–529.

Bhana, D. (2007). Childhood Sexuality and Rights in the Context of HIV/AIDS. *Culture, Health & Sexuality,* 9(3), pp. 309–324.

Bhana, D., & Epstein, D. (2007). "I Don't Want to Catch It." Boys, Girls and Sexualities in an HIV/AIDS Environment. *Gender and Education,* 19(1), pp. 109–125.

Body & Soul (2011). *Life in My Shoes.* Available at: http://lifeinmyshoes.org [Accessed November 20, 2011].

Bor, R., Miller, R. & Goldman, E. (2004). HIV/AIDS and the Family: A Review of Research in the First Decade. *Journal of Family Therapy,* 15(2), pp. 187–204.

Brashers, D. E., et al. (2002). Social Activism, Self-Advocacy, and Coping with HIV Illness. *Journal of Social and Personal Relationships,* 19(1), pp. 113–133.

Callon, M., & Rabeharisoa, V. (2003). Research "in the Wild" and the Shaping of New Social Identities. *Technology in Society,* 25(2), p. 193.

Callon, M., & Rabeharisoa, V. (2004). Gino's Lesson on Humanity: Genetics, Mutual Entanglements and the Sociologist's Role. *Economy and Society,* 33(1), pp. 1–27.

Campbell, T., et al. (2009). "Sex, Love and One-Night Stands: Getting the Relationship You Want": Evaluation of a Sexual Health Workshop for HIV+ Young People. *Education and Health,* 27(2), pp. 23–27.

CHIPS (2011). Collaborative HIV Paediatric Study (CHIPS): Summary Data to the End of March 2011. Available at: http://www.chipscohort.ac.uk/summary _data.asp [Accessed January 28, 2012].

Christensen, P. (2000). Childhood and the Cultural Constitution of Vulnerable Bodies. In A. Prout, ed., *The Body, Childhood and Society.* New York: St. Martin's Press.

Clark, C. D. (2003). *In Sickness and in Play: Children Coping with Chronic Illness.* Rutgers University Press.

Coole, D. H., & Frost, S., eds. (2010). *New Materialisms: Ontology, Agency, and Politics.* Duke University Press.

CWAC (2011). History of Children with AIDS Charity. *Children With AIDS Charity—Supporting families infected and affected by HIV/AIDS.* Retrieved from http://www.cwac.org/aboutushistory.htm

Day, E. (2011). Battling HIV Prejudice with Body & Soul. *The Observer,* p. 14.

Douglas, M. (1970). *Purity and Danger: An Analysis of the Concepts of Pollution and Taboo.* New ed., Penguin Books.

Epstein, S. (1998). *Impure Science: AIDS, Activism and the Politics of Knowledge.* New Ed., University of California Press.

Fassin, D. (2008). AIDS Orphans, Raped Babies, and Suffering Children: The Moral Construction in Post-Apartheid South Africa. In C. R. Comacchio, J. Golden, & G. Weisz, eds., *Healing the World's Children: Interdisciplinary Perspectives on Child Health in the Twentieth Century.* McGill-Queen's Press—MQUP.

Gibb, D. (2003). Decline in Mortality, AIDS, and Hospital Admissions in Perinatally HIV-1 Infected Children in the United Kingdom and Ireland. *BMJ,* 327, pp. 1019ff.

Goertzel, T. G., & Bluebond-Langner, M. (1991). What Is the Impact of a Campus AIDS Education Course? *Journal of American College Health,* 40(2), pp. 87–92.

Goffman, E. (1968). *Stigma: Notes on the Management of Spoiled Identity.* Penguin.

Hekster, B., & Melvin, D. (2006). Psychosexual Development in Adolescents Growing Up with HIV Infection in London. In *Sex, Mind, and Emotion: Innovation in Psychological Theory and Practice.* Karnac Books.

Henderson, P. C. (2006). South African AIDS Orphans Examining Assumptions Around Vulnerability from the Perspective of Rural Children and Youth. *Childhood,* 13(3), pp. 303–327.

Latour, B. (2004). *Politics of Nature: How to Bring the Sciences into Democracy.* Cambridge, MA: Harvard University Press.

Law, J. (1999). Actor network theory and after. Wiley-Blackwell, Oxford.

Laxton, R. (2011). Him & Her. *The Rollover.*

Lindau, S. T., et al. (2006). Mothers on the Margins: Implications for Eradicating Perinatal HIV. *Social Science & Medicine,* 62(1), pp. 59–69.

Mahajan, A. P., et al. (2008). Stigma in the HIV/AIDS Epidemic: A Review of the Literature and Recommendations for the Way Forward. *AIDS,* 22(Suppl 2), pp. S57–S65.

Mayall, B. (1998). Towards a Sociology of Child Health. *Sociology of Health & Illness,* 20(3), pp. 269–288.

Melvin, D. (2007). Breaking the Silence, Reducing the Stigma. *Positive Nation.*

Melvin, D., & Sherr, L. (1995). HIV Infection in London Children: Psychosocial Complexity and Emotional Burden. *Child: Care, Health and Development,* 21(6), pp. 405–12.

Michaud, P.-A., et al. (2009). To Say or Not to Say: A Qualitative Study on the Disclosure of Their Condition by Human Immunodeficiency Virus–Positive Adolescents. *Journal of Adolescent Health,* 44(4), pp. 356–362.

Mitchell, C., Walsh, S., & Larkin, J. (2004). Visualizing the Politics of Innocence in the Age of AIDS. *Sex Education: Sexuality, Society and Learning,* 4(1), p. 35.

NAM (2011, Autumn). HIV & AIDS Information, 209. Barriers to Care: Immigration Removal Centres and HIV. Retrieved from http://www.aidsmap.com/Barriers-to-care-immigration-removal-centres-and-HIV/page/2094823/

Parker, R., & Aggleton, P. (2003). HIV and AIDS-Related Stigma and Discrimination: A Conceptual Framework and Implications for Action. *Social Science & Medicine,* 57(1), pp. 13–24.

Patton, C. (1991). *Inventing AIDS.* Routledge.

PPC (2012a). Positive Parenting and Children. Retrieved from http://ppclondon.org.uk/

PPC (2012b). Positive Parenting and Children UK Family Project. Retrieved from http://ppclondon.org.uk/uk-family-project/

Prout, A. (2000). *The Body, Childhood and Society.* New York: St. Martin's Press.

Rintamaki, L. (2009). The HIV Social Identity Model. In *Communicating to Manage Health and Illness.* Taylor & Francis.

Rule, P., & Vaughn, J. (2008). Unbinding the Other in the Context of HIV/AIDS and Education. *Journal of Education,* 23(1), pp. 79–101.

Scambler, S. (2005). Exposing the Limitations of Disability Theory: The Case of Juvenile Batten Disease. *Social Theory and Health,* 3(2), pp. 144–164.

SCOPE (2001). *The Spastics Society to SCOPE: The Story of the Name Change and Re-Launch of November 1994,* Available at: http://www.scope.org.uk/help-and-information/publications/spastics-society-scope [Accessed January 7, 2012].

Shevory, T. C. (2004). *Notorious H.I.V.: The Media Spectacle of Nushawn Williams.* U of Minnesota Press.

Spirig, R. (2002). In Invisibility and Isolation: The Experience of HIV-Affected Families in German-Speaking Switzerland. *Qualitative Health Research,* 12(10), pp. 1323–1337.

Stephney, I., & Deacon, H. (2007). *HIV/AIDS, Stigma and Children: A Literature Review.* Human Sciences Research Council.

Swendeman, D., et al. (2006). Predictors of HIV-Related Stigma among Young People Living with HIV. *Health Psychology,* 25(4), pp. 501–509.

THT (2012). THT: Campaign for Fairer Benefits. Retrieved from http://e-activist.com/ea-action/action?ea.client.id=66&ea.campaign.id=13081

Treichler, P. A. (1999). *How to Have Theory in an Epidemic: Cultural Chronicles of AIDS.* Duke University Press.

U.K. Select Committee (2011). *No Vaccine, No Cure: HIV and AIDS in the United Kingdom Report, House of Lords Paper 188 Session 2010–12.* The Stationery Office.

Wiener, L., et al. (2007). Disclosure of an HIV Diagnosis to Children: History, Current Research, and Future Directions. *Journal of Developmental and Behavioral Pediatrics,* 28(2), pp. 155–166.

Wilcox (1996). Rebecca's Secret. *The Visit.* Retrieved from http://www.imdb.com/title/tt0809583/

# 15

# "We Are Not Criminals": Activists Addressing the Criminalization of HIV Nondisclosure in Canada

*Daniel Grace and Tim McCaskell*

There will be calls for "law and order" and a "war on AIDS." Beware of those who cry out for simple solutions, for in combating HIV/AIDS there are none. In particular, do not put faith in the enlargement of the criminal law. (Justice Michael Kirby, Australia, 1991; quoted in ARASA, 2007: 16)

Fundamentally unjust, morally harmful, and virtually impossible to enforce with any semblance of fairness, such laws impose regimes of surveillance and punishment on sexually active people living with HIV not only in their intimate relations and reproductive and maternal lives, but also in their attempts to earn a living. Proponents of criminalization often claim that they are promoting public health or morality. Some may even harbor good-hearted, if wrongheaded, intentions, of safeguarding the rights and health of women. But criminalization guarantees no one's well-being. There is no evidence that laws regulating the sexual conduct of people living with HIV change behavior in a positive way. Nor do such laws take into account the success of antiretroviral treatment (ART) in significantly reducing transmission risk and improving the quality of life and longevity for people with HIV. (UNDP, 2012: 20)

## GLOBAL HIV/AIDS ACTIVISM IN THE FIELD
## OF HIV CRIMINALIZATION

Not disclosing one's HIV status before the alleged exposure or transmission of HIV to another person is a legal offense in an increasing number of jurisdictions. For example, researchers have noted the intensification of HIV nondisclosure criminal cases in specific counties including Canada since 2004 (Mykhalovskiy, Betteridge, & McLay, 2010) and broader global trends toward the expansive use of the criminal law (Pearshouse, 2008; Bernard, 2010, 2011; Grace, 2012a, 2012b; see UNDP, 2012, for an updated global map of regions that have HIV-specific criminal laws against HIV transmission or exposure). For many activists, policy actors, researchers, and health professionals, these moves toward criminal models of addressing HIV and AIDS are highly problematic and undermine human rights and public health efforts (Elliott, 2002; Eba, 2008; Burris & Cameron, 2008; Cameron, Burris, & Clayton, 2008; Jürgens et al., 2009; UNAIDS Reference Group, 2009; UNDP, 2012).

A number of national and international advocacy campaigns have been working to raise public attention to the harmful aspects of criminalizing HIV transmission or exposure in alleged cases of HIV nondisclosure (OSI, 2008; ARASA, 2007; IPPF, 2012; etc.). As the global anticriminalization campaign of the International Planned Parenthood Foundation (IPPF) puts it, states must "Criminalize Hate Not HIV." We argue that a growing transnational group of actors are working to critique the idea that such forms of criminalization represent an appropriate public health response. They reject the idea that criminalizing people living with HIV/AIDS through new HIV-specific laws or existing general criminal laws is a just response that will serve as a deterrent to spreading HIV. The work they produce frequently invokes human rights claims and underscores the idea that responding to this epidemic with criminal law powers has "failed to acknowledge the fact that HIV and AIDS are, and should be understood as, public health issues first and foremost, rather than as problems necessarily capable of effective legal resolution through the criminal law" (Weait, 2007: 3). However, as the case study we present on activism in Canada makes clear, specific activist activities have been tailored to address unique issues of HIV criminalization in local and regional contexts such as activism in Ontario, Canada that has focused largely on concerns of legal unfairness rather than broader human rights claims.

Social scientists, lawyers, and policy analysis in Canada, the United States, and the United Kingdom have been contributing to research on the possible negative public health impacts of criminalizing HIV transmission or exposure (Galletly & Pinkerton, 2006; Burris, 2007; Adam et al., 2008; Galletly & Dickson-Gomez, 2009; Mykhalovskiy, 2011). Limited social science scholarship has addressed the claims made by the critics of criminalization. In a compelling consideration of how the legal concept of "significant risk" in Canada serves to coordinate modes of criminal law governance and negatively impact public health objectives, Mykhalovskiy (2011, p. 668) explains:

> Critics frame the criminal law as a blunt instrument that is ineffective at regulating the complex sexual activities that figure in HIV transmission. They emphasize that the vast majority of people with HIV (PHAs) take precautions to prevent HIV transmission and suggest curtailing the use of the criminal law, often citing conduct that intentionally and successfully transmits HIV as the relevant threshold (Burris & Cameron, 2008). A number of critics claim that criminalization disrupts access to HIV testing, education and support services (Wainberg, 2009) and erodes public health norms that support mutual responsibility for HIV prevention (Cameron, Burris, & Clayton, 2008). Others emphasize that criminalization heightens HIV-related stigma (GNP+, 2010), while undermining action on the underlying social factors responsible for HIV transmission (Open Society Institute, 2008: 668).

This passage from Mykhalovskiy (2011) begins to elucidate some of the key claims made by critics of this form of criminalization. Actors argue that not only is the application of the criminal law not an effective response to addressing (the vast majority of) alleged cases of HIV transmission or exposure, but such applications along with sensational media reporting of "HIV criminals" produce increased stigma, disproportionally impact marginalized subjects, and undermine prevention efforts including HIV-testing initiatives (Shevory, 2004; Wainberg, 2009; ACCHO, 2010; O'Byrne et al., 2012). We argue that the social and behavioral scientific research evidence of the public health impacts of criminalization must catch up with the strong rhetorical claims made in much anticriminalization activist work. The ongoing production of such research evidence may be an important tool for ongoing global activism in this field.

## "10 Reasons" x 2: Making Arguments to Oppose the Criminalization of HIV Exposure, Transmission and/or Nondisclosure

The activist text *10 Reasons to Oppose Criminalization of HIV Exposure or Transmission* (OSI, 2008) is a useful place to begin in order to provide an overview of why a global network of activists, academics, and policy actors have argued that criminalizing HIV transmission, exposure, and/or nondisclosure is problematic. In fact, the writing of this OSI document is evidence of a transnational network of national and international organizations working to address the global "creep of criminalization" (Grace, 2012a). The document is published in nine languages by the Open Society Institute (OSI) and provides a pithy and accessible enumeration of various factors that make the criminalization of HIV exposure or transmission highly problematic:

1. Criminalizing HIV transmission is justified only when individuals purposely or maliciously transmit HIV with the intent to harm others. In these rare cases, existing criminal laws can and should be used, rather than passing HIV-specific laws;
2. Applying criminal law to HIV exposure or transmission does not reduce the spread of HIV;
3. Applying criminal law to HIV exposure or transmission undermines HIV prevention efforts;
4. Applying criminal law to HIV exposure or transmission promotes fear and stigma;
5. Instead of providing justice to women, applying criminal law to HIV exposure or transmission endangers and further oppresses them;
6. Laws criminalizing HIV exposure and transmission are drafted and applied too broadly, and often punish behavior that is not blame worthy;
7. Laws criminalizing HIV exposure and transmission are often applied unfairly, selectively and ineffectively;
8. Laws criminalizing HIV exposure and transmission ignore the real challenges of HIV prevention;
9. Rather than introducing laws criminalizing HIV exposure and transmission, legislators must reform laws that stand in the way of HIV prevention and treatment; and,
10. Human rights responses to HIV are most effective. (OSI, 2008)

This text acknowledges the concerns of civil society and government actors who have pushed to apply the criminal law in cases of HIV exposure and transmission, but strongly contends that the use of such criminal law powers represents an unjust and ineffective response.

Other global activist networks have focused their energies on the specific ways in which criminalization is harmful for particular populations including women. As such, it is useful to list the enumerated claims made by ATHENA's gender-focused anticriminalization campaign called *10 Reasons Why Criminalization of HIV Exposure or Transmission Harms Women:*

1. Women will be deterred from accessing HIV prevention, treatment, and care services, including HIV testing;
2. Women are more likely to be blamed for HIV transmission;
3. Women will be at greater risk of HIV-related violence and abuse;
4. Criminalization of HIV exposure or transmission does not protect women from coercion or violence;
5. Women's rights to make informed sexual and reproductive choices will be further compromised;
6. Women are more likely to be prosecuted;
7. Some women might be prosecuted for mother-to-child transmission;
8. Women will be more vulnerable to HIV transmission;
9. The most "vulnerable and marginalized" women will be most affected; and,
10. Human rights responses to HIV are most effective. (ATHENA, 2009)

Many of these points in this gender-focused activist work link to the OSI (2008) campaign (above) while bringing issues of gender-based violence and marginality into increased focus. The campaign was developed through a process of community and NGO consultations and has been widely disseminated internationally.

The harmful role of the media has also been addressed by academics and activists concerned with this mode of public health governance (Shevory, 2004; Mykhalovskiy & Sanders, 2008). For example, in a critical examination of the prosecution of Nushawn Williams in the United States, Shevory reviews how Williams, an African American man in his early 20s, was charged in 1997 in New York for knowingly transmitting HIV to multiple sex partners. Shevory presents a complex look at how Williams's name and picture were released to the press and the subsequent media spectacle that constructed him as a "public health threat" and "AIDS monster." Rather than a movement toward the "increasingly satisfactory realization of legal and political rights" consistent with dominant (Western) narratives of progress, "[s]ociety now shows less willingness than in the past to find a balance between the rights of the infected and the interests of the community" (Shevory, 2004: 111). Recognizing the potentially harmful role of dominant media discourse of criminalization for people living with HIV and public health goals more broadly, some NGOs and collectives working on this issue have designed media talking points on criminalization (Canadian AIDS Society, 2009) and are focusing on the problematic and harmful role of the media in perpetuating gender inequities (Welbourn, 2008), stigma, and racism (ACCHO, 2010).

To conclude this section it is important to note that in 2010 UNDP/UNAIDS formed the Global Commission on HIV and the Law to "increase understanding of the impact of the legal environment on national HIV responses ... to focus on how laws and law enforcement can support, rather than block, effective HIV responses" (UNDP/UNAIDS, 2010: 1). The press release for the Global Commission states:

> ... there are many countries in which negative legal environments undermine HIV responses and punish, rather than protect, people in need. Where the law does not advance justice, it stalls progress. Laws that inappropriately criminalize HIV transmission or exposure can discourage people from getting tested for HIV or revealing their HIV positive status. Laws which criminalize men who have sex with men, transgender people, drug-users, and/or sex workers can make it difficult to provide essential HIV prevention or treatment services to people at high risk of HIV infection. In some countries, laws and law enforcement fail to protect women from rape inside and outside marriage—thus increasing women's vulnerability to HIV. (UNDP/UNAIDS, 2010: 1)

The Commission's final report is a powerful testament to the many complex ways in which the criminalization of HIV transmission, exposure, and nondisclosure is highly problematic (UNDP, 2012). Here we can see how this issue of criminalizing HIV transmission or exposure is part of a broader conversation about the ways in which the law can support or undermine human rights and HIV prevention, treatment, and care. With this brief global overview of this issue provided, we can now turn to a focused case study of anticriminalization activist work in Ontario, Canada.

## CASE STUDY: THE ONTARIO WORKING GROUP ON CRIMINAL LAW AND HIV EXPOSURE

### Background

Canada has no HIV-specific laws but in 1998, the Supreme Court of Canada found that an HIV-positive man, Henry Cuerrier, had committed fraud by not disclosing his HIV status to two women before having unprotected sex. Although neither of the women became HIV positive, since they presumably would not have consented to such sex had they known his status, the Supreme Court ruled that their apparent consent was invalid, and Cuerrier was therefore guilty of aggravated sexual assault. The Court elaborated that HIV-positive people were required to disclose their status before engaging in any behavior that involved "significant risk" of infecting others. While it was suggested that use of a condom might mean that a person with HIV did not have to disclose, the Court did not clarify what significant risk was, nor how it was to be determined (Symington, 1999; Mykhalovskiy, 2011; Grace, 2012b).

Against a background of AIDS phobia and ignorance, the result was wildly different interpretations in courts across the country. A number of people were charged and convicted of sexual assault although they had only engaged in what was generally considered very low-risk activity. After 2004, the charges themselves began to escalate both in number and seriousness (Mykhalovskiy, Betteridge, & McLay, 2010). Canada became an international leader in the prosecution of HIV nondisclosure cases (GNP+, 2010). Worse, police began publishing media alerts with the names and pictures of those accused in a hunt for other "victims," even before there had been any finding of guilt. Lurid media reports of trials exaggerated the risk of HIV transmission and represented PLHAs as irresponsible, dishonest, and criminally dangerous (Mykhalovskiy & Sanders, 2008).

The Ontario Working Group on Criminal Law and HIV Exposure (CLHE) was formed in 2007 in response to anxieties over the effect that such high-profile court cases about HIV nondisclosure were having on the lives of people living with HIV/AIDS (PLHAs), and the management of the AIDS epidemic in Canada. The group's membership was largely drawn from AIDS Service Organizations (ASOs) and included PLHAs. Its co-chairs were Ryan Peck, ED of HALCO (HIV & AIDS Legal Clinic Ontario), a legal aid clinic that focused on issues around HIV, and Anne Marie DiCenso, ED of PASAN (Prisoners HIV/AIDS Support Network). The group's purpose was to oppose the growing and expansive use of criminal law powers with respect to issues of HIV exposure and transmission.

By the time CLHE developed its position paper on the criminalization of HIV nondisclosure in 2008, over 60 people had been criminally charged across the country (Mykhalovskiy, Betteridge, & McLay, 2010). The position paper was the result of months of discussions and served as a basis of unity and collective understanding for the group. It opens by arguing that "the criminal law is an ineffective and inappropriate tool with which to address HIV exposure. HIV/AIDS is an individual and public health issue first and foremost and should be addressed as such" (CLHE, 2008: 1). The paper outlines the negative effects of the use of criminal law, including: "hindering HIV testing and access to services, spreading misinformation about HIV, increasing stigma and discrimination associated with HIV, and invasions of privacy" (CLHE, 2008: 1). It also points out the disproportionate impact of criminalization upon specific groups such as new immigrants, racialized men, Aboriginal women, and prisoners. Importantly, this text makes explicit why PLHAs might be unwilling or unable to disclose and calls for a "review of Canada's present criminal law and its application with respect to HIV exposure" (CLHE, 2008: 1).

While the process of producing the position paper helped the group understand and clarify central issues, it proved inadequate to mobilize a significant broader political collective to work for change. Although many individuals became persuaded of the problematic nature of criminalization over time, even getting endorsement for CLHE's position from boards of ASOs across the province proved difficult. It appeared that dominant notions of responsibility, romance, and intimacy around sex positioned instances of nondisclosure as a betrayal. The nuances between ethical and legally culpable behavior appeared to be lost for many people.

In retrospect, the document could be read as internally inconsistent, beginning by calling the use of criminal law "ineffective and inappropriate" (CLHE, 2008: 1)—presumably in all cases—and then opposing the "*expansive* use of criminal law," which indicated that in some cases the use of criminal law might be appropriate after all (CLHE, 2008: 1; emphasis added). The standpoint from which the text was written was that of PLHAs concerned about the social effects of criminalization on their lives, and its impact on those on the front lines trying to control the epidemic, but it did not take up the individual concerns of those who felt they had been exposed out of negligence or malice. Further, since the majority of the most high-profile cases involved heterosexual men failing to disclose to women, the document could be accused of gender bias—privileging the privacy rights of men over the physical safety of women.

Finally, the position paper's call for a review of criminal law and its application was far from a concrete demand. Who would conduct such a review? The Supreme Court had already made its position clear and the content of the Canadian Criminal Code is the responsibility of the federal government. Could anyone expect the Harper government, perhaps the most socially conservative in recent memory, to conduct a review that would not further promote its established pro-incarceration, law-and-order agenda? In reflecting on the political context in which the position paper was produced, it is germane to consider the broader question of HIV/

AIDS activism and political pragmatism: To what extant and in what circumstances must activist texts such as the CLHE position paper consider issues such as the political climate in order to frame palatable (or at least possible) solutions?

## Responding to Aziga and Getting Bloody

Weaknesses in CLHE's early work became especially evident during the Aziga trial in 2008–2009. Johnson Aziga, a Ugandan-born Canadian, was accused of infecting a number of women with HIV, two of whom had subsequently died. He was charged with and subsequently found guilty of two counts of first-degree murder and 10 counts of aggravated sexual assault (see Bernard, 2012, for a collection of global cases, including Aziga). The debate around the Aziga case was stacked against activist groups like CLHE that focused on the social and public health impact of criminalization. The character of the dominant narrative in Aziga is important to understand as it provides social context for CLHE's activist work. It was a simple and seductive story: a black man, an immigrant, who through gross negligence or malice deceived his partners and infected them with a virus that killed them. The story was congruent with popular and racist tropes about black men assaulting white women, immigrants as diseased and dangerous; binaries of guilt and innocence, love and betrayal, and notions of good and evil were constructed (see Shevroy, 2004; ACCHO, 2010).

In its media interventions at the time, CLHE tried to advance a nuanced narrative focusing on the complex effects of stigma on marginalized groups and potential subsequent effects on transmission and public health. This message proved difficult to articulate to mass media outlets and broader publics. From the perspective of those working at CLHE it appeared as if any expression of concern about the role that criminal law was playing on broader issues of transmission, any attempt to ask people to reflect on the problematic and long-term effects of criminalization, was to side with evil and against innocence and justice. Not unexpectedly then, CLHE was pilloried in the press and isolated politically. Although by this time most ASO leaders and staff were sympathetic, such service organizations were often reluctant to take a public stance on controversial issues that potentially could interfere with funding.

As noted above, there was division among those who could be traditionally expected to rally around HIV/AIDS issues. Most of those charged were heterosexual men who had failed to disclose to female partners. Several prominent HIV/AIDS physicians took the position that criminal sanctions were needed to protect women from such irresponsible predators. It is worth noting that such fears parallel a similar set of claims made in the African context in support of HIV-specific laws that criminalize HIV transmission (Grace, 2012a). Others took the opposite stance: that criminal cases and the resulting stigma drove people underground and would inflame the epidemic.

The queer community in Ontario was likewise divided. A libertarian current argued there should never be any role for criminal law in HIV infection and that criminal prosecutions illustrated AIDS phobia and homophobia. Others echoed hegemonic discourses that anyone who was positive had an unequivocal responsibility to disclose at all times. CLHE had been seriously bloodied in the public battle. If it was going to stop the damage being done, the group believed it needed an alternative strategy that would allow for a broader basis of unity and public engagement. Meanwhile the escalation in charges continued. By 2009 there were 104 charges laid across the country, slightly less than half of them in Ontario (Mykhalovskiy, Betteridge, & McLay, 2010).

## Developing Prosecutorial Guidelines as a Harm Reduction Strategy

Before noting the activism around prosecutorial guidelines in Ontario, it is important to note the work done in this field in the United Kingdom. The idea of developing prosecutorial guidelines in this field of law had been explored since (at least) 2007–2008 when the Crown Prosecution Service of England and Wales published a document of legal guidance to Crown prosecutors (Crown Prosecution Service, 2008). Since Crown prosecutors ultimately decide whether or not charges will be taken to court, the guidelines successfully reduced the number and severity of charges in England and Wales—a trend Ontario activists hoped to replicate. This work in England and Wales informed some of the strategies used in the Canadian context. Here we see an important example of how local activism in Ontario has been informed by other focused initiatives working to respond to this global trend of HIV criminalization. Furthermore, the activism and scholarship concerning guidelines in Ontario have informed persons in Quebec in their provincial work to engage stakeholders in the development of prosecutorial guidelines (Claivaz-Loranger et al., 2012).

A major advantage of the guidelines approach for CLHE activists was that while the content of the Criminal Code itself is the mandate of the federal government in Ottawa, the administration of justice is a provincial responsibility. For CLHE, Ontario's Liberal provincial government was far more accessible and likely to be open to discussion. While CLHE had found itself on the losing side of arguments that pitted notions of individual justice against concerns about the social impact of stigma and its effect on transmission, demanding prosecutorial guidelines was within the ambit of the criminal justice system and avoided this polarity. Here CLHE was fighting against an unjust application of the criminal justice system to individuals who had not put anyone at significant risk of HIV infection. This reframing of the issue permitted a discussion of the social impact of such injustice without seemingly disregarding cases where people had actually been harmed.

While a call for prosecutorial guidelines would not meet the demands of those who argued that there was no place for the use of criminal law powers whatsoever, it was thought that people would understand the harm reduction strategy of trying to reduce the number and the severity of the charges and the damage caused. Just as importantly, it was thought that making a distinction between the most egregious cases and others where actual transmission risk was insignificant might also help bring on side some of those who felt that criminal punishment for "irresponsible" behavior was justified. The strategy was therefore envisioned to be able to overcome divisions in the traditional AIDS community base and rebuild relationships, a precondition before any broader bloc could be produced.

It is important to note that CLHE members engaged in a process of reflexivity and soul searching before shifting gears to the strategy of pursuing prosecutorial guidelines. The shift in activism was facilitated by the concept of harm reduction that was already widely accepted among ASOs. Harm reduction had emerged as a response to the "War on Drugs" that focused on policing, punishment, and incarceration to discourage drug use. Harm reduction advocates argue that such a law-and-order approach has been spectacularly unsuccessful. They instead focus on how to limit the harm that drug use can cause though providing clean needles, supervised injection sites, recovery programs, and so on (Boyd et al., 2009). By the same principle, given the Supreme Court decision and the ideological position of the federal government, the deployment of the criminal justice system in cases of HIV nondisclosure was unlikely to stop. Prosecutorial guidelines, however, might limit the damage being done by restricting cases to those few that involved the significant risk of transmission and intent to harm. CLHE hoped that calling for prosecutorial guidelines would also establish a new concrete action around which to rally broader community support.

## The Call: Building Support and Rolling Out a Campaign

The Working Group drafted a call to the attorney general (AG) of Ontario, the cabinet minister in charge of the administration of justice in the province, to develop prosecutorial guidelines. The call opened by affirming that the use of criminal law needed to be compatible with attempts to prevent the spread of the epidemic. It conceded that criminal prosecutions might be warranted in some circumstances, but that the "current expansive use of criminal law" was cause for concern. It called on the AG to "undertake a process to develop guidelines for criminal prosecutors" in such cases, and to ensure that this process involved "meaningful" consultation with stakeholders (CLHE, 2011). The call purposely did not suggest what such guidelines should entail, or where the line between significant or insignificant risk should be drawn. That was an issue around which there would no doubt still be divisions within the HIV community. But what was agreed on was that a line needed to be drawn somewhere and the overly broad use of the criminal law must be halted.

Once the wording was developed, but before the campaign went public, the Working Group approached opinion leaders and leading organizations in the various sectors that needed to be mobilized, in order to ask them to publicly endorse the call. These people and organizations, listed as supporters when the campaign went online, illustrated the parameters of the bloc that CLHE was attempting to bring together. It included the traditional base of the AIDS community: AIDS researchers in the social, medical, and epidemiological sciences; physicians; AIDS activists; and ASOs. Beyond this group, CLHE felt it was important to include a broader coalition of legal experts, academics, religious figures, unions, feminist leaders, and social justice groups. CLHE believed establishing a broad network of support among diverse populations and opinion leaders was the wider collective necessary to exert pressure on the government. Beyond the call itself, CLHE developed a "Questions and Answers" document to address the kinds of questions that those struggling to understand the issue might ask (CLHE, 2011). The text provides some general legal background, explains the problems that expansive use of the law produces, the role of public health, how prosecutorial guidelines work, and their use in other jurisdictions.

For even more popular consumption and advocacy, a series of five colorful postcards was produced (for example, see Figures 15.1 and 15.2). Each conveys a different message reflecting common HIV criminalization concerns: "You shouldn't be prosecuted for oral sex" and "You shouldn't be

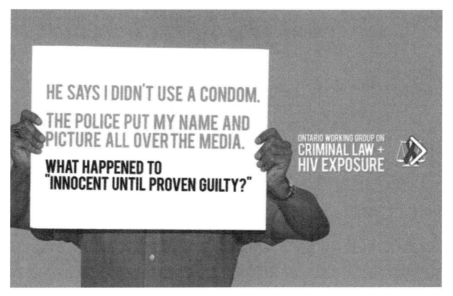

**Figure 15.1** Activism campaign materials produced by the Ontario Working Group on Criminal Law and HIV Exposure (CLHE). For more examples visit http://ontarioaidsnetwork .on.ca/clhe (Ontario Working Group on Criminal Law and HIV Exposure)

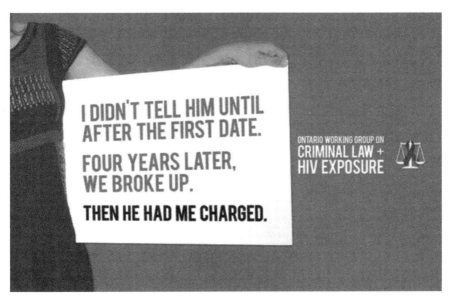

**Figure 15.2** Activism campaign materials produced by the Ontario Working Group on Criminal Law +HIV Exposure (CLHE). For more examples visit http://ontarioaidsnetwork .on.ca/clhe (Ontario Working Group on Criminal Law and HIV Exposure)

prosecuted for protected sex" touched on anxieties of those engaging in low-risk activities that they still might be caught up in the criminal justice system. "My HIV viral load is undetectable. That means I'm much less likely to pass on HIV during sex. Do I still have to disclose?" raised the question of uncertainty that was the result of ambiguities in the law. "He says I didn't use a condom. The police put my name and picture all over the media. What happened to 'innocent until proven guilty'?" addressed the questions of invasion of privacy and false accusations. Finally, "I didn't tell him until after the first date. Four years later we broke up. Then he had me charged," dealt with the issue of vindictive behavior. Here we can see the focused set of issues raised in CLHE activism. While these concerns are related to issues raised in the two "10 reasons" campaigns reviewed above, the CLHE campaign focused less on issues of human rights and more on concerns of vagueness and unfairness in the law, invasion of privacy, and dangerous public health outcomes of the criminalization of HIV nondisclosure.

The process of developing these materials was facilitated by another parallel effort that took place through the Ontario HIV Treatment Network (OHTN). The OHTN is a collaborative network of researchers, health service providers, community members, policy actors, and PLHAs who work in the field of HIV treatment, education, and research in Ontario. York University Professor Eric Mykhalovskiy spearheaded a research effort that produced a document titled *HIV Non-Disclosure and the Criminal Law: Establishing Policy Options for Ontario* (Mykhalovskiy et al., 2010). This was a more scholarly text aimed at policymakers and lawyers within the ministry of the attorney general. In a series of sections it brought together what was known about the trends and patterns of legal cases, their legal and public policy rationale, demographic data of those charged, medical research on risk of HIV infection, and social science research on the effects of criminalization, concluding with a list of policy options to address the issue. The document was soon established as the authoritative resource on the issue and underscores the importance of the diverse actors who compose the CLHE.

The campaign was officially launched at a joint forum organized by the Canadian HIV/AIDS Legal Network, the HIV & AIDS Legal Clinic Ontario, and CLHE. At the forum, the rise of prosecutions in Canada was discussed—as of the end of September 2010 there were 140 cases across the country—alongside the global "creep of criminalization" (Grace, 2012a). The keynote speaker at the launch was Edwin Bernard, a British journalist and anticriminalization activist who had been involved in the negotiations that had resulted in the UK guidelines. Bernard also runs an influential blog for international activists in this field (Bernard, 2012). The meeting was well attended, and although there were some probing questions from individuals who appeared to be closer to the "no criminal code under any circumstances" position, the vast majority seemed to be convinced by the arguments that the campaign was an important step.

A website was launched featuring the call and the names of well-known endorsers with signing-on capacity for those who wished to declare their support. One had only to enter one's name, email, and postal code, and a message was sent directly to the provincial attorney general's office. CLHE then had access to a growing list of supporters across the province that could be contacted if further political action was needed. A major conduit for outreach was the network of ASOs that make up the Ontario AIDS Network (OAN). These organizations would be key stakeholders and allies in terms of the campaign's rollout in their local communities. CLHE depended on them to conceptualize the appropriate local strategy, whether to contact local media or not, and engage their networks as they deemed appropriate.

There was also an effort to try to make the campaign "go viral." ASO clients, members, and staff were encouraged to forward the link of the campaign website to their email lists and across their various social networking sites. The idea was to help turn PLHAs themselves into educators and leaders on this issue. They would become part of a conversation with their contacts, answer questions, and engage in discussion. This conversation would in turn drive them back to the website to become more acquainted with the arguments. The fact that these conversations were happening with individuals with a personal stake in the outcome made them ideal educators. It also encouraged and empowered them to challenge the stigma that criminalization had been generating.

## The Window

Given our focus on reviewing issues of history and context, it is important to understand the window for this activist initiative (Pal, 2006). A major concern that shadowed the campaign was that a provincial election would be taking place the following autumn. CLHE had less than a year to achieve its goal before the government would be completely distracted. Worse, if the provincial Liberal government fell, it was thought that the shift would likely be to the Conservative party, which would presumably change this opportunity for effectively advocating for limiting the application of the criminal law. Even if there was no change in government, there would be a new cabinet and likely a new attorney general, and CLHE and its allies could find themselves having lost all the momentum that was building. After three months (December 2010), nearly a thousand people had signed on to the call and sent messages to the attorney general.

In March 2011 the Ministry of the Attorney General (MAG) publicly confirmed it was developing guidelines (McCann, 2011). It was a major victory, but the MAG itself was closed to public input and despite some low-level meetings, no meaningful process of consultation was announced. Finally, CLHE took the initiative and solicited support from the MAC Foundation to conduct targeted educational consultations. In the spring of 2011, eight full-day consultations were held across the province involving a range of stakeholder groups: PLHAs, communities affected by HIV, legal public health, criminal justice and scientific experts, health care providers, and women's rights advocates. An online consultation survey was also posted.

The report based on the consultations was submitted to the minister in June 2011. It argued that sexual offences involving coercion force and violence should not be equated to allegations of HIV nondisclosure and that Crown prosecutors should act with restraint in such cases. It gave specific recommendations about bail conditions, scientific/medical evidence, and screening of charges. In terms of establishing what constituted significant risk, the text maintained that charges should not proceed in situations involving oral sex alone, where the viral load of the accused was undetectable or a condom was used (CLHE, 2011).

The response from the MAG was silence. CLHE watched with increasing anxiety as the election came closer. It finally became obvious that no proposed guidelines would be issued before the vote. On the one hand this was a form of relief since no one wanted the issue to become election fodder for the Conservative opposition. There was also a rational argument to be made that the province might want to wait until the Supreme Court decided on upcoming cases from Manitoba and Quebec where the issue of "significant risk" would be central (Supreme Court of Canada, Court File Nos. 33976/34094; see CLHE, 2011). It would be the first time the Court would revisit the issue in more than a decade.

## Betrayal

Any grounds for complacency were dashed in the middle of the election campaign when the province applied for intervener status at the upcoming

Supreme Court hearing. In an outline of its arguments, the province proposed that lack of significant risk should be abandoned entirely as a defense, and that HIV-positive people would be committing fraud, and therefore sexual assault, if they failed to disclose their status, no matter how insignificant the risk. The move was an incredible disappointment for CLHE and contradicted the AG's promise to develop prosecutorial guidelines. It became clear that CLHE had been managed by the Ministry while they were preparing to move in the opposite direction from that promised by the minister. Furthermore, the internal politics of the Ministry continued to be opaque. It was unclear whether the intervention had been approved by the AG or whether Ministry lawyers had moved on their own initiative while the politicians were distracted by the election.

At this point, from CLHE's perspective, it appeared as if there was nothing to lose if the matter became an election issue. Members of the Working Group contacted an openly gay Liberal member of the provincial parliament (MPP) to express their dismay and questions were raised at the next all-candidates meeting. The MPP in turn contacted the premier and the attorney general. Although it did not become a political football, so to speak, HIV criminalization was certainly brought to the government's attention during a difficult reelection campaign. In the end the Liberals were reelected, although reduced to a minority. A new attorney general was selected. But now a new deadline imposed itself: the province's factum, the full arguments it planned to make, needed to be filed with the Supreme Court by late December. Once the factum was submitted, the province's position could not be changed.

CLHE once again moved into campaign mode, this time to demand that the province withdraw its intervention at the Supreme Court. A new letter-writing campaign to the AG went online utilizing the constituencies that had been assembled over the previous year. CLHE members across the province demanded to meet local MPPs. With the help of the sympathetic local MPP, those in Toronto insisted on a face-to-face with the AG himself. After several weeks of intense activity, CLHE members were given an audience with the AG and his deputy minister. The group did not "pull its punches" and was more than frank about what it considered a betrayal. The AG, who ruefully mentioned the number of emails and phone calls he was getting around the issue, was noncommittal, but a day later, the province withdrew its application for intervener status at the Supreme Court.

It was a stunning about-face and an important example of the success of this HIV activist work. The constituency that CLHE had assembled was not yet strong enough for its position to prevail at the MAG, but it was significantly strong to block those who wished to deepen the scope of criminalization. The Canadian HIV/AIDS Legal Network, CLHE, and a coalition of other groups were given intervener standing at the Supreme Court. Their submission argued for a scientific determination of "significant risk" and the exclusion from prosecution of those whose viral load was undetectable, those only engaging in oral sex, and those that use condoms for penetrative sex. On the other side, the province of Manitoba argued that significant risk should be dropped as a defense, and that disclosure of HIV status should be required in all circumstances.

Either way, the landscape of HIV criminalization could dramatically change in Canada in the coming months when the Supreme Court rules on this matter. No matter what the outcome, CLHE's strategy of developing a campaign around prosecutorial guidelines and working with a broad network of social actors has broken the isolation of those fighting against HIV criminalization in Ontario, Canada, and established the basis for possible progressive change on the issue. Activism in this field continues with a new AAN! "Think Twice" campaign launched in July 2012 echoing calls for the need to "Stop the witch-hunt" and demonstrate heightened restraint in the application of the criminal law (AAN!, 2012).

## CONCLUSION

This chapter represents an opportunity for an examination of a contemporary issue of local global HIV activism. We present this as a partial history of a complex, evolving story, in an effort to contribute to the scant literature on specific work in the field of anticriminalization HIV activism. We argue that it is important for activist networks and coalitions to share rich descriptions of lessons learned from past success and struggles in and beyond this contentious issue of criminalization. By contextualizing broad transnational activist activities in this area and providing a focused case study of CLHE, we have endeavored to map some of the complex work of challenging the trend to criminalize PLHAs in Canada. We have demonstrated the context-specific claims and work activities CLHE has engaged in to limit the overly broad application of criminal law to PLHAs. We underscore that instances of persons intentionally transmitting HIV are extremely rare and represent a minute fraction of the hundreds of global prosecutions to date. Prosecutions for HIV nondisclosure in Canada must be based on accurate and complete scientific and medical evidence rather than on preconceptions, fear, or prejudice. While looking at transnational activities and criminalization trends at a global level is important, focused examinations of specific, historically situated initiatives may serve as important examples in order to better understand the complexity and strategy of such HIV activism.

## AUTHORS' NOTE

At the time of publication the legislative landscape in Canada changed. To the dismay of many public health actors, the Supreme Court of Canada (SCC) ruled on October 5, 2012, that the duty for an individual with HIV to disclose his or her status to sexual partners can be dispensed only when a condom is used *and* the individual also has a low viral load. For more information about this SCC decision and ongoing activism on the implications of this regressive move, please visit aidslaw.ca.

## ACKNOWLEDGMENTS

The authors wish to acknowledge the valuable feedback of members of the Ontario Working Group on Criminal Law and HIV Exposure as well as comments from the editor of this volume and anonymous peer reviewers. The first author also wishes to acknowledge many conversations with Dr. Eric Mykhalovskiy that have helped to shape his understanding of Canadian activism in this field.

## BIBLIOGRAPHY

ACCHO (2010). *Criminal and victims: The impact of the criminalization of HIV non-disclosure on African, Caribbean and black communities in Ontario.* A. Larcher & A. Symington Toronto, Ontario.

Adam, B., et al. (2008). "Effects of the criminalization of HIV transmission in Cuerrier on men reporting unprotected sex with men." *Canadian Journal of Law & Society* 23(1), 143–159.

AIDS ACTION NOW! (2012). *AAN! pickets Ontario attorney general: "Think Twice" before you prosecute.* Retrieved from http://www.aidsactionnow .org/?p=813

ARASA (2007). *Report on the ARASA/OSISA civil society consultative meeting on the criminalisation of the willful transmission of HIV—11 and 12 June 2007.* Windhoek. Retrieved from http://www.arasa.info/publications.php

ATHENA (2009). 10 Reasons Why Criminalization of HIV Exposure or Transmission Harms Women. Retrieved from http://www.athenanetwork.org/assets/ files/10%20Reasons%20Why%20Criminalisation%20Harms%20Women.pdf.

Bernard, E. J. (2010). *HIV and the criminal law.* London: NAM.

Bernard, E. J. (2011). "HIV and criminal law: Global advocacy for justice." *HIV Australia* (8)4. Retrieved from http://www.afao.org.au/view_articles.asp?pxa= ve&pxs=103&pxsc=127&pxsgc=138&i=926

Bernard, E. J. (2012). *Criminal HIV transmission: A collection of published news stories and opinion about so-called "HIV crimes."* Retrieved from http:// criminalhivtransmission.blogspot.com

Boyd, S. C., MacPherson, D., & Osborn, B. (2009). *Raise shit!: Social action saving lives.* Halifax: Fernwood Publishing.

Burris, S., et al. (2007). "Do criminal laws influence HIV risk behavior? An empirical trial." *Az. St. L. J.* 39, 467.

Burris, S., & Cameron, E. (2008). "The Case Against Criminalization of HIV Transmission." *JAMA* 300(5), 578–581.

Cameron, E., Burris, S., & Clayton, M. (2008). "HIV is a virus, not a crime." *HIV/ AIDS Policy & Law Review* 13(2/3).

Canadian AIDS Society (2009). *Criminalization of HIV—Media speaking points.* Retrieved from http://www.cdnaids.ca/criminalizationofhivmedia

Claivaz-Loranger, S., et al. (2012). "Criminal prosecutions for non-disclosure of HIV: Engaging stakeholders for the development of prosecutorial guidelines in Quebec, Canada." *XIX International AIDS Conference.* WEPE557.

CLHE (2008). *Position paper on the criminalization of HIV non-disclosure.* Toronto. Retrieved from http://www.pasan.org/Toolkits/Criminalization_of_ HIV_Non-Disclosure_Position_Statement_-_2008.pdf

CLHE (2011, June). *Consultation on prosecutorial guidelines for Ontario cases involving non-disclosure of sexually transmitted infections: Community report and recommendations to the attorney general of Ontario.* Submitted by the Ontario Working Group on Criminal Law & HIV Exposure. Retrieved from www.ontarioaidsnetwork.on.ca/clhe/

Crown Prosecution Service. (2008). "Intentional or Reckless Sexual Transmission of Infection." Retrieved from http://www.cps.gov.uk/legal/h_to_k/ intentional_or_reckless_sexual_transmission_of_infection_guidance/

Dodds, C., Bourne, A., & Weait, M. (2009). "Responses to criminal prosecutions for HIV transmission among gay men with HIV in England and Wales." *Reproductive Health Matters,* 17(34), 135–145.

Eba, P. (2008). "One size punishes all … A critical appraisal of the criminalization of HIV transmission." *ALQ* 10/11, 1–10.

Elliott, R. (2002). *Criminal law, public health and HIV transmission: A policy options paper.* Geneva: UNAIDS.

Galletly, C. L., & Dickson-Gomez, J. (2009). "HIV seropositive status disclosure to prospective sex partners and criminal laws that require it: Perspectives of persons living with HIV." *International Journal of STD & AIDS,* 20, 613–18.

Galletly, C. L., & Pinkerton, S. D. (2006). "Conflicting messages: How criminal HIV disclosure laws undermine public health efforts to control the spread of HIV." *AIDS & Behavior,* 10, 451–461.

Global Network of People Living with HIV (GNP+) (2010). *Global criminalization scan report.* Retrieved from http://www.hivpolicy.org/Library/HPP001825.pdf

Grace, D. (2012a). *This is not a law: The transnational politics and protest of legislating an epidemic.* Dissertation. University of Victoria, Canada. Retrieved from http://hdl.handle.net/1828/3944

Grace, D. (2012b). "Reconceiving the 'problem' in HIV prevention: HIV testing technologies and the criminalization of HIV non-disclosure." In *An intersectionality-based policy analysis framework,* ed. O. Hankivsky, Institute for Intersectionality Research and Policy, Simon Fraser University. Retrieved from www.sfu.ca/iirp/ibpa

IPPF (2012). *Criminalize hate not HIV campaign—What can you do?* Retrieved from http://www.hivandthelaw.com/campaign/what-can-you-do

Jürgens, R., et al. (2009). "Ten reasons to oppose the criminalization of HIV exposure or transmission." *Reprod Health Matters* 17(34), 163–72.

McCann, M. (2011, March 2). "AIDS groups sway attorney general on nondisclosure cases." *Xtra.* Retrieved from http://www.xtra.ca/public/National/AIDS_groups_sway_attorney_general_on_nondisclosure_cases-9824.aspx

Mykhalovskiy, E. (2011). "The problem of 'significant risk': Exploring the public health impact of criminalizing HIV non-disclosure." *Social Science & Medicine* 73, 668–675.

Mykhalovskiy, E., Betteridge, G., & McLay, D. (2010). *HIV non-disclosure and the criminal law: Establishing policy options for Ontario.* Toronto. Funded by the Ontario HIV Treatment Network.

Mykhalovskiy, E., & Sanders, C. (2008). "There is no excuse for this wanton, reckless, self-indulgent behavior. A critical analysis of media representation of the criminalization of HIV non-disclosure in Canada." Presented at the November 2008 Ontario HIV Treatment Network Annual Conference. Toronto, Ontario.

O'Byrne, B., Bryan, A., & Woodyatt, C. (2012). "Nondisclosure prosecutions and HIV prevention: Results from an Ottawa-based gay men's sex survey." *JANAC,* 1–7 (in press).

OSI (2008). *10 reasons to oppose the criminalization of HIV exposure or transmission.* Retrieved from http://www.soros.org/health/10reasons

Pal, L. (2006). *Beyond policy analysis: Public issue management in turbulent times,* 3rd ed. Toronto: Nelson Education.

Pearshouse, R. (2008). "Legislation contagion: Building resistance." *HIV AIDS Policy Law Rev.,* 13(2/3), 1–11.

Shevory, T. (2004). *Notorious H.I.V.: The media spectacle of Nushawn Williams.* Minneapolis: University of Minnesota Press.

Supreme Court of Canada. Court File Nos. 33976/34094. Her Majesty the Queen and Clato Lual Mabior, and Her Majesty the Queen and D. C.

Symington, A. (2009). "Criminalization confusion and concern: The decade since the Cuerrier decision." *HIV/AIDS Policy & Law Review,* 14(1), 5–10.

UNAIDS (2002). *Criminal law, public health and HIV transmission: A policy options paper.* Geneva. Retrieved from www.unaids.org

UNAIDS. (2008). *Criminalization of HIV transmission.* Policy Brief. Accessed December 8, 2009, at http://data.unaids.org/pub/BaseDocument/2008/20080731_jc1513_policy_criminalization_en.pdf

UNAIDS Reference Group (2009). *Statement on criminalization of HIV transmission or exposure.* Retrieved from http://data.unaids.org/pub/Report/2009/20090303_hrrefgroupcrimexposure_en.pdf

UNDP/UNAIDS (2010). Press Release: *Launch of the Global Commission on HIV and the Law: "Addressing punitive laws and human rights violations blocking effective AIDS responses."* Geneva, Switzerland.

UNDP (2012) *HIV and the law: Risks, rights and health.* The Global Commission on HIV and the Law. Retrieved from www.hivlawcommission.org

Wainberg, M. (2009). "Criminalizing HIV transmission may be a mistake." *Canadian Medical Association Journal,* 180(6), 688.

Weait, M. (2007). *Intimacy and responsibility: The criminalisation of HIV transmission.* London and New York: Routledge-Cavendish.

Wellbourn, A. (2008). "Into the firing line . . . : Placing young women and girls at greater risk". ALQ 10/11: 14–19.

# 16
# Community Mobilization, Community Planning, and Community-Based Research for HIV Prevention in the United States

*William Ward Darrow*

The evolving field of public health was defined almost a century ago as "the science and art of preventing disease, prolonging life, and promoting health and efficiency through organized community effort" (Winslow, 1920). Although the field has matured and grown considerably since "the bacteriologic revolution" of the early 20th century, this definition was reaffirmed in 1988 when a committee of the Institute of Medicine (1988, p. 7) forecast the future:

> The committee defines the mission of public health as fulfilling society's interest in assuring conditions in which people can be healthy. Its aim is to generate organized community effort to address the public interest in health by applying scientific and technical knowledge to prevent disease and promote health.

Writing during the early years of the acquired immune deficiency syndrome (AIDS) pandemic, the Committee for the Study of the Future of Public Health supported "a massive media, educational, and public health campaign" of "effective education to inform the public of the danger and to describe changes in behavior that can minimize the risk of infection" (Institute of Medicine, 1988, p. 21). It recognized health education as an essential public health service and as a vital component of health promotion programs to prevent infectious and chronic diseases, disabilities, and premature deaths.

This chapter goes to the heart of public health by examining organized community efforts to prevent human immunodeficiency virus (HIV) disease by community-based organizations, federal agencies, and biomedical and social science researchers. An elaboration of three major persistent challenges and three major emerging issues follows an overview of the three major concepts central to the substance of this chapter: community mobilization, community planning, and community-based research.

## COMMUNITY MOBILIZATION

Community refers to an aggregate of people who have a shared identity, a sense of belonging, and access to collective resources (Dignan & Carr, 1992). Members are recognized by one or more common characteristics and, often, by identifiable places (Green & Kreuter, 2005). Particularly important to the concept of community is the web of social institutions and human relationships that hold a community together. Thus, we can hear people speaking of a "gay community" that is recognized by a common sexual orientation, a shared sense of belonging, and identifiable places, such as "gay bars," "gay bookstores," and even "gay ghettos" (Levine, 1979).

Community mobilization refers to the process of stimulating collective action in a community to respond effectively to a perceived threat or concern (Bracht, Kingsbury, & Rissel, 1999). Particularly important in the mobilization process are: (1) recognition of the seriousness and severity of the perceived problem by a large segment of the community, (2) accepting responsibility for addressing the problem, and (3) committing time, talent, and treasure to doing something significant to alleviate the problem. When reports of a highly unusual gay-related immune deficiency (GRID) began to circulate in the early 1980s, gay men and others concerned about this apparent threat got together and established formal organizations, such as "Stop AIDS" in San Francisco and the Gay Men's Health Crisis (GMHC) in New York City, to respond to the threat by providing educational and other services for community members.

### Stop AIDS—San Francisco

Grassroots organizing was the basis for the first and one of the most successful community mobilization efforts ever conducted in response to public health warnings about GRID (Wohlfeiler, 1997). The gay, bisexual, lesbian, and transgender community in San Francisco responded to information about the AIDS crisis through a "Stop AIDS" community mobilization campaign designed to change norms by alerting members of the community to the potential risks of sexual transmission (Puckett & Bye, 1987). A widely read "safer sex" guide, *Play Fair!*, was published and distributed by "Sister Florence Nightmare" (Bobbi Campbell, RN) and other "Sisters of Perpetual Indulgence." "Safer Sex Parties," modeled after Tupperware parties, were held in private homes to demonstrate how latex condoms should be used. An explicit videotape, *Hot, Horny, and Healthy Sex,* was distributed to teach gay and bisexual men about sexual negotiation and the skills required to use condoms properly. Rancorous debates were held in public forums about whether bathhouses and other establishments licensed by the city should remain open to provide educational opportunities in intimate settings or should be closed for facilitating the spread of an unidentified sexually transmitted agent (Bayer, 1989).

Data collected from representative samples of community residents indicated that sexual behavior changed dramatically among men who have sex with men (MSM) in San Francisco (Winkelstein et al., 1987). Annual HIV infection rates among men 25–55 years old selected at random from 19 census tracts in San Francisco decreased from an estimated 18.4 percent per year from 1982 to 1984, to 5.4 percent and 3.1 percent during the first and second halves of 1985; then to 4.2 percent during the first six months of 1986. These sharp declines in HIV incidence were associated with reductions of 60 percent or more in the prevalence of high-risk sexual practices associated with HIV transmission. Extensive changes in sexual practices among MSM occurred as a result of sexually explicit educational materials being widely disseminated and discussed throughout the community. Community mobilization served to call a community to action and provoke a highly effective collective response in the face of federal government inaction.

## Gay Men's Health Crisis—New York

In many ways, the response to AIDS among gay men in New York City and other metropolitan areas of North America parallels the response of gay men in San Francisco. Volunteerism became the most necessary and reliable response to the political problems caused by AIDS as gay communities mobilized to contain and resolve the social, psychological, and spiritual issues that the disease raised (Kayal, 1993). Gay AIDS volunteerism in New York City was a response to a lack of response by Ronald Reagan's presidential administration and Edward Koch's mayoral administration and to being ignored and inadequately served by publicly funded federal and municipal agencies.

The Gay Men's Health Crisis (GMHC) was founded in 1982 to define and contain the effects of AIDS. "GMHC was shaped by two undeniable social facts: homophobic disinterest and the rebirth of American volunteer ideology under President Ronald Reagan" (Kayal, 1993, p. 5). Over the next five years, GMHC served to turn AIDS into a broader international and humanitarian issue. By 1992, GMHC had an annual budget approaching $20 million, had an active corps of over 2,000 volunteers, and had served nearly 14,000 people living with HIV or AIDS.

An epidemiologic study of 378 homosexually active men residing in New York City showed that the prevalence of HIV infection rose from 6.6 percent in 1978–1979 to 43.7 percent in early 1984 (Stevens et al., 1986). Seroconversions among susceptible men increased from 5.5 percent before 1981, when reports about GRID began to circulate, to 10.6 percent after 1981. Although most men reported decreasing their sexual activities after they first heard about AIDS, many continued to engage in unprotected receptive anal intercourse with one or more sexual partners. As was the case in San Francisco, community mobilization efforts significantly impacted the sexual practices of gay men in New York City, but HIV transmissions continued.

## Stop AIDS—Switzerland

The United States ("America Responds to AIDS"), Great Britain ("Don't Die of Ignorance"), and Australia ("The Grim Reaper") implemented mass media campaigns in the mid-1980s to warn their citizens of the threat of AIDS (Darrow, 1997). These fear-based campaigns were not as effective in mobilizing community support for HIV prevention as the national campaign conducted in Switzerland. The Swiss STOP AIDS campaign was launched in 1985 to promulgate two major messages: (1) use a condom during any sexual contact with an "inherent risk of infection" and (2) "never swap needles" (Kocher, 1993).

STOP AIDS Switzerland was constructed on ethical principles of human dignity, autonomy, and the common good. It focused on "risk situations" rather than "risk groups." The entire population was segmented into separate audiences to receive specific messages through appropriate channels. The program was designed to (1) do everything possible to promote solidarity between the infected and the uninfected, and (2) not do anything to suggest differentiating between "those worth saving" and "those beyond help."

Education was the first step in a "three-tier information-supply and action model." In March 1986, a brochure about AIDS printed in four languages was sent to every Swiss household. Over half (56 percent) of the recipients surveyed said they had read it. Readers' knowledge clearly improved, but campaign sponsors realized that informative messages had to be repeated. Much more work had to be done to change behaviors through "exposure-oriented prevention."

One Swiss innovation was to reintroduce and market the old tired latex prophylactic as a "Hot Rubber" (Darrow, 1997). It worked. Sales jumped from 2,000 units per month in early 1985 to a steady sale of about 75,000 units per month in 1986.

Community mobilization on a national scale can be effective when guided by scientific evidence, sound social marketing constructs, and ethical principles that respect human rights, but sufficient political, economic, and social support is absolutely necessary to achieve success (Kocher, 1996). The pragmatic Swiss were able to link together all organizations that could potentially contribute to AIDS prevention by emphasizing unity and avoiding divisiveness. They sought and were able to attain social solidarity in a "climate free of fear."

## COMMUNITY PLANNING: PRINCIPLES AND PRACTICES

In the United States, AIDS was defined by the Republican Reagan and George H. W. Bush administrations as a biomedical problem that could only be solved through scientific research. With the election of Democrat William J. Clinton in 1992, community activists were able to exert considerably more pressure on the federal government to respond more vigorously to unmet needs. Community planning for HIV prevention evolved out of the conviction that "effective prevention must be community-based, ecologically dispersed, locally relevant, adequately funded, responsive to change, and sustained over time" (Roe, Roe, Carpenter, & Sibley, 2005, p. 386).

In December 1993, the Centers for Disease Control and Prevention (CDC) began requiring grantees in 65 state, local, and territorial health departments in the United States to prioritize and select HIV-prevention interventions through a participatory "community planning process" (Johnson-Masotti, Pinkerton, Holtgrave, Valdiserri, & Willingham, 2000). As the federal agency primarily responsible for developing and supporting HIV-prevention programs in the United States, CDC promulgated 13 major principles for each community planning group to follow. Principle 10 stated, "The prioritization process should take into consideration behavioral theory, population needs, intervention effectiveness and cost-effectiveness, and local values and norms."

This new initiative of the 1990s was designed to deliver evidence-based interventions culturally consistent with the needs, priorities, and values of communities at risk for HIV infection. Major goals were to involve representatives of affected communities in local decision making, increase the use of epidemiologic data to identify high-risk behaviors in local populations, and include careful consideration of the demonstrated effectiveness and efficiency of proposed interventions. Organizing principles for each planning group required "parity, inclusion, and representation." Evaluations showed that community planning groups sought to put more resources into risk-reduction education and fewer into counseling and testing services than had many of the grantees before the participatory planning process was implemented.

## The State of Florida Red Ribbon Report

Governor Lawton Chiles of Florida requested in 1992 that a panel of 11 community members advise him on how to improve HIV/AIDS prevention and education and provide better, more cost-effective care (Governor's Red Ribbon Panel on AIDS, 1993). Among the recommendations were increased funding for comprehensive HIV/AIDS education in grades K through 12, HIV/AIDS education in Florida's universities and community colleges, and culturally competent and sensitive peer education and condom skills training. It also called for "removal of legal barriers which prevent clean needle exchange" (p. 4) and expressed "an urgent need for all of us to join together in the fight against the further spread of the disease" (p. 5).

## Community Planning in Miami-Dade County

With a total of 16,105 cumulative AIDS cases reported in Miami–Dade County through 1995, the Dade County HIV/AIDS Prevention Community Planning Group (DCPG) identified as their three most effective interventions (1) targeted community-based education and related "skills-building" activities, (2) street outreach, and (3) needle exchange (DCPG, 1996). To improve HIV-prevention services, the 27 voting members of DCPG recommended that "more detailed" needs assessments of priority populations be conducted, "as well as the development and implementation of interventions that appropriately address those needs in targeted communities" (DCPG, 1996, p. ii). Furthermore, "independent evaluation mechanisms should be implemented to assess the impact of various HIV-prevention efforts in specific target communities."

Clearly, the 27 local representatives of diverse communities in Miami–Dade County expected CDC, the State of Florida, and the local health department to allocate resources in accordance with their recommendations. "Ultimately," they wrote, "this Plan is intended to form the basis for funding allocation decisions at the national, state, and local levels" (p. i). It was not. Funding in Miami–Dade County and elsewhere continued to pour primarily into the HIV-prevention services that had been mandated by CDC as "essential": (1) surveillance, (2) seroprevalence screening of pregnant women and other "high-risk groups," and (3) anonymous and confidential HIV-antibody testing of individuals with costly pre- and post-test counseling. As it became increasingly apparent that national public health officials were ignoring the input of local community planning groups regarding priorities for funding, many community representatives became frustrated and withdrew from the process. Exasperation with public health officials and disappointment in their intransigence inhibited HIV-prevention efforts in south Florida during the late 1990s to a much greater extent than "AIDS fatigue" or "burnout."

## Community Planning in Broward County

Although the impact of community planning was greatly diminished by CDC's failure to respond with adequate funding to the needs and recommendations of local community representatives, the community planning process limped along for another decade. Then, in 2005, the State of Florida announced that it would no longer support local community planning groups (Broward Community Planning Partnership, 2006). The state decided it would do what was minimally acceptable to CDC. It restricted community planning to a single entity: the State of Florida Community Planning Group.

The last Broward County Prevention Plan (p. 46) contained this confession: "Original models of HIV behavior change put far too much emphasis on individualistic approaches and failed to consider the social, cultural, and economic environment and context in which behaviors occurred. They assumed that individuals could always make informed decisions based on the information provided to them by prevention and then act on those decisions." It concluded with a recommendation for a more complex model with multiple components: "There is no 'magic bullet'" (p. 48). Prevention must take a long-term perspective. Effective prevention takes time.

## Community-Based Research

Community-based research involves systematic inquiry with community members into their relationships and practices in a community setting, and not in a laboratory, hospital, clinic, or artificially contrived experimental situation (Blumenthal & Yancey, 2004). Community-based research can be contrasted with clinical research where individuals (typically, "patients") are used as the unit of analysis. It is much more difficult to randomly assign communities to experimental treatment and control (or "placebo") conditions than it is to randomly assign "well-worked-up patients." It is also much more difficult to control forces extraneous to a "social experiment" from interfering with the observations and outcomes of community-based research (Shadish, Cook, & Campbell, 2002).

Typically, community-based research is centered on the needs of populations, partnerships, and primary, secondary, and tertiary prevention alternatives. It always occurs in natural settings, tends to be multidisciplinary, and often uses mixed methods of data collection and analysis. The purpose typically is not to isolate the effects of a single variable on an expected outcome, as is usually the case in experimental research, but to find out what is going on and what seems to work with people as they go about living their daily lives. Results should be used to guide public health decision making to improve the health of populations, just as results of clinical research are used to guide the decisions of physicians in caring for their patients.

Community-based research should not be confused with "community-focused," "community-placed," or "community-informed" research (Wallerstein & Duran, 2008). "Community based" means that members of the community are involved in the planning, conduct, and reporting of research procedures and study results. "Community-based participatory research (CBPR)" requires that members of a community affected by a public health problem be treated as equal partners with public health scientists in the discovery process of identifying and characterizing a research problem, developing and implementing appropriate research procedures, and in analyzing, interpreting, and reporting all relevant research findings.

CBPR is a partnership approach to research that equitably involves community members, organizational representatives, and researchers in all aspects of the research process (Israel, Eng, Schulz, & Parker, 2005). Its purposes are to enhance understanding of phenomena and community dynamics and to integrate the knowledge gained with action to improve health and well-being. CBPR recognizes communities as an aspect of collective and individual identity, builds on strengths and resources within a community, and promotes co-learning and capacity building. In addition, it offers mutual benefits, assumes an ecological perspective of multicausation, and involves systems development through an iterative process. Furthermore, CBPR facilitates collaborative and equitable partnerships in all phases of research. It requires a commitment to sustainability.

Action research is committed to improving community conditions so that community members are better off when a research project ends than they were when the project began (Stringer, 1999). Action researchers measure their success as scientists by the degree to which they can demonstrate that quality of life has improved among community members as a direct result of their collaborative efforts. Seeing healthier lifestyles among community members is more important to action researchers than seeing the publication of their original scientific articles in prestigious professional journals. Needless to say, very few action researchers are successful in obtaining large R01 research grants from the National Institutes of Health. Few are currently principal investigators in major HIV-prevention research projects being conducted in the United States.

## AIDS Community Demonstration Projects

Community-level interventions for high-risk, hard-to-reach populations were introduced in five U.S. cities in 1989 to assess their efficacy in increasing consistent condom use to prevent HIV infections with main and other sexual partners (O'Reilly & Higgins, 1991). Theoretically driven interventions were developed after formative evaluations were conducted to identify underlying cognitive factors. They were based on four behavior-change theories and models: health belief model, theory of reasoned action, social cognitive theory, and the stages of change continuum of the transtheoretical model. Key components of the AIDS Community Demonstration Projects (ACDP) were (1) creation of small-media materials featuring theory-based role model stories and other prevention messages, (2) increased availability of condoms and bleach kits for injection drug users, and (3) community mobilization of community volunteers to distribute and verbally reinforce prevention messages and materials among their peers.

Results showed that most populations were in the "precontemplative stage of behavior change" with respect to consistent condom use when baseline data were collected (CDC, 1996). Recent exposure to role-model stories and other materials increased in intervention communities from 5 percent during month 2 to a peak of 54 percent during month 27. Those who said they had been exposed to project materials were more likely than others to report engaging in consistent condom use for vaginal intercourse with "nonmain partners." By June 1994, a fivefold increase toward action was realized as condoms and print materials encouraging consistent and proper use were continuously delivered by project staff and community network members (CDC AIDS Community Demonstration Projects Research Group, 1999).

## REACH 2010 in Broward County

Racial and Ethnic Approaches to Community Health (REACH) 2010 was a national effort funded by CDC to reduce disparities in six major diseases adversely affecting six major minority populations (Giles et al., 2004). The Coalition to Eliminate Disparities in HIV Disease in Broward County, Florida, was one of 32 successful applicants for a cooperative agreement to conduct formative research to develop a viable community action plan (CAP) in 1999. The Broward CAP called for grassroots community mobilization to make everyone in diverse black and Hispanic communities aware of the devastating effects of HIV disease, to encourage greater community participation in HIV-prevention efforts, and to take ownership and action to solve the HIV/AIDS problem (Darrow et al., 2004).

The Broward Coalition was one of 24 coalitions in the United States to receive an award to implement and evaluate its program from fiscal year 2000 through 2007. Interventions were developed by following steps in the PRECEDE model for health promotion planning (Green & Kreuter, 2005) and by paying attention to the findings of the needs assessment (Bartholomew et al., 2011). Four interventions were chosen: (1) educational outreach to community residents, (2) educational outreach to stakeholders, gatekeepers, and other influential individuals and groups, (3) strategic communications, and (4) capacity building and infrastructure development. From the outset, the central coordinating organization (Florida International University) insisted that at least half of the available resources be committed to providing services that would directly benefit 18–39-year-old residents of the 12 (out of 53) ZIP-code areas with the highest incidence of AIDS reported for black and Hispanic populations.

Figure 16.1 illustrates the effects of CDC slashing the REACH 2010 budget for Broward County in half, from over $900,000 in fiscal year 2004 to under $500,000 in fiscal year 2005 (Darrow et al., 2010). With these drastic budget cuts, the coalition was forced to terminate contracts with the three Broward CBOs carrying out effective educational outreach to residents in the 12 ZIP-code areas of high-AIDS incidence. Immediately following these severe cutbacks, the number of new HIV cases reported for black residents rose from a low of 108.8 per 100,000 in calendar year 2006 to 133.6 per 100,000 in 2007; then it leveled off (see Figure 16.1). Rates of new HIV infections in the Hispanic and white populations of Broward County

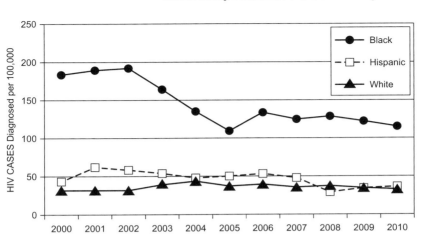

**Figure 16.1** Impact and sustainability of REACH 2010 interventions on trends in new HIV cases diagnosed among black, Hispanic, and white residents of Broward County, Florida (Note: Data for Broward County were provided on October 25, 2011, by Florida Department of Health, Bureau of HIV/AIDS [HSDHIV], Tallahassee, Florida 32399-1715, and were analyzed by Ms. Elena Sebekos, MPH, and the author. HSDHIV advised us that the apparent increase in rates per 100,000 of HIV cases diagnosed and reported in 2006 and subsequent years may have been attributable in part to changes in State of Florida reporting requirements that took effect on November 20, 2006.)

were identical in 2010, but the hope of eliminating disparities in HIV disease for black populations was not realized.

## The Test, Link to Care, Plus Treat (TLC-Plus) Approach to HIV Prevention

TLC-Plus is being conducted to test the feasibility of a "community focused enhanced test and link-to-care strategy" in the Bronx, New York, and Washington, DC (El-Sadr & Branson, 2010). The expanded HIV-testing component involves "social mobilization with targeted messaging to promote testing," coupled with universal testing in emergency departments and hospital inpatient admissions. The biomedical breakthrough driving this project is proof that viral suppression through high levels of adherence to antiretroviral therapy (ART) prevents HIV transmission (Dieffenbach & Fauci, 2009). A major objective of TLC-Plus is to identify every HIV-infected adolescent and adult residing in the two communities and immediately start them on ART, so that the chances of their infecting others will diminish to near zero, regardless of their sexual and drug-using behaviors (El-Sadr & Branson, 2010).

In Washington, DC, the Department of Public Health has formed a partnership with the Global Business Coalition and Pfizer to implement a pilot program under which Pfizer sales representatives will promote routine testing and provide toolkits to 200 DC physicians. The three-year feasibility study also has other components that will be evaluated, but written informed consent will not be obtained from study participants because TLC-Plus activities "do not constitute research." Furthermore, study teams will not report adverse events or social harms because "there is no biomedical intervention." Effectiveness of TLC-Plus will be determined by reviewing trends in routine HIV-surveillance data collected in the two communities chosen for intervention compared with HIV-surveillance data collected in "four non-intervention communities": Chicago, Illinois; Houston, Texas; Miami, Florida; and Philadelphia, Pennsylvania (El-Sadr & Branson, 2010).

Although local community-based organizations and many others in the Bronx and DC have written letters of support and community advisory boards have been created to review project procedures, TLC-Plus represents a major departure from the grassroots community mobilization efforts of the 1980s and 1990s. The entire project is top-down, conceived by NIH experts in Bethesda, Maryland, and CDC experts in Atlanta, Georgia; presented with generous amounts of federal funding to local health departments and health care providers in two carefully selected geographic areas of the northeastern United States; and delivered to every sexually active individual 15 years of age or older captured by a cooperative local medical facility or provider. The major intervention is medicinal: Provide continuous ART therapy to every HIV-infected individual to protect the entire community from HIV transmission (Mayer & Venkatesh, 2010). The idea driving the TLC-Plus demonstration project is to identify HIV-infected persons as quickly as possible, put them on ART as soon as possible, and keep them on ART as long as possible, so they can't possibly infect anyone else no matter what they do with their used needles and sexual organs.

## PERSISTENT CHALLENGES

Our overview of community mobilization, community planning, and community-based research for HIV prevention has revealed the presence of several 21st-century challenges. First and foremost is the determined devotion of public health officials to adhere to a biomedical model of reductionism that focuses primarily on the attributes of the etiologic agent, the biology of the human host, and the microenvironment where the retrovirus and host react to each other. From this perspective, the best interventions to employ are those that destroy the virus, restore the immune system, and nurture the human host through biomedical modalities. Critical components of ensuing programs include patient counseling, repeated testing, and entry into supervised medical care. The best outcomes associated with the biomedical model and its preferred interventions are those that directly contribute to carefully constructed knowledge, even if they do not necessarily benefit patients or improve human health conditions in the short run.

## A Biomedical or a Socioecological Approach to HIV Prevention

What is the best available model to guide public health decision making? Is it the dominant biomedical model or should it be something else? Before AIDS was first recognized by health authorities in 1981, Engle (1977) observed, "All medicine is in crisis," because of "adherence to a model of disease no longer adequate for the scientific tasks and social responsibilities" of the profession (p. 129). He noted that the biomedical model embraces both "reductionism" and "mind-body dualism." Reductionism is particularly harmful when it neglects the impact of nonbiological circumstances upon biologic processes. Whatever cannot be explained by the biomedical model is *excluded* from the category of disease. Engle recommended that the biomedical model be replaced by an alternative "biopsychosocial model" that takes "into account the patient, the social context in which he lives, and the complementary system devised by society to deal with the disruptive effects of illness" (p. 132). He concluded, "Systems theory provides a conceptual approach suitable for understanding the proposed biopsychosocial concept of disease and studying disease and medical care as interrelated processes" (p. 134).

Five years after AIDS was recognized, the Ottawa Charter for Health Promotion (World Health Organization, 1986) proclaimed, "The inextricable links between people and their environment constitutes the basis for a socioecological approach to health." A socioecological approach to health extends beyond the narrow focus of pathogen, human host, and cellular biology by attempting to account for people living in diverse communities, contexts, and systems. In this biopsychosocial model, health promotion action means building healthy public policy, creating supportive environments, strengthening community actions, developing personal skills, and reorienting health services away from treatment and toward primary prevention (Nutbeam & Blakey, 1990).

In a sociological approach to disease prevention, understanding the social transmission of HIV entails the location of the epidemic in its social context (Bloor, 1995). The issues of concern are not so much the biological mechanisms of transmission, but the social relationships within which HIV transmission occurs. Social relationships are more important to understand than risk behaviors, because HIV is spread from one person to another through social, not individual, actions. The task of health promotion with respect to primary HIV prevention is not to proscribe relationships, but to encourage and reinforce alterations in sexual relationships that minimize, if not eliminate, the risk of HIV transmission. Changes in sexual norms and steep declines in risky sexual practices among MSM occurred in the mid-1980s in response to community mobilization and educational efforts, but these changes could not be sustained indefinitely without additional support. The number of men engaging in unsafe sexual practices grew larger as highly active antiretroviral therapy was shown to be effective in containing the damaging effects of HIV infection. For risk reduction to occur and be sustained for long periods of time, a favorable social structural and social policy framework must be established.

A promising framework is contained within the Principles of the Ethical Practice of Public Health (Public Health Leadership Society, 2002). It maintains that public health should address principally the fundamental causes of disease and requirements for health, achieve community health in a way that respects the rights of individuals in the community, and advocate and work for the empowerment of disenfranchised community members. Public health policies, programs, and priorities should be developed and evaluated through processes that ensure an opportunity for sufficient input from community members. They should incorporate a variety of approaches that anticipate and respect diverse values, beliefs, and cultures within a community. Public health institutions and their employees should engage in collaboration and affiliations in ways that build both the public's trust and the institution's effectiveness. They should provide communities with information for decision making and obtain the community's consent for the implementation of public health policies and programs to benefit community members.

## Patient-Centered or Community-Based Strategies for HIV Prevention

What are the best interventions to employ to stop the spread of HIV: those that alter biological susceptibility or those that alter social vulnerability to infection? HIV-prevention research and programs continue to focus on persons in virtual isolation from the political, economic, and cultural realities of their lives (Beeker, Guenther-Grey, & Raj, 1998). The cause of AIDS is a retrovirus, but the societal problem of AIDS has *multiple determinants*. Therefore, communities must participate in defining and solving the societal problem of AIDS and in addressing its social, political, economic, cultural, and behavioral determinants. Community empowerment and capacity building may be necessary to assist communities in achieving effective HIV prevention.

An empowerment paradigm extends the lens of psychosocial models of behavior change. Empowerment is a social-action process that promotes the participation of people, organizations, and communities toward goals of increased individual and community control, political efficacy, improved quality of life, and social justice. Community empowerment provides a framework for developing interventions to bring about enduring community-wide change in HIV-transmission rates. Community empowerment was very much a part of earlier efforts to prevent the spread of HIV in communities. It appears to be absent in current efforts to substitute chemoprophylaxis (e.g., "Viread" and "Truvada") for social (e.g., abstinence and partner reduction) and mechanical (e.g., proper and consistent latex condom use) prophylaxis (Mayer & Venkatesh, 2010).

In their critique of "Treatment as Prevention" Holtgrave, Maulsby, Wehrmeyer, and Hall (2012) have noted that slightly over half of the new cases of HIV infection in the United States each year are transmitted by a relatively small number of persons who *are aware* of their HIV infections. Less than half are transmitted by those who have not been made fully aware of their infections. Therefore, the impact of ART on HIV incidence will accrue from only a relatively small proportion of the HIV-infected population that strictly adheres to medical care. The interplay between the risky behaviors of a relatively small group of highly likely transmitters, treatment access, and viral load suppression at the community level must be better understood for treatment as prevention to work. "The national effect of treatment availability is likely a complex function of biological, clinical, behavioral, and social factors," writes David R. Holtgrave (2009); therefore, the test and treat strategy "may not be the optimal framework to guide the National Institutes of Health HIV prevention agenda." Holtgrave and colleagues (2012) advise that "complementary prevention" should replace "combination prevention" that pits biomedical interventions against a constellation of more appropriately balanced behavioral and biomedical interventions.

## Evidence-Based or Effectiveness-Based Decision Making for Public Health

What are the best outcomes for the public's health: advances in scientific knowledge or significant improvements in human health? The U.S. government has invested more resources into biomedical research to understand pathogenesis and develop better diagnostic tests, treatments, and a vaccine than into well-designed and fully implemented HIV-prevention programs, believing that the ultimate solution to AIDS lies in the discovery of "magic bullets." Rigorous scientific research to find and test these "wonder drugs" requires patience; it takes time and can be very costly. The immediate payoff comes in the form of lessons learned. The evidence gathered is used to develop programs that may or may not be effective when implemented in U.S. communities. Another problem that continues to limit the full potential of HIV-prevention programs is the reliance on evidence produced (and not produced) from a relatively small number of randomized control trials (RCTs) designed to test *the efficacy of an intervention* instead of relying on evidence of *the effectiveness of public health programs* (Kettner, Moroney, & Martin, 1999). The *efficacy* of an intensive standardized intervention established with plentiful resources by highly motivated scientific investigators and research subjects in a carefully controlled experimental setting may not translate into program *effectiveness* when the "evidence-based" intervention is adapted and exported to "real-world" settings with great expectations, but with less highly motivated program participants, poorly trained and motivated program staff, and little or no funds for proper implementation, quality assurance, and outcome evaluation (Noar, 2008).

HIV/AIDS health promotion is always context-bound, taking place within discrete communities and in specific settings (Aggleton, 1993). An understanding of social context is essential. The communities within which interventions are introduced are not all alike. They are fragmented socially and culturally. Health promotion in the 21st century is taking place in a context of political polarization, continued and pervasive stigmatization and prejudice, and preserving the status quo rather than stimulating social change. Community-inspired health promotion initiatives often challenge the ideology and interests of modern biomedicine. Three-year feasibility programs imposed by federal agencies to test research hypotheses in vulnerable communities may be perceived by residents as patronizing and exploitive. Such top-down strategies promoted by outsiders usually prove to be less effective than those that originate from the expressed needs of communities, include extensive periods of exploratory research that engender mutual understanding and trust, and are designed to have more lasting impact by building community capacity and changing social norms (Merzel & D'Afflitti, 2003).

The current piecemeal approach to public health in the United States is to shape and reshape HIV-prevention programs on the basis of interpretations of the scientific evidence and political expediency. Decisions are almost never made on the basis of documented effectiveness in up-and-running state and municipal programs. The shaping process is controlled by carefully selected advisory committee members, bureaucrats, and political appointees in the executive branch of the U.S. government. Community input is frequently sought and used to formulate recommendations, but funding decisions that determine implementation are typically made by agency directors in line with the political priorities of the party in power. Public health in the United States currently involves a top-down process that starts in the White House (Office of National AIDS Policy), the neighboring National Institutes of Health (NIH) in Bethesda, Maryland, or, perhaps, the Centers for Disease Control and Prevention (CDC) in Atlanta, Georgia, and ends up affecting communities like the Bronx and the District of Columbia, providing there is enough money in the budget to at least partially implement a program.

## EMERGING ISSUES

The discovery of AIDS in 1981 led to HIV/AIDS awareness campaigns and biomedical interventions that included voluntary counseling and HIV-antibody testing, referral for medical care, and partner notification (CTRPN) programs in the 1980s; community planning and ART programs for persons living with HIV/AIDS in the 1990s; and a narrowly focused Serologic Approach to Fighting the Epidemic (SAFE) program to "advance HIV prevention" in the 2000s (CDC, 2006). Community mobilization, once the backbone of HIV-prevention efforts in the United States, is now regarded as an option that might or might not be included in an "enhanced comprehensive HIV-prevention program" (ECHPP) that mandates the inclusion of 14 biomedical interventions (Darrow, 2011). Community planning has become a routinized pastime that requires minimal input (but expects maximal "buy-in") from vulnerable communities. Community-based research meant to address local health problems has been subverted by the powerful interests of an HIV-Prevention Trials Network (HPTN). Emerging as critical issues from these disturbing trends are

(1) the disrupting effects of biomedical breakthroughs, (2) the dismantling of underfunded health promotion programs, and (3) an obvious disdain for population health.

## Game Changers

How do we deal with biomedical breakthroughs and their disruptive effects on organized community efforts to promote health, prevent disease, and eliminate disparities? With the election of Democrat Bill Clinton in 1992, CDC was forced to reassess its CTRPN HIV-prevention program and consider a wider range of interventions than those dictated by the biomedical model. With the election of Republican George W. Bush in 2000, CDC returned to its old ways with a vengeance. Through SAFE, CDC refocused programmatic efforts on "individuals infected with HIV" (Janssen et al., 2001). Instead of keeping their promise to help communities implement their carefully crafted HIV-prevention plans, CDC redirected federal funds away from community mobilization efforts and toward (1) diagnosing all HIV-infected persons in a community, (2) linking them to appropriate medical care and services, (3) assisting them to adhere to treatment regimens, and (4) supporting them through behavior modification interventions that address "motivation" and "psychologic barriers" (Janssen et al., 2001).

SAFE marked the beginning of the 21st century and a new era in HIV prevention. "As the number of individuals with HIV continues to increase because of ART, so does the urgency for lifelong prevention strategies customized for them," argued Janssen and his CDC colleagues (p. 1023). "Such an approach couples the traditional infectious disease control focus on the infected person with behavioral interventions that have become standard elements in HIV prevention programs." Instead of mobilizing communities for HIV prevention, CDC opted to mobilize a new public-private coalition, "X-AIDS ACT NOW! National Partnership," and welcomed medical care organizations, the pharmaceutical industry, and private industry to help address the specific needs of SAFE (Janssen et al., 2001). This new initiative opened the door to an alliance between U.S. federal health agencies, the American pharmaceutical industry, Madison Avenue, and Wall Street that would spur a biomedical research agenda to reduce "community viral load" and lead to the recommendation of a Food and Drug Administration advisory committee to approve Truvada for preexposure prophylaxis (Cahill, 2012).

With the licensing of a simple rapid HIV test, OraQuick, in November 2002, and apparent increases in the incidence of HIV and syphilis, CDC launched "Advancing HIV Prevention: New Strategies for a Changing Epidemic" to reduce barriers to an early diagnosis of HIV infection and increase access to quality medical care, treatment, and ongoing prevention services (CDC, 2003). This initiative specified the "proven public health approaches" to be included: (1) appropriate routine screening, (2) identification of new cases, (3) partner notification, and (4) increased availability of sustained treatment and prevention services for those infected (prevention case management). Missing from this announcement was any mention of the proper and consistent use of latex condoms, needle exchange, harm reduction, professional and peer educational outreach, strategic communications, role-model stories, partner concurrency, partner reduction, or capacity building to sustain HIV-prevention efforts.

## Dismantling of Community Health Promotion Programs

The current "Find, Test, Treat, and Retain" approach to HIV prevention is remarkably similar to the situation in the early 1950s when Dwight D. Eisenhower was elected president of the United States. Back then, penicillin was hailed as "the miracle cure" for syphilis and gonorrhea (Parascandola, 2008). With the availability of this "magic bullet" to treat cases, there was no need to continue a program of health promotion for venereal disease prevention. Congress cut funding in half and the newly created Department of Health, Education, and Welfare began to dismantle the Division of Venereal Disease (VD). Components of the VD program were disassembled and staff were either sent to the Communicable Disease Center in Atlanta, Georgia, or assigned elsewhere.

Initially, AIDS was defined as an infectious disease, just like syphilis and gonorrhea (Fee & Krieger, 1993). Once the etiologic agent was identified, scientists turned their attention away from the societal factors propelling transmission and toward laboratory studies of the virus that could lead to patents and profits: highly sensitive and specific diagnostic tests, a safe and effective vaccine, and a cure. The serostatus approach of dividing a community into those who were positive and those who were negative ignored the complex power dynamics of interpersonal relationships and assumed that health behaviors were solely a function of rational calculation. The costly case management model of today pours more and more dollars into screening, early case detection, and lifelong treatment. Finding the right pharmaceutical product represents the epitome of successful disease management.

As enthusiasm for supporting basic scientific research mounted in the United States, few research dollars were expended on studies designed to improve social interventions for HIV prevention. The biomedical model placed the onus of staying healthy on the individual, not the community. It limited explanations of disease to narrowly defined proximate causes. Distal societal factors, such as poverty and discrimination, were either deemed irrelevant or ignored. Patients were seen as willing and compliant participants in "cutting-edge" biomedical research and treatment programs. Community activists were not regarded as equal partners in seeking a solution to the societal problems of AIDS. Only physicians and biomedical scientists had the wisdom and expertise to design, develop, and implement prototypical programs. Scientific knowledge was held to be outside the bounds of social context (Fee & Krieger, 1993).

## Private Medical Care and the End of Population Health

The United States spends more on health care than any other country, provides fewer of its citizens with insurance coverage, and has "so enriched the health-care industry as to make change extraordinary difficult" (Starr, 2011, p. 2). The Patient Protection and Affordable Care Act was passed by Congress in March 2010 and signed into law by President Barack Obama, but its future remains tenuous. The constitutionality of one of its major provisions was upheld by the U.S. Supreme Court, but its implementation is left in large measure to governors and state legislatures. The U.S. Congress has been reluctant to support the act's "public health and prevention fund," making it extremely difficult to carry out health promotion and disease prevention programs in the United States. And the unsuccessful presidential nominee of the Republican Party, Mitt Romney, pledged to do everything in his power to repeal "Obamacare" if he were elected in November 2012.

In a climate of fiscal austerity and accountability, public health is finding it increasingly difficult to provide essential services and meet obligations to promote health, prevent disease, and eliminate health disparities. Discretionary funding for preventive care is disappearing from budgets. Health departments in Florida and elsewhere are eliminating positions, consolidating services, and cutting back to make ends meet. Fewer Americans can afford private medical care and costly health insurance coverage while public health services are being cut to the bone. Twentieth-century concerns about the need for population health are giving way to 21st-century concerns about reining in a massive public debt.

## SUMMARY, CONCLUSION, AND RECOMMENDATION

A socioecological model for HIV prevention has been proposed as an alternative to the biomedical model, because "AIDS is at once a social and biological disorder; its course cannot be understood or altered without attention to its social and political context" (Fee & Krieger, 1993, p. 1477). A socioecological model can accommodate features of the biomedical model by including attributes of the etiologic agent, human host, and cellular environment into its robust architecture (Coates, Richter, & Caceres, 2008). Whereas the biomedical model demands adherence to the laws of nature, the socioecological model allows flexible choices for different populations, different social, cultural, political, economic, and geographic environments, and different combinations of interventions to maximize program effectiveness and efficiency while minimizing costs. The socioecological model is localized and particularistic, not generic and monolithic. It is bottom-up, not top-down.

Nothing has been more damaging to ongoing community-level HIV-prevention efforts in the last decade than announcements of biomedical breakthroughs. With each new report of scientific efficacy, limited funds are diverted away from community health promotion programs and toward the purchase and distribution of simpler and quicker tests for seronegatives and more potent and expensive pills for seropositives. Clearly, increasing numbers of HIV-infected persons are living longer due to the availability of more effective biomedical products, but the price paid by promising community demonstration projects, such as REACH 2010 in Broward County, and the 65 state, municipal, and territorial public health programs in the United States has been exceedingly steep.

AIDS is, in essence, a social disease. Above all else, AIDS is about people in personal and social relationships. Critical characteristics of successful programs appear to be: (1) an ecological approach to problem identification, understanding, and solving, (2) tailoring of interventions to meet the specific needs of at-risk individuals and vulnerable communities, and (3) participation and influence of those affected by a problem in designing, implementing, and evaluating the effectiveness of interventions (Israel et al., 2005). The emphasis should be on a collective rather than an individualistic approach to HIV-disease prevention and control. Unfortunately, now it is not.

## BIBLIOGRAPHY

Aggleton, P. (1993). Promoting whose health? Models of health promotion and education about HIV disease. In G. L. Albrecht & R. S. Zimmerman (eds.),

*Advances in medical sociology: The social and behavioral aspects of AIDS* (pp. 185–200). Greenwich, CT: JAI.

Bartholomew, L. K., Parcel, G. S., Kok, G., Gottlieb, N. H., & Fernandez, M. E. (2011). *Planning health promotion programs: An intervention mapping approach* (3rd ed.). San Francisco, CA: Jossey-Bass.

Bayer, R. (1989). *Private acts, social consequences: AIDS and the politics of public health.* New York: Free Press.

Beeker, C., Guenther-Grey, C., & Raj, A. (1998). Community empowerment paradigm drift and the primary prevention of HIV/AIDS. *Social Science and Medicine, 46*(7), 831–842.

Bloor, M. (1995). *The sociology of HIV transmission.* London: Sage.

Blumenthal, D. S., & Yancey, E. (2004). Community-based research: An introduction. In D. S. Blumenthal & R. J. DiClemente (eds.), *Community-based health research* (pp. 3–24). New York: Springer.

Bracht, N., Kingsbury, L., & Rissel, C. (1999). A five-stage community organization model for health promotion: Empowerment and partnership strategies. In N. Bracht (ed.), *Health promotion at the community level* (2nd ed.) (pp. 83–104). Thousand Oaks, CA: Sage.

Broward Community Planning Partnership (2006). *2007–2009 Broward County HIV prevention plan.* Retrieved from http://cfbroward.org/cfbroward/media/Documents/HIVPrevPlan2007-2009.pdf

Cahill, S. (2012). *Policy focus—Pre-exposure prophylaxis for HIV prevention: Moving toward implementation.* Boston, MA: The Fenway Institute. Retrieved from http://www.fenwayhealth.org/site/DocServer/PolicyFocus_PrEP_v7_02.21.12.pdf?docID=9321

CDC AIDS Community Demonstration Projects Research Group (1999). Community-level HIV intervention in 5 cities: Final outcome data from the CDC AIDS community demonstration projects. *American Journal of Public Health, 89*(3), 336–345.

Centers for Disease Control and Prevention (1996). Community-level prevention of human immunodeficiency virus infection among high-risk populations: The AIDS community demonstration projects. *MMWR Recommendations and Reports, 45*(RR-6), 1–24.

Centers for Disease Control and Prevention (2003). Advancing HIV prevention: New strategies for a changing epidemic—United States, 2003. *Morbidity and Mortality Weekly Report, 52,* 329–332.

Centers for Disease Control and Prevention (2006). Evolution of HIV/AIDS prevention programs—United States, 1981–2006. *Morbidity and Mortality Weekly Report, 55,* 597–603.

Coates, T. J., Richter, L., & Caceres, C. (2008). Behavioural strategies to reduce HIV transmission: How to make them work better. *Lancet, 372,* 669–684.

Dade County HIV/AIDS Prevention Community Planning Group (1996). *A plan for hope: 1996/1997 State of Florida District XI-A HIV prevention plan.* Miami, FL: Health Council of South Florida.

Darrow, W. W. (1997). Health education and promotion for STD prevention: Lessons for the next millennium. *Genitourinary Medicine, 73,* 88–94.

Darrow, W. W. (2011). President Obama's national HIV/AIDS strategy for the United States: Change we can believe in or more of the same [Abstract]? *Journal of Sexual Medicine, 8* (Suppl. 3), 219. doi: 10.1111/j.1743-6109.2011.02325.x

Darrow, W. W., Kim, S., Montanea, J. E., Uribe, C. L., Sánchez-Braña, E., & Gladwin, H. (2010). Summative evaluation of a community mobilization program to eliminate disparities in HIV disease. *International Public Health Journal, 2,* 301–311.

Darrow, W. W., Montanea, J. E., Fernández, P. B., Zucker, U. F., Stephens, D. P., & Gladwin, H. (2004). Eliminating disparities in HIV disease: Community mobilization to prevent HIV transmission among black and Hispanic young adults in Broward County, Florida. *Ethnicity and Disease, 14*(Suppl. 1), S108–S116.

Dieffenbach, C. W., & Fauci, A. S. (2009). Universal voluntary testing and treatment for prevention of HIV transmission. *Journal of the American Medical Association, 301,* (22) 2380–2382.

Dignan, M. B., & Carr, P. A. (1992). *Program planning for health education and health promotion* (2nd ed.). Philadelphia, PA: Lea & Febiger.

El-Sadr, W., & Branson, B. (2010). *TLC-plus: A study to evaluate the feasibility of an enhanced test, link to care, plus treat approach for HIV prevention in the United States (HPTN 065).* Washington, DC: Division of AIDS, U.S. National Institute of Allergy and Infectious Diseases, U.S. National Institutes of Health.

Engle, G. L. (1977). The need for a new medical model: A challenge for biomedicine. *Science, 196,* 129–136.

Fee, E., & Krieger, N. (1993). Understanding AIDS: Historical interpretations and the limits of biomedical individualism. *American Journal of Public Health, 83*(10), 1477–1486.

Giles, W. H., Tucker, P., Brown, L., Crocker, C., Jack, N., Latimer, A., … Harris, V. B. (2004). Racial and ethnic approaches to community health (REACH 2010): An overview. *Ethnicity and Disease, 14*(3 Suppl. 1), S5–S8.

Governor's Red Ribbon Panel on AIDS (1993). *Report: Governor's red ribbon panel on AIDS.* State of Florida: Department of Health and Rehabilitative Services, AIDS Program.

Green, L. W., & Kreuter, M. W., (eds.) (2005). *Health promotion planning: An educational and ecological approach* (4th ed.). New York: McGraw-Hill.

Holtgrave, D. R. (2009). Strategies for preventing HIV transmission [Letter]. *Journal of the American Medical Association, 302,*(14). 530. doi:10.1001/jama.2009.1442

Holtgrave, D. R., Maulsby, C., Wehrmeyer, L., & Hall, H. I. (2012). Behavioral factors in assessing impact of HIV treatment as prevention. *AIDS and Behavior, 16*(5), 1085–1091. doi 10.1007/s10461-102-0186-1)

Institute of Medicine (1988). *The future of public health.* Washington, DC: National Academy Press.

Israel, B. A., Eng, E., Schulz, A. J., & Parker, E. A. (eds.).(2005). *Methods in community-based participatory research for health.* San Francisco, CA: Jossey-Bass.

Janssen, R. S., Holtgrave, D. R., Valdiserri, R. O., Shepherd, M., Gayle, H. D., & DeCock, K. M. (2001). The serostatus approach to fighting the HIV epidemic: Prevention strategies for infected individuals. *American Journal of Public Health, 91,* 1019–1024.

Johnson-Masotti, A. P., Pinkerton, S. D., Holtgrave, D. R., Valdiserri, R. O., & Willingham, M. (2000). Decision-making in HIV prevention community planning: An integrative review. *Journal of Community Health, 25*(2), 95–112.

Kayal, P. M. (1993). *Bearing witness: Gay Men's Health Crisis and the politics of AIDS.* Boulder, CO: Westview.

Kettner, P. M., Moroney, R. M., & Martin, L. L. (1999). *Designing and managing programs: An effectiveness-based approach* (2nd ed.). Newbury Park, CA: Sage.

Kocher, K. W. (1993). *Stop AIDS: The stop AIDS story 1987–1992.* Basel, Switzerland: The Swiss AIDS Foundation and Federal Office of Public Health.

Kocher, K. W. (1996). *Stop AIDS: The stop AIDS story,* Part 2, *1993–1995.* Basel, Switzerland: The Swiss AIDS Foundation and Federal Office of Public Health.

Levine, M. P. (1979). Gay ghetto. *Journal of Homosexuality, 4*(4), 363–377.

Mayer, K. H., & Venkatesh, K. K. (2010). Antiretroviral therapy as HIV prevention: Status and prospects. *American Journal of Public Health, 100,* 1867–1876. doi: 10.2105/AJPH.2009.184796

Merzel, C., & D'Afflitti, J. (2003). Reconsidering community-based health promotion: Promise, performance, and potential. *American Journal of Public Health, 93,* 557–574.

Noar, S. M. (2008). Behavioral interventions to reduce HIV-related sexual risk behavior: Review and synthesis of meta-analytic evidence. *AIDS and Behavior, 12,* 335–353. doi: 10.1007/s10461-007-9313-9

Nutbeam, D., & Blakey, V. (1990). The concept of health promotion and AIDS prevention: A comprehensive and integrated basis for action in the 1990s. *Health Promotion International, 5*(3), 233–242.

O'Reilly, K. R., & Higgins, D. L. (1991). AIDS community demonstration projects for HIV prevention among hard-to-reach groups. *Public Health Reports, 106*(6), 714–720.

Parascandola, J. (2008). *Sex, sin, and science: A history of syphilis in America.* Westport, CT: Praeger.

Public Health Leadership Society (2002). *Principles of the ethical practice of public health,* Version 2.2. Retrieved from http://www.apha.org/NR/rdonlyres/1ced3cea-287e-4185-9cbd-bd405fc60856/0/ethicsbrochure.pdf

Puckett, S. B., & Bye, L. L. (1987). *The Stop AIDS Project: An interpersonal AIDS-prevention program.* San Francisco: Stop AIDS Project.

Roe, K. M., Roe, K., Carpenter, C. G., & Sibley, C. B. (2005). Community building through empowering evaluation. In M. Minkler (ed.), *Community organizing and community building for health* (2nd ed.) (pp. 386–402). New Brunswick, NJ: Rutgers University Press.

Shadish, W. R., Cook, T. D., & Campbell, D. T. (2002). *Experimental and quasi-experimental designs for generalized causal inference.* Boston, MA: Houghton-Mifflin.

Starr, P. (2011). *Remedy and reaction: The peculiar American struggle over health care reform.* New Haven, CT: Yale University Press.

Stevens, C. E., Taylor, P. E., Zang, E. A., Morrison, J. M., Harley, E. J., Rodriguez de Cordoba, S., … Rubenstein, P. (1986). Human T-cell lymphotropic virus type III infection in a cohort of homosexual men in New York City. *Journal of the American Medical Association, 255*(16), 2167–2172.

Stringer, E. T. (1999). *Action research* (2nd ed.). Thousand Oaks, CA: Sage.

Wallerstein, N. B., & Duran, B. (2008). The theoretical, historical and practice roots of CBPR. In M. Minkler & N. Wallerstein (eds.), *Community based participatory research for health* (2nd ed.) (pp. 25–46). San Francisco, CA: Jossey-Bass.

Winkelstein, W., Jr., Samuel, M., Padian, N. S., Wiley, J. A., Lang, W., Anderson, R. E., & Levy, J. A. (1987). The San Francisco men's health study: III. Reduction in human immodeficiency virus transmission among homosexual/bisexual men. *American Journal of Public Health, 76*(9), 685–689.

Winslow, C. E. A. (1920). The untilled field of public health. *Modern Medicine, 2,* 183–191.

Wohlfieler, D. (1997). Community organizing and community building among gay and bisexual men: The STOP AIDS project. In M. Minkler (ed.), *Community organizing and community building for health* (pp. 230–243). New Brunswick, NJ: Rutgers University Press.

World Health Organization (1986). *Ottawa charter for health promotion.* Geneva, Switzerland: World Health Organization. Retrieved from http://www.who.int/hpr/NPH/docs/ottawa_charter_hp.pdf

# 17

# Diversifying AIDS Activism: Lessons Learned from ACT UP/Philadelphia

*Jeff Maskovsky*

It is nearly impossible to overstate the importance of the last quarter-century of radical AIDS activism. Yet, with a few noteworthy exceptions (Chambré, 2006; Stockdill, 2003; Gould, 2009), surprisingly little has been written about the inner workings of AIDS activists groups. This chapter describes the diversification of the Philadelphia chapter of the radical AIDS activist group, ACT UP. Famously, ACT UP, the AIDS Coalition to Unleash Power, is a nonviolent direct action group that launched a powerful, politically militant response to the AIDS crisis. Its media-savvy demonstrations and dramatic acts of civil disobedience have been remarkably effective in combating homophobia and the stigma against AIDS; challenging governmental inaction in the face of a growing epidemic; contesting the power of medical expertise; demanding more effective treatments and better research; inventing more participatory models of research, social service provision, treatment, and prevention; and promoting the people-first language of people with AIDS (PWA) empowerment, not victimhood, among many other accomplishments. Remarkably, 70 ACT UP chapters have formed since the group was founded in New York City in 1987, including ACT UP/Philadelphia.

Managing diversity has been a persistent challenge for ACT UP since its inception. The group has always valued diversity. Its charter emphasizes diversity and nonpartisanship, and it maintains a leaderless, ultra-democratic political structure that places everyone interested in a militant response to the AIDs crisis on equal footing, in contrast to hierarchical organizations with appointed or elected leadership or organizations that become associated with political parties or benefactors. Yet it has sometimes been easier for ACT UP chapters to manage diverse political points of view than it has been for them to diversify across race, class, gender, sexuality, nationality, and other axes of difference and inequality. An important exception to this is ACT UP/Philadelphia, which became one of the most vibrant and diverse ACT UP chapters to have formed in the 25-year history of militant AIDS activism.

This chapter explores lessons learned from ACT UP/Philadelphia's experiments in diversification. It focuses in particular on the group's activities during the period from 1997 to 2012. Although militant AIDS activism in the United States was in many respects in decline during this period, ACT UP/Philadelphia thrived. Participation by low-income African Americans reinvigorated the group and sustained it as a political force. In this chapter, I emphasize two interconnected aspects of the group's diversification process. The first is the internal dilemmas that diversity posed for the chapter, and the concrete changes that its members made to their radical democratic practice in order to overcome them. The second is the extent to which low-income African Americans enhanced the political effectiveness of ACT UP/Philadelphia's grassroots campaigns. My broader argument is that, although ACT UP/Philadelphia was unable to overcome entrenched race- and class-based inequalities, it managed them in ways that helped to sustain the AIDs activist movement. This, in turn, created an important space of political participation for low-income African Americans, for whom movement participation restored essential civil rights, a sense of social value, and, for many, life itself.

Drawing on ethnographic fieldwork (1995–2011) and on my own work and activism in the AIDS community, the chapter begins with a historical account of the increase in participation of the most vulnerable and marginalized segments of Philadelphia's African American population—the group that pundits and social scientists typically refer to as the "underclass"—in AIDS activism. Mainstream U.S. poverty scholarship, exemplified by the work of William Julius Wilson (1987) and others (e.g., Small & Newman, 2001), directs disproportionate attention to the poorest of the black inner-city poor, the so-called "underclass," and their rates of illegitimate births, female-headed households, and participation in the informal economy. Critics of the underclass concept emphasize not the "behaviors" of the inner-city poor, but their modes of survival, resistance, and political participation (see di Leonardo, 1998; Goode & Maskovsky 2001; Reed, 1999; and Steinberg, 1995). This chapter follows in this critical vein. I then turn to three brief examples of recent campaigns that highlight ACT UP/Philadelphia's political challenges and successes. The chapter concludes with a brief critical discussion of the strategies and tactics that emerged for managing unequal power relationships, differences, and inequalities inside and outside of a radical AIDS activist group.

## REMAKING ACT UP/PHILADELPHIA

The conventional wisdom among activists, pundits, and students of social movements is that radical AIDS activism crested during the period of direct action protest of the late 1980s and early 1990s, and that what followed was a protracted period of movement decline brought on by the lessening of stigma associated with AIDS, activist deaths, and political burnout; the arrival of effective antiviral therapies and the attendant redefinition of AIDS from a "death sentence" to a "manageable disease"; the advent of postgay AIDS politics; the professionalization and bureaucratization of the AIDS community; state repression; and public and political disparagement of street protest tactics, among other factors (Altman, 1994; Singer, 1998; Gould, 2009). So intensely felt is this sense of decline that in some quarters a concerted effort has been made to preserve and archive movement history (see the ACT UP Oral History Project). Furthermore, newer generations of queer activists—those who came of age politically in the mid-1990s and beyond—frequently express more nostalgia for ACT UP itself than they do interest in or identification with its ongoing campaigns (e.g., Hilderbrand, 2006).

As is usually the case with conventional wisdom, this story of AIDS activism's rise and fall contains just enough truth to be misleading. For, although involvement in radical AIDS activist groups such as ACT UP has certainly decreased, as is evidenced, for example, by the declining size and number of active ACT UP chapters across the country since 1997, participation by low-income African Americans has actually increased dramatically during this same period. Focusing too narrowly on movement decline thus risks relegating low-income African Americans to the margins of AIDS activist history. It treats them as having arrived late to the cause and minimizes their political impact. Building on scholarship that acknowledges the contributions of people of color and low-income people in AIDS activism's earlier phases (e.g., Chambré, 2006; Stockdill, 2003), one of my main points here is to encourage a rethinking of the last 15 years as well. In fact, it may be more useful to think of this "late" phase of AIDS activism as not exclusively a postgay period of demobilization, as it is sometimes described, but instead as the period during which the AIDS mobilization effort achieved its zenith in terms of diversity across race and class lines. This perspective upends much of the conventional wisdom about what it takes to sustain a movement while also making it more diverse. Let me now turn to the specific case of ACT UP/Philadelphia to flesh out these points.

ACT UP/Philadelphia's early history was in many respects very similar to that of other ACT UP chapters in the United States. At its founding in 1988, most of its members came from the local gay community, and it took on many of the same political struggles and used many of the same political strategies and tactics for which ACT UP as a whole has become famous as a unique and vital political force (Crimp & Rolston, 1990; Shepard & Hayduk, 2002; Chambré, 2006; Stockdill, 2003).

Yet ACT UP/Philadelphia was also somewhat unique in its early years. The gay community in Philadelphia was smaller than in New York, Los Angeles, or San Francisco, where other ACT UP chapters thrived. Philadelphia's Quaker tradition, with its emphasis on peace and conflict resolution, also shaped the group's internal culture and helped it to avoid the factionalism that divided militant AIDS activists from one another in other cities. For example, treatment activists in Philadelphia never left ACT UP, as they did in New York, where they split off from ACT UP/New York to form the Treatment Action Group in 1992. And the gulf between radical activism on the one hand and AIDS service organizations and the city on the other was narrower and less antagonistic than it was in other cities, in part because of the pervasiveness of nonprofit and government employment in a city with a chronic shortage of capital investment and a frequently troubled private sector. In fact, many radical AIDS activists, including Kiyoshi Kuromiya (1943–2000), undoubtedly one of the most committed radicals in the AIDS movement, ran programs at local AIDS service organizations, held public- and nonprofit sector consultancies, worked for the city health department, or served on local AIDS planning council boards. Taken together, these differences made ACT UP/Philadelphia somewhat precarious and even compromised; yet they also ensured a high level of political, social, and ideological flexibility and made it open to change.

As in other cities, the diversification of ACT UP/Philadelphia occurred in a context of demographic shifts that placed people of color, especially black and also Latino gay men, at the center of the epidemic (AACO, 2012). Yet demography alone does not account for the significant increase in participation by low-income people of color in ACT UP/Philadelphia. This occurred for three interconnected reasons: subtle changes in ACT UP's informal leadership, an active and successful effort to diversify the group, and internal cultural changes that enabled broader participation in the deliberation process across race and class lines.

With respect to informal leadership, during the early years of ACT UP/ Philadelphia, most of the activists were gay liberation–, New Left–, antiwar–, and civil rights–influenced "gay white men" and their allies, as they were in other cities across the United States. As in other cities, ACT UP/Philadelphia also had a people of color caucus. It was formed by Kiyoshi Kuromiya and John Paul Hammond (1950–2010), among others. People of color were a relatively small minority in ACT UP/Philadelphia until the mid-1990s, when their numbers began to increase. This was in part because most African American and Latino/a activists in Philadelphia became involved in other organizations, especially We the People with AIDS/HIV, the city's PWA coalition (for a detailed history of We the People, see Maskovskya, 2000).

After the first wave in ACT UP/Philadelphia was depleted by burnout, professionalization, and death, a second wave comprised of anarchist Gen-Xers became involved, in large measure because they were attracted to the militancy of the movement and because they viewed it as a very hospitable political space to express anarchist ideas about the corruptive and oppressive nature of the family, capitalism, and the state. Somewhat unique to Philadelphia, the second wave's ranks came mostly from the city's nationally recognized anarchist community. This wave was somewhat queerer than the first, in two senses: It embraced non-normative sexuality writ large (and not exclusively that which was same-sex identified), and it was not invested formally in lesbian and gay identity politics. Accordingly, it had slightly different ideas about the intersection of sexual and AIDS politics. Whereas many of the activists in the first wave viewed homophobia and antigay bigotry as primary causes of the AIDS crisis, activists in the second wave saw sexuality as but one axis of inequality that shaped it. They saw it operating alongside other axes of inequality, such as gender, race, and class. In other words, although they did not ignore sexuality, they also did not prioritize it. The second wave thus embraced what is now widely called a "postgay" politics of identity (Ghaziani, 2011), much to the consternation, I might add, of some first-wavers. Prominently, the second wave was no less white, nor less privileged along class lines, than the first.

The second wave put a great deal of time and energy into recruiting new members, and they did so with the explicit intention of diversifying the group. The push for diversity was inspired by many factors: an ideological commitment to racial justice and to diversity, the desire to have the group's demographics reflect those of the local epidemic, and a response to pressure from prominent local AIDS community leaders who criticized the group for being unreflective—and hence out of step politically—with the vast majority of HIV-positive people in the city. Recruitment of new members took place mainly at local AIDS service organizations, HIV clinics, recovery houses, homeless shelters, drug and alcohol programs, and mental health treatment programs.

One of the most fruitful sources of new recruits, for example, was a community-based treatment education program for "hard to reach" consumers of AIDS services called Project TEACH (Treatment Education Activists Combating HIV), which was housed at Philadelphia FIGHT, a large multiservice agency. Longtime AIDS activist Julie Davids founded Project TEACH with help from the leadership of Philadelphia FIGHT and of We the People, a local people-with-AIDS (PWA) coalition founded in the 1980s that ran a drop-in center for impoverished and homeless people with HIV and AIDS. Project TEACH was designed to serve HIV-positive people from low-income communities and communities of color. Although its participants were somewhat diverse across the lines of race and class—and accordingly included some middle-income African Americans and Latino/as as well as some low-income whites—the vast majority of its participants were low-income African Americans. Importantly, this was a population that had been marginalized from respectable black community politics because of drug use, sexual minority status, poverty, or AIDS (cf. Cohen, 1999). The founding premise behind Project TEACH was that HIV-positive people from these communities did not have access to the independent, up-to-date treatment information that they needed to make sound medical decisions, and that they would benefit if this information were delivered via a formal community education program. This contrasted greatly to the way that first-wave activists disseminated information about HIV treatments, which in the early years of the epidemic famously took place in informal, nonmedical settings and through ACT UP's "medical updates." Project TEACH consisted of an eight-week intensive HIV treatment and prevention education program, after which "graduates" were placed in "peer education" jobs in AIDS service and care organizations. Its founders also established ancillary programs specifically for Latino/as and for the formerly incarcerated. Significantly, as an early example of a "secondary prevention" program designed to reduce the spread of HIV by bringing "hard to reach" HIV-positive populations into care, it received several hundred thousand dollars annually in CDC and Ryan White Care Act funding. This level of public support allowed Project TEACH to train hundreds of HIV-positive people each year.

Davids and her collaborators had a somewhat unique take on "secondary prevention," however. They designed Project TEACH as a Paulo Freire–inspired, Midwest Academy–style activist training school. In their minds, the two goals of secondary prevention and mobilizing against AIDS went hand in hand. Participants, they reasoned, would better understand and commit to secondary prevention practices—including safe sex, adherence to anti-HIV drugs, and other life-sustaining measures—if these individual practices were embedded in the collective struggle for social equality and justice. The entwined histories of AIDS activism, civil rights, and gay liberation were thus an essential part of the Project TEACH curriculum. This was, of course, precisely the perspective that animated the gay community response to AIDS in the early years of the epidemic, although in this case it was repackaged for a majority black constituency, only some of whom were gay. Davids frequently informed Project TEACH participants about ACT UP campaigns and other activist efforts, but she and others were careful not to engage in explicit recruitment activities while the program was officially in session. In fact, Davids was cautious about recruiting Project TEACH participants to join ACT UP directly, and frequently encouraged them instead to observe ACT UP demonstrations and other activities before making a decision to join.

For their part, many Project TEACH participants were inspired by the prospect of learning how to harness political power to gain control over the domain of medical research and treatment. For example, John Bell was a new recruit who told me that he was inspired by early AIDS activists' efforts to reform the anti-HIV drug approval process. He simply could not believe, he told me, that a small group of people could force a government that he viewed as indifferent, inept, and prejudiced to change the way that it dealt with people who were suffering with a life-threatening illness. He joined ACT UP immediately after graduating from Project TEACH.

ACT UP's diversification across race and class lines created new challenges inside the group. For example, new recruits were often put off by the group's nonhierarchical culture and its consensus decision making. This was not because they were averse to egalitarian political practices. On the contrary, it was because these practices were clearly not egalitarian enough. In fact, from many a new recruit's perspective, consensus decision making helped to produce and secure an informal leadership hierarchy based on race and class. John Bell also remembered feeling very alienated at his first meeting, not only, as many new members felt, because a group of insiders was talking about things he did not understand, but also because of the way that this lack of understanding was racialized. He explained,

I'd be in this room with all these white, gay people. The gay thing was not an issue. The race thing was. And I couldn't understand. I couldn't understand. (personal interview with Julie Davids, November 2004)

This exemplifies the dilemmas that ensue when race- and class-blind radical democratic practices guide the internal decision making of activist groups. That new participants often experienced race and class not just as social differences but also as sites of inequality is a problem that threatened to undermine the group's recruitment efforts. Of equal importance, that ACT UP's gay orientation did not bother Bell and many other low-income African Americans who were new recruits complicates our understanding of homophobia in the African American community. For although homophobia certainly exists in African American communities, as it does in many other communities as well, the fact that many African Americans are not homophobic, and that, in this case, many impoverished and homeless urban African Americans felt comfortable joining a pro-gay political group with a large and highly visible LGBT presence is almost never mentioned in popular and political discussions about homophobia in the black community.

To overcome race and class dynamics that threatened to undermine these recruitment efforts, ACT UP/Philadelphia reinvented "consensus decision making" in ways that favored long-term participation by less affluent people of color. For example, it sometimes enacted "go-arounds" at the end of Monday night meetings. This entailed going around the room, one person at a time, so that each person had his or her chance to comment on the discussion and to express approval or disapproval about a proposed plan of action. Go-arounds are an explicit borrowing from the recovery movement with which most new recruits were familiar. By using them, new members were thus no longer obligated, as with Robert's Rules of Order, to raise their hands to assert themselves, a practice that many found, understandably, to be very intimidating. Although this did not change new recruits' perspectives that white middle-class members had disproportionate influence over the decision-making process, it created a new sense of responsibility among them, for the go-arounds made them feel obligated to lay out their concerns when given the chance or to accept the group's decisions fully as their own.

The group also provided financial and social support to new members. For example, public transportation tokens were distributed at Monday night meetings. This was controversial, even among new recruits themselves. Whereas some saw the transit tokens as a way of defraying the financial cost of going to and from meetings, others saw their distribution as tantamount to a bribe that encouraged attendance by individuals who otherwise would not be interested in the group's activities. Fascinatingly, the group has been engaged in a more than decade-long conversation about the politics and ethics of giving out tokens, and it has decided several times to suspend their distribution, though never permanently. The controversy is itself instructive: It points to the careful balance that the group attempted to achieve between offering forms of social and financial support that might enhance participation by the less affluent on the one hand and maintaining an overall sense of pure, selfless, unremunerated political participation on the other.

Finally, and perhaps most important, is the significance of the agency of low-income African Americans themselves in managing racial hierarchies and class differences within the group. For them, part of becoming more experienced AIDS activists entailed learning to navigate and exploit the whiteness and middle-classness of many of their fellow activists. For example, Cliff Williams, a formerly homeless African American with HIV, practically spearheaded ACT UP/Philadelphia's AIDS housing campaign of 2010 (about which I will say more below). He was quite explicit about his belief that city officials take ACT UP's demands more seriously when his more affluent and white counterparts are present in meetings with city officials. This example makes clear that it would be a colossal mistake to assume that low-income African Americans are simply dupes of their more affluent white counterparts. To the contrary, they cultivated their own readings of privilege and unequal power relations and sought to use them to their advantage. Clearly, low-income African Americans not only understood quite clearly the power of white middle-class authority and expertise; they were also willing to manipulate it to achieve their own political ends.

These arrangements enabled ACT UP/Philadelphia to become a new cross-race and cross-class political assemblage. And despite the pronounced race and class divisions within it, this configuration was surprisingly resilient: it held together for longer than the entire political life span of most ACT UP chapters and played an important role in several of the most important AIDS activist campaigns of the last 15 years. Of equal importance, over time, its leadership also diversified. In fact, many low-income African Americans assumed informal leadership positions within the group. These activists sustained the group as the second wave of activists who recruited them left ACT UP (many to form or work for new AIDS advocacy organizations elsewhere), and as an even younger generation of anarchist and queer activists found their way to ACT UP. I now turn to three campaigns to flesh out further what this newly diverse group was able to achieve.

## "WE CANNOT SEPARATE OURSELVES FROM THESE PEOPLE": ACT UP/PHILADELPHIA'S PURSUIT OF GLOBAL JUSTICE

One noteworthy campaign in which the newly remade ACT UP/Philadelphia chapter participated was the campaign for global AIDS drug access. One of the most galvanizing AIDS activist campaigns of the late 1990s and 2000s, it was an international effort to expand HIV treatment and care in the global South. The contours of the issues at stake are generally well known: Whereas anti-HIV drugs and other life-saving medical treatments became available in the advanced industrialized countries of the global North by the mid-1990s, they were withheld from many of the developing countries in the global South, including many of the countries in sub-Saharan African, where HIV infection rates are among the highest. Instead, the World Health Organization and many developing countries focused narrowly on HIV prevention efforts, in part because they did not consider treatment to be cost-effective and in part because they believed these countries lacked a sufficient public health "infrastructure" to provide effective anti-HIV drug therapies. In response, activists forged transnational networks across the North–South divide to fight for global access to AIDS drugs. Arguing that access to HIV treatments is a basic human right, they forced reluctant governments to provide people infected with HIV with anti-HIV drugs, pressured the World Health Organization to change its policies, and challenged U.S. and World Trade Organization trade policies that favored pharmaceutical company profits and patent rights over access to affordable generic AIDS drugs. Through these efforts, AIDS activists thus established themselves as pioneers in the global justice movement.

What I wish to highlight here is the practical and symbolic importance of low-income African American participation in these efforts. For ACT UP/Philadelphia, including its low-income African American members, played a crucial role in helping to organize some of the earliest U.S.-based demonstrations protesting U.S. government and global pharmaceutical policies that impeded AIDS drug access in the global South. On April 19, 1999, for example, activists blocked the entrance to the headquarters of the Pharmaceutical Research and Manufacturers of America in downtown Washington, DC, and rallied to protest the Africa Growth and Opportunity Act. This Clinton-era legislation, drafted at the behest of the pharmaceutical industry, would have created a NAFTA-like free trade zone in Southern Africa, punishing area governments and corporations for producing discounted anti-AIDS treatments or for importing them from third-party generic producers. HealthGAP (Global Access Project), formed less than a year earlier, partnered with ACT UP/Philadelphia to organize the demonstration, which complemented campaigns occurring in South Africa and elsewhere (for a detailed account of the campaigns that occurred in South Africa, see Susser, 2009).

For the April 19, 2012, demonstration, busloads of protestors—perhaps the largest contingent, in fact—came from Philadelphia. They were there because ACT UP/Philadelphia member John Bell and others spent months organizing in recovery houses, AIDS service organizations, and in prisons in and around Philadelphia. Carrying signs reading "Human Rights, Not Corporate Rights" and "Just Say No to Drug Lobbyists," this contingent joined protestors from other ACT UP chapters and from U.N.I.T.E., Rainforest Action Network, Public Citizen, and Treatment Action Campaign of South Africa. Preceding the famous anti-WTO Battle of Seattle by six months, this was one of the first demonstrations in which organized labor, consumer groups, community-based health advocacy groups, and environmental NGOs joined AIDS activist groups to attack U.S. AIDS policy. A contingent from ACT UP/Philadelphia also showed up at the World Bank protests in Washington, DC, in 2000, and they continued to be involved in similar campaigns during the Bush and Obama eras. Importantly, ACT UP/Philadelphia was a training ground for global justice activism. Among the many global justice activists who have joined or partnered with the group, HealthGAP staffers and board members Paul Davis, Asia Russell, and Jose DeMarco all got their start in ACT UP/Philadelphia.

In addition to mobilizing protestors, ACT UP/Philadelphia also helped to provide symbolic rhetoric that linked activists in the global North to those in the global South. For example, before he was arrested for blocking the PRMA trade center entrance, John Bell made public comments that established connections between U.S. domestic and international policies and, perhaps more importantly, asserted a nonpaternalistic moral imperative on the part of African Americans to act on behalf of fellow activists in Southern Africa. Directing his comments toward the large contingent of African Americans at the demonstration, he said:

> I want you all to know why we are here: the fact that folks [in Southern Africa] aren't getting their medication and the fact that some of them are not victims. Some of them know the same information that we

do. . . . they know about the United States and its policies. They know about how the cities function here. I had gone to Vietnam to fight for freedom, freedom by any means. I fought for democracy and for freedom. To do that, to be African American, and to see what is going on in the continent of Africa, and ... to have an African background by being an African American, there is no way we can separate ourselves from these people, and they are dying.

Bell's comments demonstrate a level of political sophistication that goes way beyond the kind of "local" self-interested politics that is normally ascribed to low-income inner-city residents, particularly African Americans. Indeed, ACT UP/Philadelphia's participation in the global AIDS drug access campaign challenges the idea of poor urban African Americans as passive, ungovernable, or engaged defensively only in "local" level struggles, isolated from political ideologies and transnational political movements. Instead, what developed was a global perspective on freedom, empowerment, and human rights combined with an in-depth understanding of the broader issues of international trade, global manufacturing, health inequalities, and survival that are of central concern to the global justice movement (on the local/global split in urban activism, see Maskovsky, 2003).

## PRISONS AND HIV PREVENTION: EXPANDING THE SOCIAL SAFETY NET IN THE INNER CITY

A similar level of political savvy is on display in ACT UP/Philadelphia's Condoms in City Jails campaign, which used similar grassroots tactics to contest the dominant urban and health policy agendas that have been in place in major U.S. cities like Philadelphia since the 1970s. These agendas combine fiscal austerity with welfare state retrenchment, privatization, cost-containment policy reform, and law and order policies. Among the many deleterious consequences of these developments for cities as a whole and for low-income urbanites in particular has been the undermining of many of the gains of the black civil rights movement through the mass incarceration of urban African Americans. Mass incarceration interferes in many ways with HIV prevention and treatment efforts targeting urban African Americans: It disrupts or strains survival networks in black communities, blocks access to parts of the social safety net for the incarcerated and formerly incarcerated, forces large numbers of urban African Americans to rely on prisons and other penal institutions for health care, blunts the political power of African Americans (prisoners often lose the right to vote, even after they are released), and on the whole complicates urban African American's access to HIV treatment and prevention programs.

ACT UP/Philadelphia launched its Condoms in Philadelphia Jails campaign to address this situation. On July 31, 2006, ACT UP/Philadelphia met with Philadelphia Prison System Commissioner Leon King to demand condom access for all inmates in Philadelphia county jails. The activists presented King with proof, in the form of an AIDS Prevention Program memorandum, of a longstanding policy, pushed through by AIDS activists in 1988, authorizing condom distribution to inmates. They also gave him a new report documenting the high rate of HIV among the currently and formerly incarcerated, as well as proof—largely in the form of recorded testimony from the formerly incarcerated—of the lack of condom access inside Philadelphia jails, and of correctional officers' *de facto* policy of treating condoms as contraband and of their routine confiscation. These efforts were facilitated in part by ACT UP/Philadelphia's partnership with a New York City–based national AIDS advocacy group called CHAMP (Community HIV/AIDS Mobilization Project), which had received funding from the Ittleson Foundation and the Public Welfare Foundation to provide technical assistance in support of local AIDS activist campaigns across the country.

In the months following the meeting, ACT UP/Philadelphia published attention-grabbing press releases, set up press interviews with HIV-positive ex-offenders, held meetings with public officials, and threatened direct action protests. Through these actions, the group overcame popular, bureaucratic, and political opposition to condom access in jails. Importantly, they used arguments emphasizing the synergistic effects of the twin epidemics of mass incarceration and HIV on "at-risk" communities, as well as the life-saving benefits and cost-effectiveness of science-based public health policies such as condom distribution. As ACT UP member Waheedah Shabazz-El told a *City Paper* reporter, "Our prisons, like it or not, have become primary health-care providers to our husbands and fathers, wives and mothers, brothers and sisters, and condoms are scientifically proven to be the first and cheapest defense against this disease ravaging our communities" (Pasquariello, 2006). A year after the campaign began, ACT UP/Philadelphia succeeded in expanding condom access in the Philadelphia jails. They have been less successful, however, at scaling up this campaign to state and federal levels, a major activist goal since the majority of inmates are incarcerated by the state, not the city.

This campaign exemplifies the kind of social welfare gains that become possible when AIDS activists rely on purportedly "apolitical" scientific criteria as their basis for calculating risk and for elaborating political demands for the preservation of life, and it is all the more remarkable given the hostile, anti-welfarist, punitive climate in which this victory occurred. Importantly, AIDS activists in this case also went beyond the practical policy-oriented argument that inmate access to condoms is a sensible public health measure because it slows the spread of disease in "at-risk" communities by blocking transmission among individuals who will one day leave the prison system and resume sexual activity "outside," as prison abolitionists and AIDS activists often put it. At symbolic and political levels, the campaign also represents an effort to restore rights, recognition, and dignity to inmates in city jails, a population that has for decades been treated as dangerous, undeserving, disposable, and unworthy of basic civil or political rights. Further, this campaign exemplifies the extent to which the fight against AIDS is now thoroughly enmeshed in the fight for racial and economic justice.

## FIGHTING "ALMOST DEADNESS": MOBILIZING FOR AIDS HOUSING IN PHILADELPHIA

A third important campaign for ACT UP/Philadelphia was the campaign for AIDS housing in Philadelphia. This campaign built on 20 years of AIDS housing activism by ACT UP and other local groups that pressured city, state, and federal governments to expand housing opportunities for people with HIV and AIDS. Unsurprisingly, the AIDS housing crisis intensified in the late 2000s as a consequence of budget cuts and other fallout from the 2007 global economic downturn. In 2010, with more than 200 eligible people on a two-year-long waiting list, ACT UP/Philadelphia began a series of actions to draw attention to the fact that Philadelphia's housing programs were not meeting the needs of homeless people with HIV. In December of that year, for example, the group went Christmas caroling at City Hall and at Philadelphia Mayor Michael Nutter's house, where they sang their own unique version of "The Twelve Days of Christmas." They sang:

> On the twelfth day of Christmas,
> The mayor gave to me,
> Lines for food and showers,
> Expensive city clinics,
> No beds to sleep on,
> Rules for being sober,
> Cold nights on the street,

TB in the shelters,
Less library hours,
Years on waiting lists,
ID requirements,
Foreclosed homes,
Shelters taking meds,
And no money for AIDS housing.

For a follow-up, they disrupted Nutter's annual budget address, on March 3, 2011, by shouting "Homes Not Graves for People with AIDS" from the balcony of the city council chambers in City Hall. The press release ACT UP issued before the demonstration featured the story of ACT UP/Philadelphia member Carla Fields, who was also a homeless person with HIV who was eligible for AIDS housing. In 2010, she was forced to rely on the city shelters system because no housing was available. In the press release, she was quoted as saying, "I have had 75 percent of my body eaten up by bedbugs in the shelter. . . . the mayor apologized to me personally for having to suffer and get sick in the shelter system, but I don't want his apology. I want him to end the AIDS housing waiting list!"

Significantly, in this campaign, ACT UP/Philadelphia sought not just to gain concrete resources for people with HIV. Mirroring previous campaigns, they wanted also to change the way that city bureaucrats, politicians, policy-makers, and the public thought about poverty, homelessness, and illness. The overall motto for this campaign was, "Housing Equals Prevention, Treatment and Justice." Again, they also used moral arguments declaring "AIDS housing is a right." And they embedded this rights talk in a broader science-based public health argument about effective HIV treatment and prevention. With slogans such as "AIDS housing saves lives," they insisted that housing is as vital to people with HIV as is anti-HIV drug therapy. In a policy brief that they wrote with the assistance of students at the University of Pennsylvania, they provided scientific evidence for the claims that shelters threatened the health of homeless people with HIV, that housing is just as important as drug treatment in improving health outcomes and in preventing the spread of HIV, and that AIDS housing reduces city expenditures on health care and shelters. These points, in turn, became activist talking points. For example, at the budget speech demonstration, ACT UP member Antonio Davis said, "It would save the city money and save lives, plain and simple. But instead, the mayor is taking the easy way out."

It might be tempting to assume that, in the context of a steep economic downturn and revenue shortfall, the city gives no value at all to the lives of homeless people with HIV and AIDS; that it treated them as a disposable population that has been shorn of civil and political rights, and that now survive in a state of "bare life," to use Agamben's useful phrase (Agamben, 1998), on the margins of the city, in it, but not of it. But the situation is more complicated, thanks in large measure to the efforts of ACT UP/Philadelphia. For a cornerstone of ACT UP/Philadelphia's campaign is the demand for an expanded definition of life itself. Today, in Philadelphia, as in other cities, biomedical distinctions between an HIV and an AIDS diagnosis are used in housing policies so that the more precarious the life of a homeless person with HIV, the easier it is for him or her to get access to housing. In other words, it is only those who are "advanced" enough in their disease progression—in particular, those with an AIDS diagnosis, not just those who are HIV positive—who are eligible for AIDS housing. The logic here follows longstanding ethical guidelines for organ donation and other protocols for health care rationing that are widely enforced across our health care and social services systems. ACT UP/Philadelphia members contested the logic underlying this arrangement. They argued that it produces a catch-22 for homeless people with HIV and AIDS. It gives them a choice between homelessness with HIV and housing with AIDS. Indeed, they complained that the city uses a threshold of "almost deadness" to calculate who is deserving of scarce resources. What activists were fighting for, therefore, was the revaluation of life itself so that a broader, more diverse group beyond the "almost dead" could receive AIDS housing.

ACT UP/Philadelphia has also challenged the underlying logic of Philadelphia's homeless service provisioning system. The city's current model to end homelessness, the continuum of care model, makes psychiatric and substance abuse treatment and sobriety a prerequisite for permanent housing. As a result, more than 10 percent of the city's homeless population uses shelters, which are viewed as the proper entry point in the continuum of care for the most vulnerable populations (ACT UP Philadelphia, 2010). The logic here is that homeless people with acute psychiatric or substance abuse problems are too unstable for permanent homes. Yet activists point out that this model has dangerous public health implications for homeless people with HIV and AIDS, and for the homeless in general. As mentioned above, they point out that homelessness itself increases an individual's inability to safely manage illness, leaving those living with HIV at an increased risk for becoming sicker. ACT UP/Philadelphia has formally presented the city with an alternative housing plan based on a Housing First model that offers immediate access to independent housing without requiring psychiatric treatment or sobriety (National Alliance to End Homelessness, 2006).

This, they say, will prevent the spread of AIDS and enhance the health of those who are already infected.

And this campaign has been effective. The city has abandoned all moral pretense that homeless people with HIV are not deserving of housing. This in itself marks an important activist victory. For in addition to revaluing life, it also undermines longstanding distinctions between who is deserving or undeserving, who is morally virtuous and who is discredited by vice. These distinctions have been essential in setting health and welfare policy priorities for well over a century in urban America (Katz, 1990; Goode and Maskovsky, 2001). ACT UP/Philadelphia's housing campaign thus achieves an important ideological victory. It blocks the city from vilifying some of the weakest segments of the urban population—in this case, the overlapping populations of homeless people, people with HIV and AIDS, and drug users—in order to justify and legitimate the denial or withdrawal of resources and services from them.

Unfortunately, in this era of economic crisis and fiscal austerity, the new sense of inclusion and belonging that this kind of activism helps to bring about does not necessarily correspond with increased resources for homeless people with HIV and AIDS or other vulnerable populations. Mayor Nutter, for his part, expressed great sympathy for the plight of homeless people with HIV in a meeting he held with ACT UP/Philadelphia members and their allies in November 2010. But he refused to commit city funds to AIDS housing because, activists report, he "doesn't know where the resources would come from." As in most major metropolitan areas in the United States in recent years, Nutter is pursuing a fiscally conservative budget strategy in order to create a "leaner, smaller, smarter government," as he put it (Nutter, 2012), perhaps channeling Bill Clinton, or Michael Bloomberg, or any other technocratic reformer from the last 30 years, for a city with a 23 percent poverty rate, the fifth highest HIV infection rate among major metropolitan areas in the country, a growing homelessness crisis, and a long-running shortage of investment capital. In other words, although municipal leaders like Nutter are more willing than ever to embrace sound, public health– and science-based policies, they are not likely to back fiscal policies that will generate the funds to pay for them.

ACT UP/Philadelphia responded to the city's budget woes by pushing for innovative revenue-generating policies. For example, it pressured the mayor to require the city's nonprofit hospital systems and scientific and medical research facilities to make payments to the city in exchange for the city resources that they use. In policy circles, this redistributive model is called payments in lieu of taxes or PILOT. PILOTs have been used effectively in other cities to make sure large, financially secure nonprofits are a boon, rather than a burden, to cities (Brody, 2002). In Philadelphia, the rationale for using PILOTs to pay for AIDS housing is very compelling: Tax-exempt nonprofit and educational institutions occupy a disproportionate presence in the city's economy, and this limits its business tax base. Indeed, the University of Pennsylvania, with its large hospital system and academic research facility, is the largest private employer in the city. Because these nonprofit institutions have embraced bold growth strategies and profit-oriented approaches to financing in recent decades, it makes sense for them to contribute revenue to the city in exchange for the city services and resources that they consume. Ironically, ACT UP/Philadelphia members learned about PILOT models and about city financing in general through a long-term collaboration they forged with University of Pennsylvania graduate students in the Urban Studies Program and with students at the Penn Medical School; that is, with people who are a part of the very institution that has been targeted by activists. For now, Philadelphia has not yet adopted the ACT UP/Philadelphia–recommended PILOT model of "taxation."

## CONCLUSION: LESSONS LEARNED

This chapter describes how the most impoverished and vulnerable segments of the racialized, inner-city population became meaningful participants in ACT UP/Philadelphia, and how they, in turn, helped to revitalize and sustain the chapter. As well, they used their participation to make claims for essential civil rights, the right to health care, global justice, and for the revaluation of life itself. Accordingly, I see ACT UP/Philadelphia as an important example not just of AIDS activism, but of the kind of inclusive, transformational politics that is possible when different vulnerable segments of the urban population come together to challenge larger forces and to decide their own conditions of life.

The case of ACT UP/Philadelphia also confounds many commonsensical ideas about radical protest movements. For a major component to ACT UP/Philadelphia's long-term sustainability is the fact that it was forged through the unconventional use of the service delivery and community health care system. There is no denying that, for the group, access to the nonprofit sector enabled and sustained political action across race and class divides at key moments of political uncertainty and risk. We should therefore rethink political perspectives that view the AIDS community, NGOs, the nonprofit sector, and civil society more generally as exclusively demobilizing or depoliticizing spaces. At the same time, the case also makes clear the importance of political groups that are not wholly incorporated into the professionalized AIDS and nonprofit communities (cf. Brown, 1997; Piven and Cloward, 1977). The blurred boundary between the two, it turns out, was important to sustaining ACT UP/Philadelphia's momentum and facilitating its diversification, especially in this period of relative left political quiescence.

Along similar lines, sustaining ACT UP/Philadelphia also required the group to invest in and embrace complex coalition-building strategies that linked the local chapter with local, national, and international service, advocacy, and activist partners that were in many cases unusual or unexpected. For example, without its collaboration with CHAMP, the Condoms in Philadelphia Jails campaign would not have gotten off the ground. The AIDS Housing campaign relied on a unique collaboration between the chapter and students from the University of Pennsylvania. And the demonstrations for the global AIDS drug access campaign would not have been as large and well organized as they were without the involvement of Philadelphia-area recovery houses and AIDS service organizations, and of HealthGAP, of course. Often, these groups had vastly different social, institutional, professional, and political orientations and bases. Yet ACT UP/Philadelphia's focus on winnable campaigns and its human rights orientation enabled it to forge short- and long-term alliances that were vital to its political success while they did not require the group to make unholy sacrifices around moral and political issues.

The group's approach to managing racial inequalities and class divisions is also novel and important. Whereas many political groups that seek to diversify in similar ways may imagine that they can transcend race- and class-based inequalities in the course of political action itself, ACT UP/Philadelphia had no such illusions, and its members expressed a willingness to work together in the uncomfortable organizational spaces that unequal power dynamics produce on a near-constant basis. Indeed, the group as a whole was well aware of the intractable power of white middle-class expertise and comportment, and no one—not the second-generation anarchists or the homeless African American Project TEACH graduates, or anyone else—imagined that these power dynamics were not always present in the work that was done. But formal and informal efforts to encourage participation across race and class divides enabled the group to manage these dynamics effectively enough to hold itself together. Moreover, the unique history of AIDS activism and anarchism in Philadelphia was, in the end, more a catalyst than an impediment to ACT UP/Philadelphia's cross-race and cross-class organizing, since some seasoned activists from these communities came to ACT UP/Philadelphia with experience with cross-race and cross-class coalition building.

Despite its track record, the long-term sustainability of ACT UP/Philadelphia is by no means guaranteed. The group faces many challenges: a chronic scarcity of resources, internal tensions, and the inability to build a leadership structure beyond a small core of committed members whose ranks, per usual, will not be easy to replace. Beyond these internal dynamics, external factors continue to threaten the group. Today's political environment is more hostile to the kind of welfarist policy solutions on which ACT UP/Philadelphia, and AIDS activism more generally, tend to rely, even though economic and social inequality is markedly on the rise in the United States and worldwide. The 2008–2012 embrace of austerity policies in the context of the global economic crisis only exacerbates an already difficult situation. And the decline of radical AIDS activism elsewhere isolates the group further and limits its ability to build coalitions and mobilize resources.

None of these challenges are a surprise to ACT UP/Philadelphia's members, however, and they try their best to create opportunities to extend and expand their activist visions and practices. For example, on April 25, 2012, 25 years after its founding, ACT UP/New York, joined by Occupy Wall Street, staged a demonstration in New York City calling for a financial speculation tax "to raise revenues needed for urgent social needs, domestically, as well as to address global health issues," as the flyer distributed at the event explained. ACT UP/Philadelphia was there in full force. It joined the ACT UP/New York/OWS contingent, and together they marched through Lower Manhattan, displaying once again the resilience of this movement and its unique capacity to adapt to political circumstances, old and new.

## ACKNOWLEDGMENTS

I thank Julie Davids for her help in preparing this chapter. Davids is Director of National Advocacy and Mobilization at AIDS Foundation, Chicago. She was a longtime member of ACT UP/Philadelphia and was founding director of CHAMP, the Community HIV/AIDS Mobilization Project. This chapter also benefited from comments by Ray Smith, Sidney Donnell, Max Ray, José De Marco, John Bell, Jane Shull, Walt Senterfitt, Waheedah Shabazz-El, and Paul Davis.

Research was supported by the PhD Program in Anthropology at the Graduate Center and by the Department of Urban Studies, Queens College, CUNY.

## BIBLIOGRAPHY

ACT UP Philadelphia (2010). Dying For Homes. Philadelphia, PA: ACT UP Philadelphia. URL:http://www.kayteeriek.com/documents/housingreport.pdf (last accessed, August 22, 2012).

Agamben, G. (1998). *Homo sacer: Sovereign power and bare life.* Stanford, CA: Stanford University Press.

AIDS Activities Coordinating Office (AACO) (2012). *Surveillance report: HIV/ AIDS in Philadelphia.* Philadelphia, PA: Department of Public Health.

Altman, D. (1994). *Power and community: Organizational and cultural responses to AIDS.* London: Taylor & Francis.

Brody, E. (2002). *Property-tax exemption for charities: Mapping the battlefield.* Washington, DC: The Urban Institute Press.

Brown, M. (1997). *Replacing citizenship: AIDS activism and radical democracy.* New York: Guilford Press.

Chambré, S. (2006). *Fighting for our lives: New York's AIDS community and the politics of disease.* New Brunswick, NJ: Rutgers University Press.

Cohen, C. J. (1999). The boundaries of blackness: AIDS and the breakdown of black politics. Chicago: University of Chicago Press.

Crimp, D., & Rolston, A. (1990). *AIDS demographics.* Seattle: Bay Press.

Di Leonardo, M. (ed.). (1991). *Gender at the crossroads of knowledge: Feminist anthropology in the postmodern era.* Berkeley: University of California Press.

Di Leonardo, M. (1998). *Exotics at home: Anthropologies, others, American modernity.* Chicago, IL: University of Chicago Press.

Ghaziani, A. (2011, February). Post-gay collective identity construction. *Social Problems,* 58, (1): 99–125.

Goode, J., & Maskovsky, J. (2001). *New poverty studies: The ethnography of power, politics, and impoverished people in the United States.* New York: New York University Press.

Gould, D. (2009). *Moving politics: Emotion and ACT UP's fight against AIDS.* Chicago: University of Chicago Press. http://public.eblib.com/EBLPublic/ PublicView.do?ptiID=471870.

Hilderbrand, L. (2006). Retroactivism. *GLQ: A Journal of Lesbian and Gay Studies,* 12 (2): 303–317.

Katz, M. (1990). *The undeserving poor: From the war on poverty to the war on welfare.* New York: Pantheon Books.

Maskovsky, J. (2000a). *Fighting for their lives: Poverty and AIDS activism in neoliberal Philadelphia.* Dissertation. Philadelphia, PA: Temple University, Department of Anthropology.

Maskovsky, J. (2000b). "Managing" the poor: Neoliberalism, Medicaid HMOs and the triumph of consumerism among the poor. *Medical Anthropology: Cross-Cultural Studies in Health and Illness.*

Maskovsky, J. (2003). Global justice in the post-industrial city: Beyond the local/ global divide. In *Reclaiming Cities,* ed. Jane Schneider and Ida Susser. Berg Press, pp. 149–172.

Mullings, L. (1997). *On our own terms: Race, class, and gender in the lives of African American women.* New York: Routledge.

National Alliance to End Homelessness (2006). What is Housing First? Washington DC: National Alliance to End Homelessness (November 9, 2006).

URL: http://b.3cdn.net/naeh/b974efab62feb2b36c_pzm6bn4ct.pdf (last accessed, August 22, 2012).

Novas, C., & Rose, N. (2000). Genetic risk and the birth of the somatic individual. *Economy and Society,* 29 (4), 485–513. ISSN 0308-5147.

Nutter, Mayor M. A. (2012). 2012 Budget Address. Philadelphia, PA: City of Philadelphia (March 8, 2012). URL: http://www.phila.gov/pdfs/2012-budget -Address.pdf (last accessed, September 3, 2013).

Parenti, C. (2001). *Lockdown America: Police and prisons in the age of crisis.* London: Verso.

Pasquariello, A. (2006, December 20). Rubbers stomped: The city said it would provide prisoners with condoms. Why haven't they? In *City Paper,* Philadelphia, PA. http://www.citypaper.net/articles/2006/12/21/rubbers-stomped (retrieved March 5, 2011).

Patton, C. (1990). *Inventing AIDS.* New York: Routledge.

Piven, F. F., & Cloward, R. A. (1977). *Poor people's movements: Why they succeed, how they fail.* New York: Pantheon Books.

Reed, A. L. (1999). *Stirrings in the jug: Black politics in the post-segregation era.* Minneapolis: University of Minnesota Press.

Rose, N. S. (2007). *Politics of life itself: Biomedicine, power, and subjectivity in the twenty-first century.* Princeton: Princeton University Press.

Sacks, K. B. (1989). Toward a unified theory of class, race, and gender. *American Ethnologist,* 16 (3): 534–550.

Shabazz-El, W. (2008). *ACT UP Philadelphia condoms in Philadelphia jails campaign, Think piece for Project UNSHACKLE meeting.* Presented at the John M. Lloyd AIDS Project at Stony Point Center, May 16–18, 2008.

Shepard, B. H., & Hayduk, R. (2002). *From ACT UP to the WTO: Urban protest and community building in the era of globalization.* London: Verso.

Shilts, R. (1987). *And the band played on: Politics, people, and the AIDS epidemic.* New York: St. Martin's Press.

Singer, M. (1998). The *political economy of AIDS.* Amityville, NY: Baywood.

Small, M. L., & Newman, K. (2001). Urban poverty after the truly disadvantaged: The rediscovery of the family, the neighborhood, and culture. *Annual Review of Sociology,* 27: 23–45.

Steinberg, S. (1995). *Turning back: The retreat from racial justice in American thought and policy.* Boston, MA: Beacon Press.

Stockdill, B. C. (2003). *Activism against AIDS: At the intersection of sexuality, race, gender, and class.* Boulder, CO: Lynne Rienner.

Susser, I. (2009). AIDS, sex, and culture: Global politics and survival in southern africa. Chichester, West Sussex, U.K: Wiley-Blackwell.

Wilson, W. J. (1987). *The truly disadvantaged: The inner city, the underclass, and public policy.* Chicago: University of Chicago Press.

# Index

# About the Editors
and Contributors

Raymond A. Smith, PhD (Editor), is an Adjunct Assistant Professor of Political Science at both Columbia University and New York University. He is also an investigator in the Division of Gender, Sexuality, and Health at the Columbia University Medical Center and Director of Communications at the HIV Center for Clinical and Behavioral Studies at the NYS Psychiatric Institute. In addition, Smith has served as Associate Program Director of the MAC AIDS Fund Leadership Initiative, an HIV prevention fellowship program in South Africa. Smith is editor of the award-winning *Encyclopedia of AIDS* (Fitzroy-Dearborn, hardcover 1998; Penguin, paperback 2001); editor of *The Politics of Sexuality* (Greenwood, 2010), a collection of primary documents with commentary about the politics of sexuality in the United States since 1965; and co-author (with Patricia Siplon) of *Drugs into Bodies: Global AIDS Treatment Activism* (Praeger, 2006). Previously, Smith served as editor of the community-based HIV/AIDS magazine *Body Positive* and as Research Director of the National Alliance of State and Territorial AIDS Directors (NASTAD) in Washington, DC. He has co-authored HIV/AIDS-related articles in academic journals including *The American Journal of Public Health, Women and Health, The AIDS Reader, Journal of AIDS,* and *The American Journal of Community Psychology.* Smith holds an MA in international relations from Yale University and a PhD in political science from Columbia University, with an emphasis on American politics, and is a senior fellow with the Washington, DC–based think tank, the Progressive Policy Institute.

Brandon Aultman, MA (Associate Editor), is an Instructor in Political Science at Baruch College and a doctoral student in political science at the Graduate School of the City University of New York.

He also holds a master's in politics from New York University. He has served in a number of editorial capacities, co-authored two book chapters and several encyclopedia articles, and was assistant editor of *The Politics of Sexuality.* Currently, he is engaging in research on the theoretical and empirical effects of law on both gender transgressive identities and mobilization efforts in America. He was a Mellon Sawyer Student Fellow for the 2012–2013 academic year for the seminar series entitled "Democratic Citizenship and the Recognition of Cultural Differences" held at the City University of New York.

## ABOUT THE CONTRIBUTORS

**Emily Bass, BS, MFA,** is an activist, advocate, and writer focused on the right to health for all the world's citizens. She is the Program Director of AVAC: Global Advocacy for HIV Prevention, an international nongovernmental organization that uses education, policy analysis, advocacy, and a network of global collaborations to accelerate the ethical development and global delivery of new biomedical prevention strategies. Bass has worked extensively as a writer, serving as senior writer for *IAVI Report,* the newsletter of the International AIDS Vaccine Initiative, as well as *HIV Plus Magazine* and *The amfAR Treatment Insider*; her AIDS reporting has also appeared in *Salon, The Lancet Infectious Diseases,* and *Out Magazine*; and she is the recipient of a Fulbright Award for reporting on AIDS treatment rollout in Uganda. She has been part of the global AIDS treatment access movement for nearly 15 years.

**Richard Boulton, MA, PhD,** is a visiting tutor of sociology at Goldsmiths College, University of London in the United Kingdom. He is based in the Centre for the Study of Innovation and Social Process where he recently completed his PhD on pediatric HIV and clinical practice.

**Julien Burns, BA,** is a Program Assistant at AVAC: Global Advocacy for HIV Prevention. He works on new media communications and program coordination, and provides logistical and administrative support for a variety of AVAC projects. Burns has interned with PATH and the Global Health Council, and spent the spring of 2009 working in an orphanage in Kenya and overseeing the building of a school library.

**Catherine Campbell, PhD,** is Professor of Social Psychology at the London School of Economics. A community health specialist, she has a particular interest in the role of community mobilization in promoting sexual, reproductive, and maternal health and in facilitating smoother interfaces between health services and service users in Zimbabwe, South Africa, and India. Much of her research has been generated through her involvement in the design and implementation of large community-led HIV/AIDS management projects in marginalized settings. She has published over 100 peer-reviewed articles and several co-edited volumes on related topics. Her most well-known publication is her book *Letting Them Die: Why HIV Prevention Programmes Fail* (2003). She was recently awarded a Career Contribution Award by the ASA's Sociologists AIDS Network (SAN) for her lifelong contribution to understandings of the social dynamics of HIV/AIDS, and she is a Fellow of the British Psychological Society.

**Susan M. Chambré, PhD,** is a Professor of Sociology and the editor of the Working Papers Series of the Baruch Center for Nonprofit Management and Strategy. Her research and publications focus on civic engagement, nonprofit organizations, and public policy. She has been studying AIDS advocacy since 1988. Her current research is a historical study that focuses on the emergence of a consumer consciousness and the nature of disease advocacy for tuberculosis, polio, and HIV. She is the author of *Fighting for Our Lives: New York's AIDS Community and the Politics of Disease,* published by Rutgers University Press, and she co-edited *Patients, Consumers and Civil Society* (with Melinda Goldner), which was published by Emerald.

**Christopher J. Colvin, PhD, MPH,** is an anthropologist living and working in Cape Town, South Africa. He has a PhD in sociocultural anthropology from the University of Virginia and an MPH from the University of Cape Town (UCT) in epidemiology. He has lectured in anthropology and public health at Columbia University and several South African universities, and he was a UCT postdoctoral fellow in health and human rights. Colvin is currently Senior Research Officer at UCT's School of Public Health and Family Medicine. He also serves as the Program Director for the Health and Community Study Abroad Programs of the International Honors Program. During 2012, he was a fellow in Global Public Health at the University of Virginia in the departments of Anthropology and Public Health Sciences. His research areas include HIV/AIDS and masculinity, health systems and health system reform, community mobilization and health activism, community health workers, and qualitative research methodology.

**William Ward Darrow, PhD,** is a Professor of Public Health at the Robert R. Stempel College of Public Health and Social Work at Florida International University (FIU) in Miami, Florida. Darrow has served the South Florida community as a member of the Dade County HIV/AIDS Prevention Community Planning Group (1995–1997), Miami–Dade County AIDS Prevention Task Force (1994–1999), South Florida Syphilis Coalition (2003–2005), Florida Department of Health HIV/AIDS Epidemiology Work Group, and the South Beach AIDS Project Advisory Board (1995–2001). Darrow has led HIV-prevention and research efforts in South Beach and other areas of high HIV incidence in south Florida. From 1999 to 2008, he served as project leader and principal investigator for the REACH 2010 community mobilization project to eliminate disparities in HIV disease in Broward County. To date, he has published 125 articles in peer-review journals, chapters in books, and research monographs; has presented more than 100 scientific papers at national and international meetings; and has consulted with many professional and service organizations, including the Global Program on AIDS, the World Health Organization, and the European Union.

**Jocelyn DeJong, MPhil, PhD,** has worked on reproductive health and HIV/AIDS in the Arab region for over 20 years. She has a BA in Social Anthropology (Harvard University), MPhil in Development Studies (University of Sussex), and PhD in Health Policy in Developing Countries (London School of Hygiene and Tropical Medicine). She ran a regional grants program in reproductive health in the 1990s at the Ford Foundation's regional office for the Middle East and North Africa in Cairo. DeJong currently teaches at the Faculty of Health Sciences, American University of Beirut in Lebanon, where she was involved in a major HIV bio-behavioral study on at-risk groups and organized two regional workshops that resulted in a special issue on HIV in the Middle East in the journal *AIDS*. She coordinates two regional research networks, the Reproductive Health Working Group and the Choices and Challenges in Changing Childbirth research network. Her current main research interests include HIV and maternal health.

**Carlos Guilherme do Valle, PhD,** is Senior Lecturer in Social Anthropology at the Universidade Federal do Rio Grande do Norte. He obtained his MSc in Social Anthropology at the National Museum/ UFRJ and his PhD at the University of London. Earlier he taught at the Universidade Federal do Rio de Janeiro and the Universidade Federal da

Paraíba. He has written on Brazilian HIV/AIDS activism as well as on biomedical technologies, sexuality, and identity formation in relation to health and illness.

**Jonathan Garcia, PhD,** is a political anthropologist focused on the cultural and political determinants of global health and social movements. His areas of expertise include sexual and reproductive health and faith-based interventions. He has conducted over nine years of mixed-methods research on AIDS social movements in Brazil, publishing in both English and Portuguese. He was a postdoctoral fellow at Yale University's Center for Interdisciplinary Research on AIDS, with which he is still affiliated through the Community Research Core. He currently works in the Department of Sociomedical Sciences at the Columbia University Mailman School of Public Health as project coordinator for a study on Latino male bisexuality in New York City.

**Daniel Grace, PhD,** completed his doctorate in 2012 in sociology from the University of Victoria, British Columbia, Canada. Trained in institutional ethnography, his ongoing research interests include global health, HIV/AIDS, critical policy studies, and social inequality. He is currently a postdoctoral research fellow at the University of British Columbia, Faculty of Medicine as part of a Canadian Institutes for Health Research (CIHR)–funded multidisciplinary investigation exploring the use of new HIV testing technologies for early detection and response among gay men in British Columbia. Grace has held a number of scholarships and fellowships to support his HIV/AIDS research, including a Canadian Graduate Scholarship (CGS) from the Social Sciences and Humanities Research Council of Canada (SSHRC) (2007–2010), a University Without Walls (UWW) Fellowship (2010), a Global Health Fellowship through Duke University (2010), and a CIHR Doctoral Training Fellowship (2011–2012).

**Deirdre Grant, BA,** has worked in HIV/AIDS advocacy, communications, and program management for over six years. She is currently a Senior Program Manager at AVAC: Global Advocacy for HIV Prevention. At AVAC she contributes to the management of its U.S.- and EU-focused advocacy leadership programs, works on AVAC's multistakeholder initiatives around key issues in HIV prevention, and supports writing and editing of the full array of AVAC materials and publications. Her writing has appeared in *Treatment Issues,* a quarterly magazine produced by GMHC, and featured in *POZ* and in *Achieve,* a joint publication of ACRIA and GMHC. Prior to joining AVAC, Grant worked as an independent consultant on U.S.-China relations.

**Rana Haddad Ibrahim, MPH,** holds a master's in Public Health–Health Behavior and Education from the American University of Beirut (AUB). She worked as a project coordinator for capacity building of primary health care workers in Lebanon, a project involving the AUB and the Save the Children Fund, then as a technical officer for the Lebanese National AIDS Control Program, as well as a teacher of an undergraduate course at AUB. Since 2003, she has been working as a health behavior and education consultant on public health issues including reproductive health, HIV/AIDS/STIs, drug use, smoking tobacco, healthy lifestyles, and approaches to peer education, life skills, and children and youth participation. She has collaborated with various UN agencies, ministries, and NGOs throughout the Middle East and North Africa.

**Robert Lorway, PhD,** is a medical anthropologist and assistant professor at the University of Manitoba who studies the intersections of sexual minority rights, culture, and health, particularly with respect to global health interventions in Africa and Asia. In 2009, he received a Canadian Institutes for Health Research (CIHR) New Investigator Award in the area of HIV/AIDS Population Health/Health Services. He is the nominated principal investigator of an HIV vaccine acceptability team research program, sponsored by the Canadian HIV Vaccine Initiative. This program works closely with communities of sex workers and MSM in Kenya, China, and India to help advance their concerns related to the anticipated release of new HIV prevention technologies.

**Joanne Mantell, PhD,** is a public health researcher, a Professor of Clinical Psychology in the Department of Psychiatry at Columbia University, and a research scientist at the HIV Center for Clinical and Behavioral Studies. She has worked extensively in the United States as well as in Nigeria, South Africa, and China. Currently, Dr. Mantell is the principal investigator of studies on the integration of sexual and reproductive health and HIV care and medical male circumcision in South Africa, and a co-investigator on studies of women in antenatal clinics and men in Lesotho and men who have sex with men in South Africa. Current research interests focus on the integration of sexual/reproductive health and HIV care services, fertility intentions of HIV-positive women and men, acceptability and uptake of biomedical HIV prevention strategies (female condom, microbicides, medical male circumcision, PrEP), HIV prevention for transgender women, and structural interventions to reduce the risk of HIV acquisition or transmission, especially for female and male sex workers.

**Jeff Maskovsky, PhD,** is Associate Professor of Urban Studies at Queens College and of Anthropology and Environmental Psychology at the Graduate Center, City University of New York (CUNY). His research and writing focus on poverty and grassroots activism in the urban United States. Maskovsky was an ACT UP/New York member from 1990 to 1992 and an ACT UP/Philadelphia member from 1992 to 1995. He helped to found, and served as co-lead instructor for, Project TEACH (Treatment Education Activists Combating HIV) from 1996 to 1999 in Philadelphia. He also served on the board of directors for CHAMP, the Community HIV/AIDS Mobilization Project, from 2003 to 2010.

**Tim McCaskell, MEd,** is a long-time Toronto writer, activist, and educator. He was a collective member of *The Body Politic,* Canada's first national magazine for lesbian and gay liberation, from 1974 to 1986; chair of the Public Action Committee of the Right to Privacy Committee, which fought back against police raids on gay baths in the early 1980s; and part of the Simon Nkodi Anti-Apartheid Committee: Lesbians and Gays Against Apartheid in the late 1980s. He was a founding member of AIDS ACTION NOW! (AAN!), an activist group that won access to experimental treatments and funding for medications in the 1990s. Working in conjunction with various organizations across Canada, AAN! helped to organize the National Days of Action Against the Criminalization of HIV in 2012.

**Iman Mortagy, MSc,** is a social scientist who holds a degree in social anthropology from the American University in Cairo and an MSc in public health from the London School of Hygiene and Tropical Medicine in the United Kingdom. Mortagy has worked in the field of reproductive and sexual health for Save the Children, USA; the United Nations Programme for HIV/AIDS; and more recently the Centre for Maternal and Child Enquiries in London. She currently works as a freelance researcher and spends her time between the United Kingdom and Egypt.

**Nicoli Nattrass, PhD,** is professor of economics and director of the AIDS and Society Research Unit at the University of Cape Town. She has published widely on the political economy of AIDS policy and was actively involved in the Treatment Action Campaign's struggle for antiretroviral treatment in South Africa. Her work showed that it was cheaper to introduce mother-to-child transmission prevention than to cope with the large numbers of HIV-positive babies that would be born in its absence, and she was instrumental in forcing the government to change its policy stance. Her most recent book is *The AIDS Conspiracy: Science Fights Back* (Columbia University Press, 2012). It analyzes the roots of AIDS conspiracy beliefs in the United States and South Africa, reports on the harm associated with them (e.g., unsafe sex and the rejection of scientific evidence), and argues that the broader struggle for evidence-based medicine should be supported.

**Richard G. Parker, PhD,** is Professor of Sociomedical Sciences and Anthropology, Director of the Center for the Study of Culture, Politics and Health, and a member of the university-wide Committee on Global Thought at Columbia University in New York City. He is also the editor-in-chief of the journal *Global Public Health,* the director and president of the Brazilian Interdisciplinary AIDS Association (ABIA), and the founder and current co-chair of Sexuality Policy Watch, a global coalition of researchers, policymakers, and activists from a wide range of countries and regions that has secretariat offices in Rio de Janeiro and New York City.

**San Patten, MSc,** is a health research and evaluation consultant in Halifax, Nova Scotia, Canada, and is also an adjunct professor in Sociology at Mount Allison University and a co-investigator of the Centre for HIV Prevention Social Research based at the University of Toronto. After working for the AIDS Calgary Awareness Association and for the Alberta Community Council on HIV, Patten started her own consulting practice specializing in HIV/AIDS policy development, program evaluation, facilitation, capacity building, and community-based research. Her international work experience includes projects in India, Mexico, Zambia, Kenya, Moldova, Serbia, Cambodia, Pakistan, Uganda, and South Africa, with much of her work focused on new HIV prevention technologies.

**Amy S. Patterson, PhD,** is Professor in the Department of Political Science at the University of the South, Sewanee, Tennessee. She is editor of *The African State and the AIDS Crisis* (Ashgate, 2005) and author of *The Politics of AIDS in Africa* (Lynne Rienner Publishers, 2006) and *The Church and AIDS in Africa: The Politics of Ambiguity* (First Forum Press, 2011). She has published articles on HIV and AIDS, civil society, and gender in Africa in *Africa Today, Journal of Modern African Studies, Canadian Journal of African Studies, African Journal of AIDS Research,* and *African Studies Review.* She has conducted fieldwork in Senegal, Ghana, and Zambia. As a Fulbright Scholar in 2011, she conducted research on political empowerment and social capital development among members of secular and religious support groups for people living with HIV and AIDS in Zambia.

**Dean Peacock, MSW,** is co-founder and Executive Director of Sonke Gender Justice in Cape Town, South Africa. He is also co-founder and co-chair of the Global Men Engage Alliance. In addition to his work at Sonke Gender Justice, Dean is a member of the United Nations Secretary General's Network of Men Leaders formed to advise Ban Ki-Moon on gender-based violence prevention and of the Nobel Women's Advisory Committee on ending sexual violence in conflict settings. His writing has been published in many books and peer-reviewed journals, including *The Lancet, the Journal of AIDS, American Journal of Public Health, International Journal of Men's Health, Journal of Men and Masculinities,* and *Gender and Society.*

**Robert H. Remien, PhD,** is Professor of Clinical Psychology (in Psychiatry) at Columbia University and a Research Scientist at the HIV Center for Clinical and Behavioral Studies at Columbia University and the New York State Psychiatric Institute. Dr. Remien is Director of the HIV Center's Global Community Core, faculty mentor for HIV Center postdoctoral fellows, and clinical supervisor to psychiatric residents in training. He has served as chair for the New York State Psychological Association's Task Force on AIDS, a member of the New York City Department of Health Prevention Planning Group, senior faculty for the American Psychological Association's HIV training program for psychologists, and serves on several journal editorial boards and national advisory groups for NIH and the CDC.

**Tim Shand, MPH,** is the International Programs Manager at Sonke Gender Justice in Cape Town, South Africa. He works with Sonke's partner organizations within the Men Engage Africa network to scale up programs and policies across the region that seek to engage men and boys in achieving gender equality, preventing HIV and gender-based violence, and promoting human rights. Prior to working with Sonke, Tim was based in London with the International Planned Parenthood

Federation (IPPF) and has also worked with the World Health Organization in Geneva, where he helped to initiate WHO's work on men, gender, and health equity.

**Morten Skovdal, PhD,** works as a research fellow for the Department of Health Promotion and Development at the University of Bergen in Norway. A community health psychologist, he has a particular interest in children's health and community responses to HIV and AIDS in sub-Saharan Africa. He is a trustee and co-founder of a nongovernmental organization in Western Kenya that funds local community initiatives in support of vulnerable children. He is also affiliated with the Manicaland HIV/STD Prevention Project in Zimbabwe. Currently Skovdal works as the primary investigator of research projects investigating how schools can help HIV-affected children cope with the impacts of poverty and disease in Kenya and Zimbabwe.

**Zena Stein, MB, BCh, DSc (Hon),** is the Co-Director Emerita of the HIV Center for Clinical and Behavioral Studies at the New York State Psychiatric Institute and Columbia University. Previously, Dr. Stein was Professor of Public Health and of Psychiatry at Columbia University. She was also Associate Dean of Research and Academic Affairs of the Columbia University Mailman School of Public Health and the Director of the Department of Epidemiology of Brain Disorders at New York State Psychiatric Institute. Stein has been a leader worldwide in the movement to provide women with methods for protection against transmission of HIV that are under their control, including vaginal microbicides and the female condom. Stein has consulted frequently for international organizations such as WHO and UNICEF and has served on the study sections of NIMH, NIEHS, NIOSH, NICHD, and on several committees of the National Academy of Sciences.

**Antonio Torres-Ruiz, MA, PhD,** has taught at the University of Toronto in the Department of Political Science and the Latin American Studies Program for the last four years. He more recently joined York University's new program in Human Rights and Equity Studies as full-time faculty. His publications include articles and book reviews for *International Journal* (Canada), *História, Ciencias, Saude* (Brazil), *Journal of Latin American Studies* (UK), *Working Papers Series, CIDE* (Mexico), and the *Latin American Research Review* (United States), as well as book chapters and an edited volume on contentious politics in North America. His doctoral dissertation, "An

Elusive Quest for Democracy and Development in a Globalized World: The Political Economy of HIV/AIDS in Mexico," is being revised for publication as a monograph.

**Wessel van den Berg, MPhil,** is Integrated Projects Manager at Sonke Gender Justice in Cape Town, South Africa. In this capacity he ensures effective implementation of complex projects requiring the simultaneous involvement of each of Sonke's work units, especially the Global Men Care Fatherhood Campaign. Van den Berg worked within the social change environment in a variety of contexts. These include youth development, health, gender equality, and sustainable development. As a counselor and group facilitator he worked actively with men's personal development, and through his work in sustainable development, he has explored the wider relationships and environments that impact upon health and access to human rights.

**Mitchell Warren, BA,** is the Executive Director of AVAC, an international nongovernmental organization that uses education, policy analysis, advocacy, and a network of global collaborations to accelerate the ethical development and global delivery of AIDS vaccines, male circumcision, microbicides, PrEP, and other emerging HIV prevention options as part of a comprehensive response to the pandemic. Previously, he was the Senior Director for Vaccine Preparedness at the International AIDS Vaccine Initiative (IAVI) and also a Vice President and Director of International Affairs for the Female Health Company (FHC), the manufacturer of the female condom. Warren also spent six years at Population Services International (PSI), designing and implementing social marketing, communications, and health promotion activities in Africa, Asia, and Europe, including five years running PSI's project in South Africa.